THE MALLEABLE BRAIN: BENEFITS AND HARM FROM PLASTICITY OF THE BRAIN

THE MALLEABLE BRAIN: BENEFITS AND HARM FROM PLASTICITY OF THE BRAIN

AAGE R. MØLLER

Nova Biomedical Books
New York

For permission to use material from this book please contact us:
Telephone 631-231-7269; Fax 631-231-8175
Web Site: http://www.novapublishers.com

NOTICE TO THE READER

The Publisher has taken reasonable care in the preparation of this book, but makes no expressed or implied warranty of any kind and assumes no responsibility for any errors or omissions. No liability is assumed for incidental or consequential damages in connection with or arising out of information contained in this book. The Publisher shall not be liable for any special, consequential, or exemplary damages resulting, in whole or in part, from the readers' use of, or reliance upon, this material. Any parts of this book based on government reports are so indicated and copyright is claimed for those parts to the extent applicable to compilations of such works.

Independent verification should be sought for any data, advice or recommendations contained in this book. In addition, no responsibility is assumed by the publisher for any injury and/or damage to persons or property arising from any methods, products, instructions, ideas or otherwise contained in this publication.

This publication is designed to provide accurate and authoritative information with regard to the subject matter covered herein. It is sold with the clear understanding that the Publisher is not engaged in rendering legal or any other professional services. If legal or any other expert assistance is required, the services of a competent person should be sought from a declaration of participants jointly adopted by a Committee of the American Bar Association and a committee of publishers.

LIBRARY OF CONGRESS CATALOGING-IN-PUBLICATION DATA

Møller, Aage R.
 The malleable brain : benefits and harm from plasticity of the brain / Aage R. Moller.
      p. ; cm.
 Includes bibliographical references and index.
 ISBN: 978-1-60692-881-3
 (hardcover : alk. paper)
 1. Neuroplasticity. I. Title.
 [DNLM: 1. Neuronal Plasticity--physiology. 2. Brain--physiology. 3. Central Nervous System Diseases--physiopathology. 4. Central Nervous System Diseases--rehabilitation. WL 102 M7263m 2009]
 QP363.3.M655 2009
 612.8--dc22
                                                                      2008054760

Published by Nova Science Publishers, Inc. ✝ *New York*

CONTENTS

ACKNOWLEDGMENT

I have had help from many individuals in writing this book. The idea to write this book came from teaching courses on "Neural Plasticity and Disorders of the Nervous System' and a course on "The Neuroscience of Pain" in the School of Behavioral and Brain Sciences at The University of Texas at Dallas. Many of my students have provided valuable feedback and comments.

I thank Amanda Miller for her improvements to my writing. Dhirj Gupta helped with illustrations.

I would not have been able to write this book without the support I received of the School of Behavioral and Brain Sciences at the University of Texas at Dallas.

Last but not least I thank my wife, Margareta B. Møller, MD; DMedSci. for many suggestions and for her encouragement during writing this book.

Dallas, October 2008
Aage R. Møller, Ph.D. (D.Med.Sci.)

INTRODUCTION

I wrote this book because I wanted to share some exciting aspects of the brain that are not generally known. The brain is plastic and that has many implications. One is that it can adapt to changing demands and it can reorganize itself when some parts become damaged. These are beneficial aspects of what we call neural plasticity, but the plasticity of the brain and spinal cord can also be harmful; it can cause symptoms and signs of diseases, which we will call plasticity diseases. Examples are chronic pain and tinnitus (ringing in the ears). This side of plasticity is less known and lack of understanding of these aspects of neural plasticity causes incorrect treatment of many patients.

The brain explores the environment by the signals it receives from the environment after it has analyzed the content of these signals. It creates an image of the world and issue commands to the executive parts to engage muscles to react. Not to forget, the brain store information and create a "self".

There are many ways these functions of the brain and the spinal cord can be altered or changed. Trauma, lack of oxygen, and other injuries can damage the brain and the spinal cord causing mostly negative changes in how the brain functions, which in turn produces symptoms of disease. Strokes are common injuries to the nervous system and are caused by blockages in blood vessels (ischemic strokes) or bleeding (hemorrhagic strokes). However trauma from various kinds of accidents also causes damage to the brain and the spinal cord. It is well known that ingestion of chemical substances can affect how the central nervous system functions while they are in the body and the effect may remain after they have been broken down or excreted. Alcohol is probably the most common example of chemicals but there are many other substances that can affect brain function. Many of these have an immediate impact and some have a long-term, irreversible effect.

There is another less obvious and lesser known way that the function of the spinal cord and the brain can change, and that is because both the spinal cord and the brain are plastic (malleable). Plasticity is a property of the brain and the spinal cord that is only apparent when turned on. The basic functions of the nervous system and the nature of neural plasticity are discussed in the first two Chapters of this book.

Activation of plasticity can have many effects on the function of the senses and the systems controlling movement (the motor system), and it can affect intellectual skills. It can help the brain recover from trauma and it can help adapt to changing demands, enhance some reflexes and suppress other. It can also cause diseases that I will call "plasticity diseases". Plasticity becomes harmful when it is activated incorrectly or if it is turned on when it should not have been activated.

Activation of neural plasticity can help to better serve new situations and when parts of the brain get damaged from strokes or trauma, plasticity can shift the tasks that have been done by the damaged parts before the injury to areas in the brain that function properly. This is what is called recovery from trauma and strokes. While there is little that can be done to repair brain damage after a certain time has passed, many functions can be shifted to other regions that are intact through activation of neural plasticity. Getting use to using prostheses depends on expression of neural plasticity. The use of cochlea and brainstem implants for restoring hearing in deaf people would not be possible without the help from activation of neural plasticity. These kinds of neural plasticity are beneficial to the individual person and it is the topic of Chapter III.

The organization ("blueprint") of the brain is laid down through inherited genes passed down through many generations. These genes provide a program that control how the nervous system develops before birth. It controls and guides nerve fibers when they grow out and proceed so they reach their correct target. This means that genes supply the "recipe" or program for how to build the nervous system.

Neural plasticity plays an important role in the development of the brain and the spinal cord after birth and is important during the entire span of life without activation of neural plasticity the development of the nervous system is incomplete.

There are many unanswered questions about how the billions of nerve cells in the spinal cord and the brain manage to connect to each other in the correct way during development. Only a part of this development occurs before birth but the development continues for many years after birth. In fact the development of the brain is not finished until about the age of 20. Shortfalls in the re-organization that normally occurs after birth (the "midcourse correction") may prevent the brain to develop normally.

After completion of this "midcourse correction" that takes place during the first years of life, further development of the brain is necessary to arrive at its final organization and function. This correction is not programmed in the same way as the "midcourse correction" but is instead guided by signals from the sense organs and by signals from different parts of the body. Lack of such guidance causes deficits of various kinds.

We have all experienced how it takes some training to pronounce unfamiliar words and we have to concentrate when speaking such words. However, after some training we can speak the words without much thought. The main effect of various kinds of training is that it can facilitate the activation of plasticity. Many aspects of our senses are created through activation of neural plasticity.

The development of normal vision and hearing also depends on activation of these senses after birth. I will call that experience. The brain can change its organization throughout life through activation of neural plasticity, but it is more plastic at a young age than in adult life. There is a "critical age" above which it is more difficult to cause plastic changes. There is a period just after birth that is called the "critical period" (or "sensitive period") where such skills can best be acquired. After the end of the critical period it is still possible to learn many skills but not as easy and it takes longer time to acquire certain skills than during the critical period.

There are many other examples of how plastic changes induced by experience can alter the function, and even the structure of the nervous system. Mental exercise can help maintain cognitive skills. The saying "use it or lose it" is applicable to many aspects of human life. These effects are achieved through activation of neural plasticity.

The example of the effect of neural plasticity given above all provided benefits of one kind or another but plastic changes can also be harmful as discussed in Chapter IV. One common example of harmful plastic changes is central pain, which is pain caused by changes in the function of the spinal cord and the brain. Some forms of tinnitus ("ringing in the ears"), are also caused by harmful activation of neural plasticity. Phantom limb symptoms (pain and other sensations felt in an amputated limb) are other examples of symptoms caused by plastic changes. Several other ailments are plasticity diseases that are caused by changes in brain function. Plasticity diseases are caused by plastic changes going wrong or by changes that normally occur after birth that are not carried out correctly (such as some forms of autism and probably other disorders).

Treatment of pain is very important in clinical medicine and therefore understanding neural plasticity is important for physicians. It is also important that individuals who have chronic pain understand neural plasticity because understanding their diseases can reduce the emotional components of pain.

Plasticity of the brain and spinal cord are involved in creating the symptoms of some movement diseases such as spasm and synkinesis[1] of muscles. The "phantom limb" symptoms, where people can have pain and tingling sensations that are felt as though they come from the limb that has been amputated, are also caused by activation of neural plasticity. Removal of a limb from the body sends signals to the spinal cord and the brain, and these signals cause changes of the function of the brain because it is plastic. The change in function causes nerve cells to generate abnormal neural activity. It is this abnormal neural activity that is perceived as pain, tingling and other abnormal sensations.

Plasticity diseases that are caused by changes in the function of the brain and the spinal cord have received much less attention than they deserve. One reason is that no tests have yet been designed that can detect and measure the changes that cause plasticity diseases such as pain, tinnitus and phantom limb symptoms. Plastic changes in the brain may give many clear symptoms and signs but the changes in the brain that cause these symptoms cannot be studied using common imaging methods such as magnetic resonance imaging (MRI). There are few clinical tests that can detect and evaluate the plastic changes in the spinal cord and the brain.

Much research has been driven by what could be seen and measured, and that is also the case for diagnosis of diseases. Because plasticity diseases have no detectable physical signs, diagnosis of these diseases must rely on the patients' description of their symptoms. Nevertheless progress in treatment of most plasticity diseases must be evaluated by what the patient tells. Since many physicians and surgeons are not familiar with diagnosis of and treatment of plasticity diseases, many patients receive inadequate treatment for diseases caused by activation of neural plasticity.

---

[1] Synkinesis is the unintended contractions of muscles occurring when making voluntary muscle contractions.

Patients with plasticity diseases must therefore learn as much as possible about their disease, make their own diagnose, and take their treatment in their own hands. It is, however, a general impression that ordinary people cannot comprehend medical matters and only (licensed) physicians have that ability. This is far from correct. The informed patient usually gets the best treatment [1]. Physicians and surgeons who fiercely protect their authority and monopoly on knowledge about diseases and how to treat them have not disputed this unfortunate impression. However, it is indeed possible for ordinary people to understand the nature of many common diseases and how they can best be managed and how some may be cured.

Understanding diseases and what 'is known about treatment is not that difficult – it is definitely not the same as understanding Einstein's relativity theory. The educated patient who understand his or hers ailment has a much better chance of getting the best treatment and at a much lower cost than those who solely do as advised by physicians and drug companies. This is particularly important for diseases discussed in this book, which are poorly understood by many physicians and surgeons. People would therefore benefit from acquiring sound and unbiased knowledge about their disease and how best to treat it (or not to treat it).

Most textbooks limit their description of neural plasticity to the ability to adapt the nervous system to changing demands and how it makes it possible to regain function after damage to the spinal cord and the brain. Some books will also mention the role of neural plasticity in development of the nervous system, but few books discuss that neural plasticity can cause harm in the form of diseases (plasticity diseases) which I will discuss in detail in this book.

Neural plasticity has many similarities with learning and memory but there are many differences as well. Both memory and plasticity are based on changes in the brain that occur because of experience and practice. Memory may be defined as something that can be consciously recalled, whereas changes in functions that are caused by activation of neural plasticity occur unconsciously. Examples of plasticity are increasing the ease with which muscle reflexes can be elicited or training of physical skills. Training to speak uncommon words is a physical skill that is acquired by activation of neural plasticity. What to say, on the other hand, is learned and requires awareness and thought and it requires memory; it must be recalled.

That the brain is plastic means that it can be molded or that it is malleable. Many materials are plastic such as clay. One cannot know if a material is plastic until some force acts upon the material – just looking at it does not tell if it is solid or plastic. For example, clay does not look any different from solid material and only when pressed upon does it become apparent if a material is plastic or solid. The same for the brain and spinal cord: Only when turned on, or induced, does the effect of plasticity become apparent, hence, like genes the functions of which are not apparent unless they are expressed.

The brain does not change its form as plastic material can do but it changes the way it functions and the way different parts of the brain are connected to each other. Neural plasticity is possible because the connections between nerve cells (synapses) can change their function, new synapses can be created and existing synapses can disappear. Change in synaptic efficacy is the main way that changes in function is accomplished but other changes may occur—such as elimination of connections (axons) and creation of new ones, or even cell death occurs as a part of plastic changes.

The first two Chapters of this book concern some basics about the central nervous system (brain and spinal cord) and how it develops before and after birth (Chapter I) and the anatomical and physiological basis for neural plasticity is discussed in Chapter II. Chapter III discusses the beneficial effect of activation of neural plasticity. This Chapter also discusses why neural plasticity is necessary for the developing organism and why it is beneficial to the mature organism to change the function of specific parts of the central nervous system to suit changing demands or compensate for the effect of injuries and diseases. Chapter IV discusses plasticity diseases and treatments of plasticity diseases are discussed in Chapter V. These Chapters also speculate about the role of neural plasticity in other diseases such as addiction and depression.

That the function of the brain can change during life is a form of evolution that is different from heredity of traits and Darwinian evolution of the species. The brain's ability to change its organization and function according to circumstances has progressed during the development of species. The brain is assumed to be *purposive*, which means that it changes its function to serve the best possible purpose. Therefore, the ability to change function through neural plasticity may also be assumed to have a purpose of some kind.

We can therefore ask the question: Does the brain act with purpose when its function is changed through activation of neural plasticity? Is activation of neural plasticity purposeful? The answer depends on how purpose is defined. Many purposes can certainly be discerned and among those are the main ones, namely survival and reproduction. Being purposive is different from being beneficial to an individual person. For example, some forms of pain, such as from injury to the body or from inflammation such from arthritis, can be thought of as having the purpose of telling us something is wrong. However, if there is no effective treatment for the pain or illness it is of no benefit to the individual to receive that constant reminder that something is wrong. Central neuropathic pain does not seem to have any purpose or benefit at all.

It is easy to point to the usefulness of some forms of expression of neural plasticity but there are other forms where it is not easy to find any purpose. Tinnitus is one such expression that does not seem to have any reason. This supports the notion that purposefulness is the same as beneficial to an individual person. These questions are discussed in Chapter VI.

There are three appendices that describe the basic anatomy and physiology of acute pain, Appendix A, hearing Appendix B, and the third, Appendix C, discusses the anatomical and physiologic basis for autism.

I hope this book can contribute to enlightenment about the enormous power of neural plasticity that can cause such a wide range of effects both beneficial and harmful to individuals.

REFERENCES

[1] Møller AR. *A new epidemic: Harm in Medicine*. Nova Science Publishers; 2007.

Chapter I

VITAL FUNCTIONS OF THE BRAIN AND THE SPINAL CORD

ABSTRACT

The different parts of the brain and the spinal cord were earlier thought of having dedicated functions. It is now known that many of the brain's functions are not located in one place but in fact occur in several different parts of the brain. Interpretation of sensory signals, such as speech, is complex and may use mimicking ("analysis by synthesis"). The spinal cord processes information from the brain for control of muscles and it performs complex processing of the information. Some kinds of movements such as walking can be controlled by the spinal cord where the "central pattern generator" can control the muscles that are used for walking. It is stressed in this Chapter that the different parts of the brain are interconnected. The basics of sensory pathways and parallel and sequential processing is discussed as well as the basic building blocks and connections of the brain and spinal cord.

1. INTRODUCTION

The human brain is incredibly complex. The more we learn about the brain the more complex and sophisticated it seems. One of the more fascinating aspects of the central nervous system (brain and the spinal cord) is its plasticity. The brain can change the way it functions and the actual arrangement of cells can also change because of its plasticity.

In order to understand the implications of neural plasticity, it is necessary to consider some basic properties of the brain and the spinal cord. I will first describe building blocks of the central nervous system consisting of the brain and the spinal cord. It is also important to understand how the senses work and how the spinal cord and brain control the muscles in hands, arms and legs. The development of the nervous system before and after birth is discussed in a section of this Chapter. I will also discuss some basic neuroscience matters that are important for understanding the plasticity of the brain and the spinal cord.

1.1. The Different Parts of the Brain and Spinal Cord are Interconnected

It was earlier thought that each part of the brain had dedicated functions; for example, vision would use one part, hearing another, muscle control yet another part of the brain, and so on. In a similar way, memory was thought to be located in certain regions of the brain. It was also believed that higher thought processes and memory only involved limited and dedicated parts of the brain. Pain was assumed to only activate nerve cells in certain regions known as the pain pathways. We know now that this is not the way the brain functions. Different parts are involved in many different functions and, for example, when we hear a sound many parts of the brain become active. Other sensory signals also activate many regions of the brain. Not only do sensory pathways participate in interpretation of sensory information, but regions of the brain involved in the control of muscles also participate.

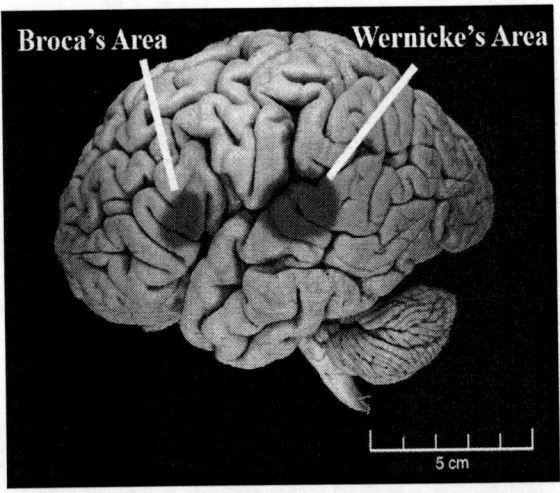

Figure 1.1. Picture of the brain (Courtesy of Dr. Edwin Rubel) with speech regions marked.

Interpreting sensory signals involves motor functions. Many sensory signals are interpreted by the brain issuing motor commands generated in the parts of the brain that normally control muscles, but without causing any muscle contractions. This means sensory signals such as speech sounds are interpreted with help from mimicking speech sounds using brain commands to muscles. Morris Halle, a speech researcher at Massachusetts Institute of Technology, first described this theory of "analysis by synthesis". People with lesions in a certain area of the brain that has to do with formulating coherent speech, known as Wernicke's area (or the posterior speech area) (see Figure 1.1), have difficulties in comprehending speech. People with lesions in a different area of the brain, known as Broca's area (or the anterior speech area) (see Figure 1.1), on the other hand, can understand speech but cannot speak because Broca's area has to do with sending commands to the muscles that are used for speaking. Wernicke's area is therefore an example of a brain area that is used for at least two different tasks, namely for controlling spoken words and for comprehending speech.

Interestingly, people who are deaf and use sign language for communication seem to use the same parts of the brain for interpreting signs as hearing people use for interpreting spoken language. Neural plasticity has made visual signals play the same role as spoken words have for hearing individuals. The same areas that are involved in spoken language usage and comprehension are also involved in reading. Therefore, losing the ability to speak (aphasia) or understand language, which often occurs after a stroke or head trauma, also causes problems with reading and writing [3].

Memory is distributed to many parts of the brain, even to the cerebellum, which was earlier associated with movement control now is known to store some kinds of information. Likewise, it is now known that acquiring knowledge, intuition, and other thought processes does not only involve parts of the forebrain but also other parts of the brain, even the cerebellum participates in thought processes.

The finding that each task is distributed over many parts of the brain has brought new insight into how the brain works but has also made it more difficult to get a comprehensive understanding of functions of the nervous system.

The fact that many parts of the brain are involved in most tasks can also explain why medications that are given to correct neural transmitters in a certain part of the brain will inevitably affect many other regions and therefore affect other functions than those anticipated. This is what we call side effects of medications. I will discuss that in Chapter V. The place in the brain where a certain task is performed can change as a result of neural plasticity, as I will discuss later, and many tasks can be carried out in different parts of the brain. This *redundancy* (duplication of function) is important for making it possible to replace functions that have been lost to trauma or strokes (through neural plasticity).

2. THE BUILDING BLOCKS OF THE BRAIN AND THE SPINAL CORD

The gray matter of the brain is composed of nerve cells that form clusters known as nuclei and the cerebral cortex. In the spinal cord, nerve cells are located in what is known as the horns of the spinal cord (Figure 1.2).

Nerve cells are complex structures and there are many different kinds. A typical nerve cell has extensions known as *dendrites* and *axons*; dendrites being the receiving organ and the axon of a nerve cell sends signals from a nerve cell to other nerve cells or to muscles and glands. The cell itself has all the common parts of a cell, such as a *nucleus*[2]), mitochondria, and organelles such as endoplasmatic reticulum, Golgi apparatus, etc. Signals from sensory receptors and from other nerve cells reach a nerve cell through *synapses*[3]). Most synapses terminate on the dendrites of cells but some terminate on the cell's membrane. Most nerve cells have many synapses terminating on them and the number of synapses on a single cell ranges from a few to several thousand.

---

[2] The name nucleus is also used for a cluster of nerve cells.

[3] The word synapse comes from "synaptein" coined by a pioneer in neuroscience, the British scientist Sir Charles Scott Sherrington (1857-1952), by combining the Greek word "syn" meaning "together" with the word "haptein" meaning "clasp".

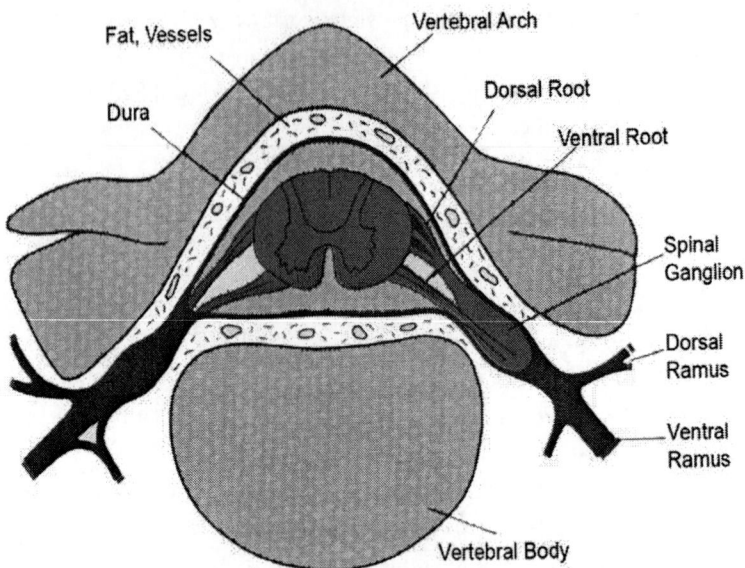

Figure 1.2A. Cross-section of the spinal cord, showing gray matter (collection of nerve cells) that has the shape of "horns". The white matter is fiber tracts, bundles of nerve fibers. (Modified from Brodal, A. 2004. *The Central Nervous System Third Edition* Oxford University Press, New York, with permission by Oxford University Press) [1].

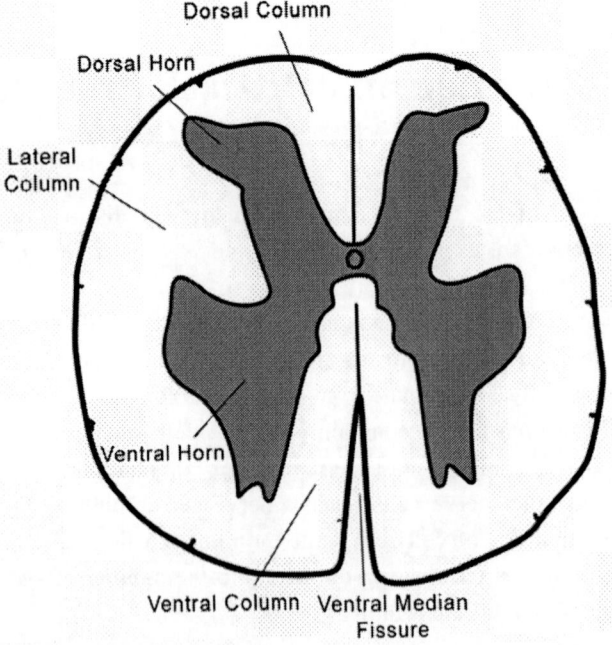

Figure 1.2B. Gray matter of spinal cord outlined.

The drawing in Figure 1.3 gives a much simplified description of a typical nerve cell – many details are omitted to keep the description comprehensible.

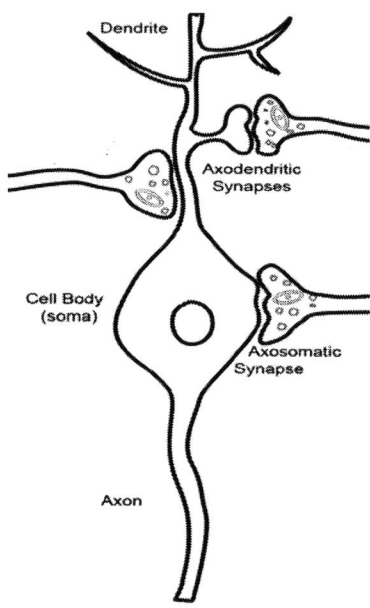

Figure 1.3. Schematic drawing of a typical nerve cell as found in the brain and the spinal cord. It is shown how synapses can be located on different parts of a cell.

Axons (or nerve fibers) are the transmission lines of the nervous system through which the sensory organs send messages to the brain and through which muscles receive commands. In the brain and the spinal cord, nerve cells communicate with each other through axons. Some axons are covered by an insulating substance known as myelin (an electrical insulating substance), some are not. Different axons have different diameters and the velocity with which messages travel in axons is proportional to the diameter of axons. The diameter of axons that are covered by myelin varies between 1 and 15 micron (thousands of a millimeter) and the corresponding velocity vary between 3 and 75 meter/second. Axons that are not covered by myelin (often referred to as C-fibers) conduct much slower, between 0.5 and 2.0 meter/second. Nerve fibers are classified according to the diameter of their axons, as Aα for those fibers that have the largest axons, Aβ fibers are smaller, and Aδ having the smallest axons. Nerve fibers that have no myelin are classified as C fibers.

Axons can have very different lengths. In the brain some axons are only a few millimeters long. Axons from cells in the motor cortex can reach cells in the spinal cord and axons from nerve cells in the spinal cord can reach muscles even as far away as the foot. Axons can therefore be very long – 5-6 feet long. Axons often have branches (bifurcate), often many branches, as discussed in connection with the description of sensory and motor pathways.

The word nucleus can have several meanings: In medical terminology a nucleus (plural nuclei) can be a part of a cell, and in neuroscience (anatomy) the term is used for a group (cluster) of nerve cells in the brain. Sometimes the term ganglion (plural ganglia) is used for a nucleus, but the word ganglion is more commonly used for the collection of cell bodies of nerves, such as dorsal root ganglia and autonomic ganglia.

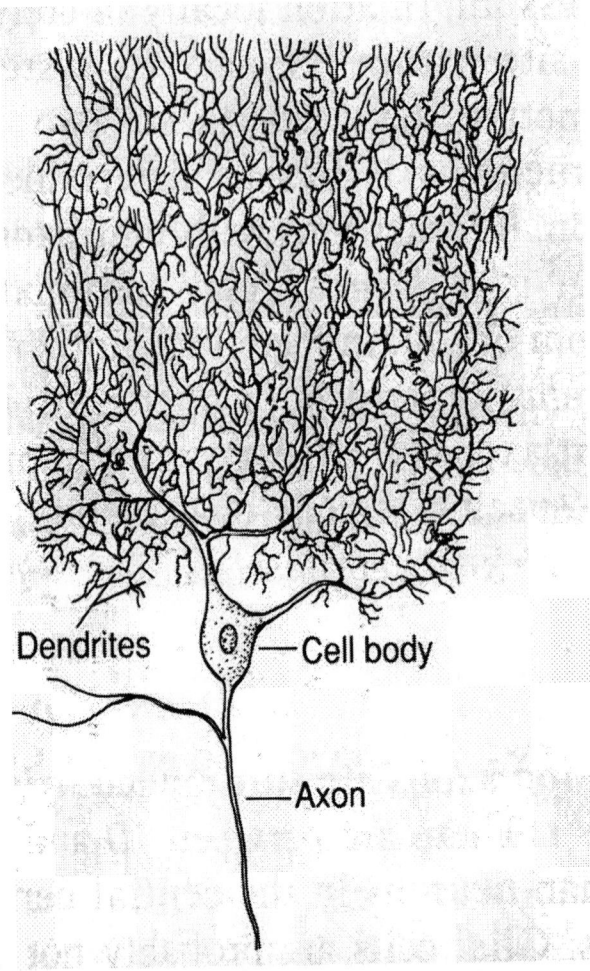

Figure 1.4. A nerve cell that has an exceptionally large dendritic tree (a Purkinje cell from the cerebellum). Reproduced from "Principles of Neural Science" Third Edition, Kandel, Schwartz Jessell, published by Appleton and Lange 1991, with permission from McGraw-Hill Companies).

Nerve cells differ much, many nerve cells have thousands of synapses and some have very large dendritic trees (Figure 1.4).

2.1. Connections between Nerve Cells (Synapses)

Synapses are the contact organ between an axon and the membrane of a nerve cell. There are two main kinds of synapses, chemical and electrical synapses. Chemical synapses use chemical substances (known as transmitter substances) to increase, or decrease the activation of the nerve cells with which they contact (see Figure 1.5) Electrical synapses work by injecting an electrical current into a nerve cell. That current can activate the nerve cell or the opposite; it can reduce the activity of a cell.

Synapses are the junctions between nerve fibers (axons) and nerve cells. There are different kinds of synapses, some are chemical and others are electrical. Synapses make the signals that are carried in the axons to activate the target nerve cell. Synapses also are the junction between a motor nerve and muscles, and synapses connect axons with glands. There are three kinds of chemical synapses, axo-dendritic synapses that terminate on a nerve cell's dendrites, axo-somatic synapses that terminate on the membrane of a cell, and axo-axonic synapses which can also modulate the impulse traffic in an axon.

In chemical synapses, small packets of special chemicals are shuttled over a small space between the ending of an axon and the membrane of nerve cells or its dendrites. When the chemical enters through the membrane of the cell the signals in the axons may activate the target cells so that it can send the message further on in the axon that leaves the cell (Figure 1.5).

It has been estimated that young children have about 10^{16} synapses (10 quadrillion). The number decreases with age and adults have about 10 times fewer synapses (1-5 times 10^{15}).

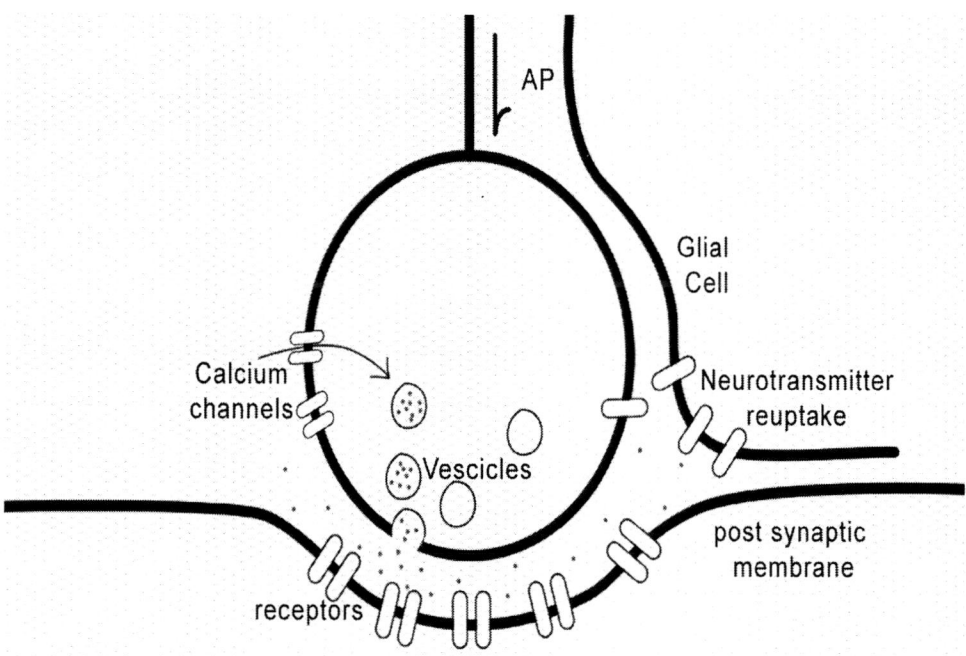

Figure 1.5A. Activation of the connections between nerve cells (synaptic transmission) is incredibly complex as shown in the picture below. Much simplified, it involves one or, more often, several substances known as transmitter substances. These chemicals are shuttled over the space between the termination of the axon, the synapse, and the membrane of the cell or, more often, the cells' dendrites. This space is very small, about 20 nanometers (20 millionth of a millimeter).

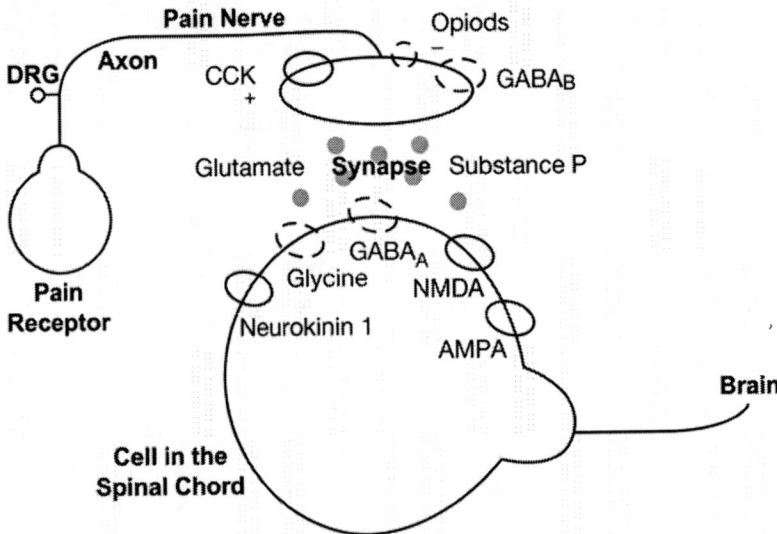

Figure 1.5B. Illustration of the involvement of many transmitter substances in synaptic transmission of pain signals in the spinal cord.

One axon can make contact with more than one cell (Figure 1.6) (known as divergence), and a cell in a neural network may receive signals through axons from many different cells (known as convergence).

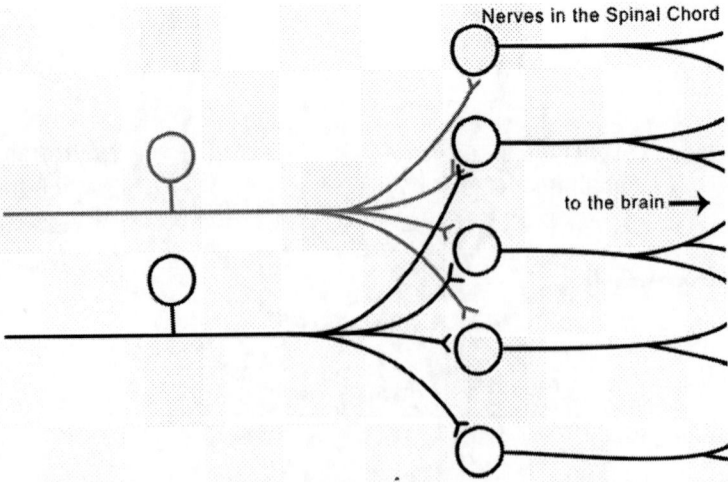

Figure 1.6. Schematic drawing of how axons connect to the next nerve cells in a typical chain of nerve cells. The picture shows that an axon may terminate on more than one nerve cell (divergence).

The picture does not show how many contacts (synapses) each nerve cell receives; it can vary between a few to several thousand, and the number of synapses varies with age. It has been estimated that in the adult brain an average cell and their dendrites receive about 1000 contacts. During development there is a competition for synaptic space on a target nerve cell. Synapses are more abundant in some parts of the brain than in others.

2.1.1. Synaptic Transmission

There are two main types of synapses, excitatory synapses that increase the likelihood of activating the target cell and inhibitory synapses that decrease the likelihood of activating the cell into sending impulses further through its axons. This makes it possible for signals that arrive at nerve cells to either accelerate or decelerate the firing in the axon that leaves the nerve cell. Altering the relation between inhibition and excitation can determine how much a cell responds and even whether it will respond or not to an incoming signal.

The signals a cell receives through the synapses that terminate on its dendrites or on its membrane controls the membrane potential of a cell. When the membrane potential exceeds the threshold, an action potential is generated in the cell's axon. That action potential propagates to the end of the axon where it may influence the next nerve cell in a chain of nerve cells. Inhibitory signals can make a cell not respond to excitatory signals at all. It is therefore the balance between excitation and inhibition that determines whether or not the signals a nerve cell receives through its connections will activate the cell. For example, most nerve cells in the pathways of sensory systems also receive signals from other parts of the brain and, in particular, from more central parts of the same sensory system. These descending connections are known to their structure but very little is known about their function.

2.1.2. Synaptic Transmission can be Modulated

The connections between axons and nerve cells are not all active. The ability of impulses in axons to activate the target nerve cells depends on the efficacy of the synapse that connects the axon with the cell. Anatomical studies can provide information about which pathways are available, but not whether they can be used. Many synapses cannot be activated and are said to be dormant. Activity that arrives at a dormant synapse will not activate the target cell. Axons that have dormant synapses cannot activate their target cells. This means anatomical studies that show axons in the brain give the impression of the existence of far more pathways than are functional. I will discuss that in detail in Chapter II.

The fact that transmission of signals by synapses can change and can be modulated are some of the bases for neural plasticity, and therefore important to consider when discussing the different aspects of neural plasticity in the Chapters of this book that follows.

Inactive synapses are "dormant" and cannot transfer signals from axons to the cell on which they terminate.

We often use information about the anatomy of the nervous system to understand how it functions. However, many connections between nerve cells in the central nervous system (axons) that are identified using anatomical methods of study are not functional because the connections between the fibers and their target nerve cells cannot be activated. We call such contacts "dormant". Such normally unused connections can be activated by different means such as novel activation; absence (deprivation) of activation or other factors may make it possible for activity in the nerve fibers to open ("unmask") such normally closed connections (see Chapter I). Connections that are not conducting (dormant) are common in all parts of the CNS. This means that we need to distinguish between anatomical connections that are functional and those that are not. Anatomical studies only provide information about which pathways are available and physiological studies are required to determine if pathways are open for neural traffic. Studies of (anatomical) connections therefore give the impression that there are many more connections than what actually have importance, because anatomical connections that are not functional have no importance.

Chemicals of various kinds can modulate the way synapses work. Many complex processes are involved in what we call plastic changes of synaptic efficacy. Activation of neural plasticity may cause "unmasking" of dormant synapses, activating new circuits in the brain and spinal cord. Active circuits are established every time we learn something, and these circuits very much stay active for the lifetime.

3. DEVELOPMENT OF THE NERVOUS SYSTEM

The basic structure of the nervous system is developed before birth, but further maturation is necessary to complete the development of the nervous system. The organization of the brain and spinal cord is only roughly laid out before birth (see figure 1.7). The basic development is normally completed after birth through activation of neural plasticity (see Chapter II). Activation of senses and use of the motor system is necessary for achieving the final organization of the nervous system.

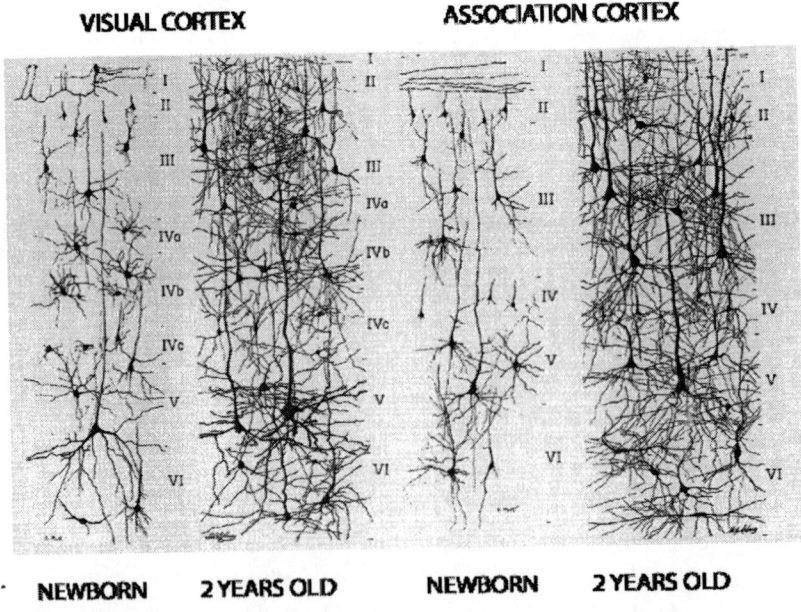

Figure 1.7. Development of the human cerebral cortex after birth. The two left hand pictures are from the visual (striate) cortex and the two other are from the parietal (association) cortex. The drawings are based on Golgi stain, is commonly used to visualize nerve cells, their dendritic trees and axons (2). (Reproduced from Brodal, A. 2004. The Central Nervous System Third Edition Oxford University Press, New York, after Conel JL. *The postnatal development of the human cerebral cortex*. Cambridge, MA: Harvard University Press; 1939, with permission by Harvard University Press).

3.1. Development of the Brain and Spinal Cord before Birth

The development of the nervous system occurs in phases that follow each other. In each phase the development is guided by certain factors. The earliest different molecules are secreted and provide targeting cues for outgrowing axons. In the next phase, neural activity guides the establishment of neural networks.

The first step concerns creation of the first neural tissue; after which cells begin to divide and multiply. These primitive cells must move around to find their correct position in the brain and the spinal cord of the fetus. Clusters of nerve cells, known as nuclei, are formed by groups of cells. This is the third step in the development of the nervous system. Later, cells begin to differentiate and get outgrowths such as axons and dendrites. This may be regarded as the fourth step in the development of the brain. During that time the cell membranes begin to become diverse in different cells and neural transmitters develop. Connections between nerve cells develop in this stage. The next step includes outgrowth of axons and the establishment of contacts between axons and membranes of nerve cells with their dendrites – sometimes also with axons. At this stage the axons must find the right cell to make contact with. There are substances secreted from cells that "attract" axons and direct the outgrowth of the axons to make synaptic contact with their target nerve cells (Fig 1.8).

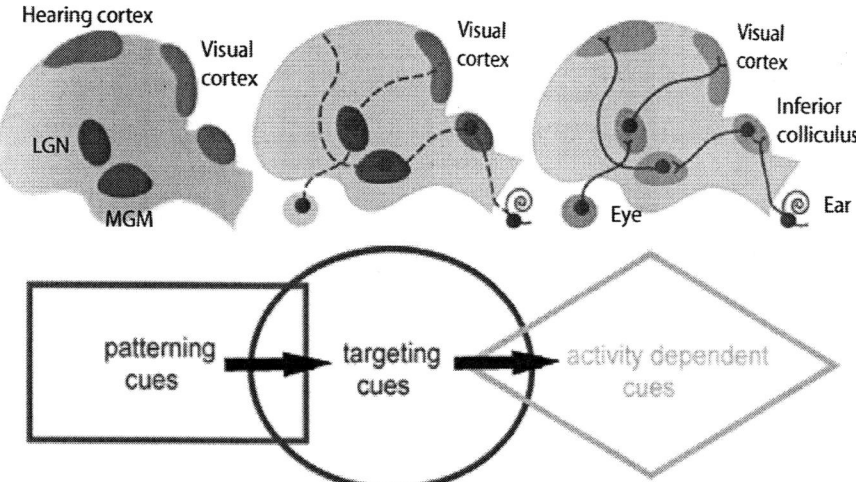

Figure 1.8. Illustration of how the neural pathways of senses (hearing and vision) develop before birth. LGN: Lateral geniculate nucleus, visual thalamic nucleus; MGM: Medial geniculate nucleus, hearing thalamic nucleus. (Reproduced from Horng, S.H., Sur, M. 2006. Visual activity and cortical rewiring: Activity-dependent plasticity of cortical networks. In: Møller, A.R., (Ed.), *Reprogramming the brain*, *Progress in Brain Research* Vol. 157. Elsevier, Amsterdam. pp. 3-11, with permission from Elsevier.

When axons arrive at nerve cells they establish synaptic contacts in a somewhat orderly fashion, but meaningful sensory signals are necessary to achieve the organization of the nervous system that is normal.

Many more nerve cells are created during the early part of the development than there are in the brain at birth. (Nerve cells are created at a rate of 250,000 per minute during early pregnancy).

Individual structures of the brain are laid out early in pregnancy. For example, the hemispheres start to develop in the fifth week and the development of the cerebral cortex starts in the eighth week.

Axons begin to get their normal myelin covering within the fourth month of pregnancy, but this process is slow and is not completed until 2-3 years after birth – progressing through the spinal cord in the direction toward the brain.

The growth and development of the brain (maturation) is controlled by mainly two factors. Our genes control a part of the development, which means genetics (and epigenetics[4])) are important for development before birth. Environmental factors also play a role as do unknown factors. The way the brain and the spinal cord develop can be affected by chemicals the mother is exposed to, diseases she may have, or her lack of adequate nutrition [5]. Until recently, these factors have been overlooked when developmental disorders such as autism are discussed (see Appendix C).

3.1.1. Development of Sensory Areas of the Brain

The networks of nerve cells in the brain and the spinal cord are first created by transcription of genes. As these networks form, target cues are generated to attract outgrowing axons so they find their correct target. For the visual system, axons from the eyes grow towards unique targets in the visual nuclei in the thalamus, and these nerve cells in turn send axons towards the visual areas of the cerebral cortex. The hearing system is somewhat more complex, but in principle, similar events occur to develop the pathways from the ear to the cerebral hearing cortex. From there the neural circuits become more complex, with axons branching and making connections to more nerve cells. These developments are guided by information from genes. After birth, development is guided by a combination of cues, such as chemical attractants and neural activity.

3.2. Development of the Brain and Spinal Cord after Birth

The brain and the spinal cord undergo extensive development after birth. Many nerve cells die during a period of a few years after birth in what is known as programmed cell death (PCD). Also many connections (axons) are eliminated. The "pruning" that reduces the connections is more extensive than the cell death and it goes on for a longer time than the cell deaths. Probably as many as 90% of nerve cells in the cerebral cortex die, whereas only 50% of the motor nerve cells in the spinal cord die during these processes. Many hypotheses have been presented to explain why we start out with too many synapses and entire nerve cells.

---

[4] Epigenetics: The word epigenetics means "above or over genetics" and it describes processes that cause changes in heredity without changing genes (DNA structure). Epigenetics, which is a way that environmental factors can change the way genes work, is one of the most exciting branches of biological science. More than 2500 articles about epigenetics were published during 2006.

The changes are controlled by programs laid out before birth, and by activation of neural plasticity. The changes that occur in the cerebral cortex after birth are considerable, as seen in Figure 1.7. Connections from the visual system to the spinal cord are eliminated and connections from the brain to circuits in the spinal cord that control reflexes are established. Neural circuits in the spinal cord can control movements, such as locomotion, and they are developed before birth. However, the brain's control of these circuits is established after birth, starting with the arms and later including the legs.

The programmed cell death, and in particular, the pruning of axons continue after birth. (Programmed cell death is also called apoptosis and it is different from cell death caused by injuries to cells such as from lack of oxygen). Development becomes guided by meaningful sensory signals such as speech, visual images, etc. that activate changes in the organization of various parts of the brain and the spinal cord (see Chapter II).

In the hearing system, nerve cells that respond to different sound frequencies are organized according to the frequency of the sounds because the basilar membrane of the cochlea separate frequencies with low ones represented at the tip of the cochlea and high ones at the base (known as tonotopic maps, se Chapter II). Also, the systems of nerve cells that control muscles are arranged according to their location on the body, but also here, use of the muscles are necessary to achieve the normal organization.

The development of the brain that occurs after birth therefore has many aspects and it stretches over long time. It seems as the development of the regions of the brain that are involved in such complex tasks as decision making are not fully developed before the age of 18-20 years.

4. ORGANIZATION OF THE BRAIN AND SPINAL CORD

It is especially sensory and motor functions that can be modified through neural plasticity. In this Chapter, I will therefore focus on how these are organized. In the discussion of sensory systems I will include pain circuits in the spinal cord and the brain, although pain is not normally regarded as a sense.

4.1. Sensory Pathways

Each of the four senses; hearing, vision, touch, and taste have two different pathways that climb from the sensory receptors to the cerebral cortex, and two that go down towards the receptors.

Sensory information as well as information about pain is carried to higher centers of the brain in these two climbing pathways that we call the classical and the non-classical pathways (Appendix A and B). These pathways are strings of nerve cell clusters (nuclei). Axons from the receptors in the ear, eye, nose, tongue, and the skin make synaptic contact with cells in the first of these nerve cell clusters (nuclei) that are located on the same side of the body as the receptors. The cells in these nuclei send axons to the next cluster of nerve cells, usually located on the other side of the brain. There can be several such clusters that information from receptors passes before it reaches the cerebral cortex. The clusters of nerve cells in these climbing pathways process (transform) the information that arrives by sensory cells before the information reaches the cerebral cortex.

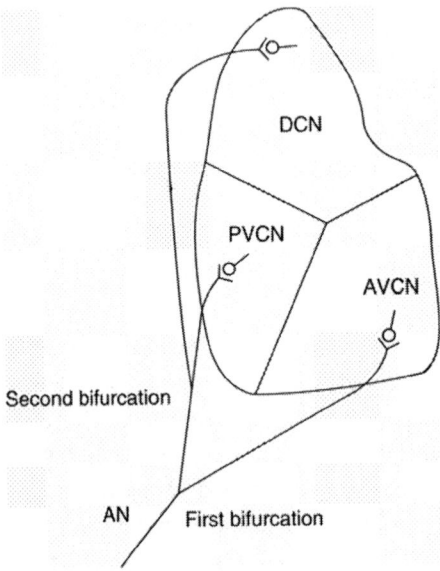

Figure 1.9. Schematic illustration of parallel processing of information in sensory system. (Reproduced from: Møller, A.R. 2006. *Hearing: Anatomy, Physiology, and Disorders of the Auditory System*, 2nd Ed. Academic Press, Amsterdam, with permission from Elsevier).

Information is processed sequentially in the sensory systems as well as in parallel (parallel processing). Sequential processing means that information is processing in one after another of a chain of nuclei. Parallel processing means the same information is processed in different structures of the brain. In the hearing pathways, parallel processing begins already when nerve fibers of the hearing nerve reach the first nucleus of the hearing pathways (the cochlear nucleus). Here nerve fibers from the ear branches out so that each nerve fiber makes connection to cells in all three of the main divisions of the cochlear nucleus (Figure 1.9). Nerve fibers from each of these groups of nerve cells connect to nerve cells in different parts of the hearing pathways.

Signals from sense organs can reach the cerebral cortex through two main routes, known às the ascending (climbing) sensory pathways. These ascending pathways consist of a chain of several nuclei that are connected by nerve fibers. Different senses have different nuclei, but the pathways of all senses pass through separate nuclei in a part of the brain known as the thalamus. The ascending pathways for all senses reach their own part of the cerebral cortex (the primary sensory cortex), from where signals travel to common parts of the cerebral cortex known as the association cortices and from there to other parts of the brain. There are also descending pathways that pass signals from the cortex and nuclei of the ascending pathways downwards to other nuclei and even as far as sensory cells in the sense organs such as the ear.

Sensory systems are often shown in a way that gives the impression that the primary cerebral cortex is the end-station. This is not the case. The signals that reach the cerebral cortex are conveyed further to secondary and association cortices after being processed in the primary cortex. We do not know where in this long chain of structures the nerve signals are perceived as sounds, visual images, taste, or touch. We know the signals that reach the structures that give perceptions are constructed on the basis of not only the sensory signals that reach the sensory receptors, but these signals are also influenced by different parts of the brain such as those that control wakefulness and attention.

There are two parallel pathways in which sensory information travels to the cortical regions of the brain. The best known of the two I will call classical pathways (also known as the lemniscal pathways or "precise" pathways); the other, much less known pathway, I call the non-classical pathways (also known as extra-lemniscal pathways or the diffuse pathway). Figure 1.10 shows a simplified drawing of the classical pathways of the hearing system and Figure 1.11 shows a simplified drawing of the non-classical pathways

One important difference is related to the thalamus, where the classical pathways use one side of the thalamus (the ventral part) while the non-classical pathways use the other side (the dorsal part). There are other differences between these two different pathways. The nerve cells in the nuclei of the classical hearing pathways can only be activated by sound, where as many nerve cells in the non-classical pathways can also be activated by signals from receptors in the skin and in the eye.

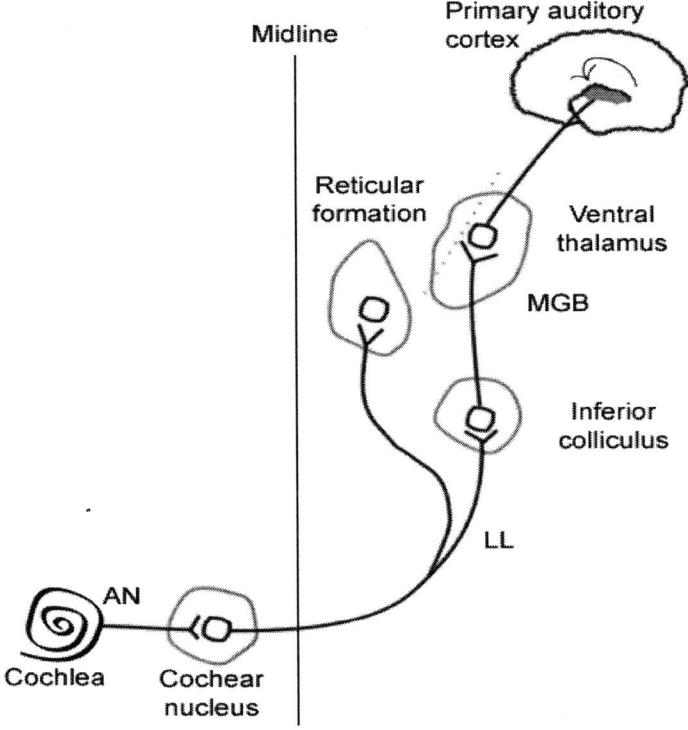

Figure 1.10. Very simplified classical hearing pathways from one ear to the primary cortex

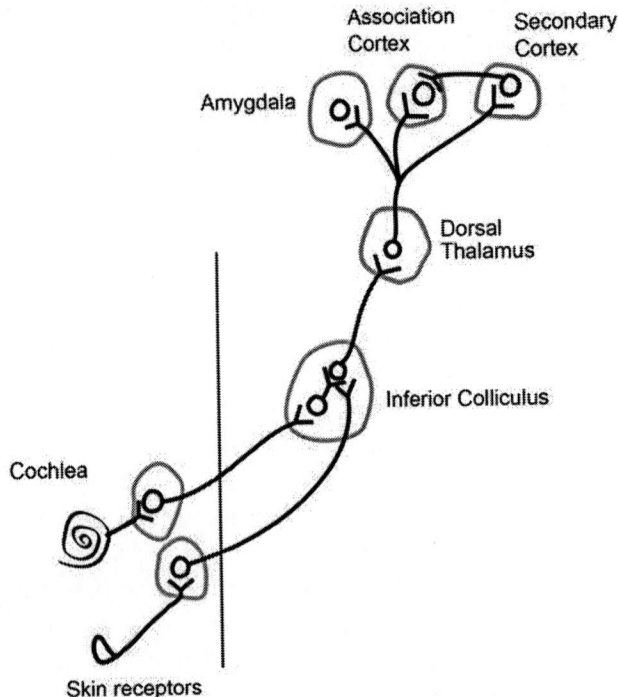

Figure 1.11. Schematic diagram of the non-classical hearing pathways from one ear.

Connections from the dorsal-medial thalamus in the non-classical pathway bypass the primary cortex and project directly to association cortices; the signals that travel in the non-classical pathways join the signals from the classical pathways (see Figure 1.11). The processing that occurs in these two different pathways is different. The non-classical pathways process signals in a less sophisticated way ("fast and dirty") than what occurs in the classical pathways ("slow and accurate") [9].

Classical and non-classical pathways make it possible for some information to reach the "emotional brain", known as the limbic system but in different ways (see Appendix B).

> The receptors for our sense of balance are in the inner ear and they are reacting when a person turns their head. The function is to assist in keeping balance (posture) and move the eyes so that a steady image is maintained on the retina in the eye when the head is turned. A reflex known as the vestibular-ocular reflex moves the eye in the opposite direction to keep an image steady on the retina. This reflex normally works without causing conscious awareness.

4.2. The Cerebral Cortex

The cerebral cortex has many parts and the different parts form a chain of complex networks of nerve cells. The primary sensory cortices are the first that are reached by sensory information. Signals that reach the primary cortices are conveyed to other parts of the cerebral cortices (secondary and, the association cortices), where information from different senses and from other parts of the brain are coordinated.

The first stage of the cerebral cortex, the primary sensory cortices, has often been regarded to be the end station of the sensory pathways, but it is by no means the end station for processing information. Sensory information progresses from the primary sensory cortices to the association cortex, where information from different sensory systems is coordinated and joined together. It is not exactly known where in the brain sensory information causes awareness and where interpretation of sensory messages occurs. It is now believed that perception of sensory information is processed in large parts of the cerebral cortex, and also in many other parts of the brain. For example, the sense of smell has very little representation in the cortex and most of the signals go to the emotional brain (the amygdala, which is a part of the emotional brain).

It is known, however, that signals can take two different paths in the association cortices. Information about the place from where sensory information comes (such as direction to a visual object or a sound source, "where") is processed in dorsal parts of the cerebral cortex, and object information ("what" kind of information) is processed in ventral parts of the cerebral cortex. This separation of different information in "where" and "what" path is known as stream segregation (see Figure 1.12).

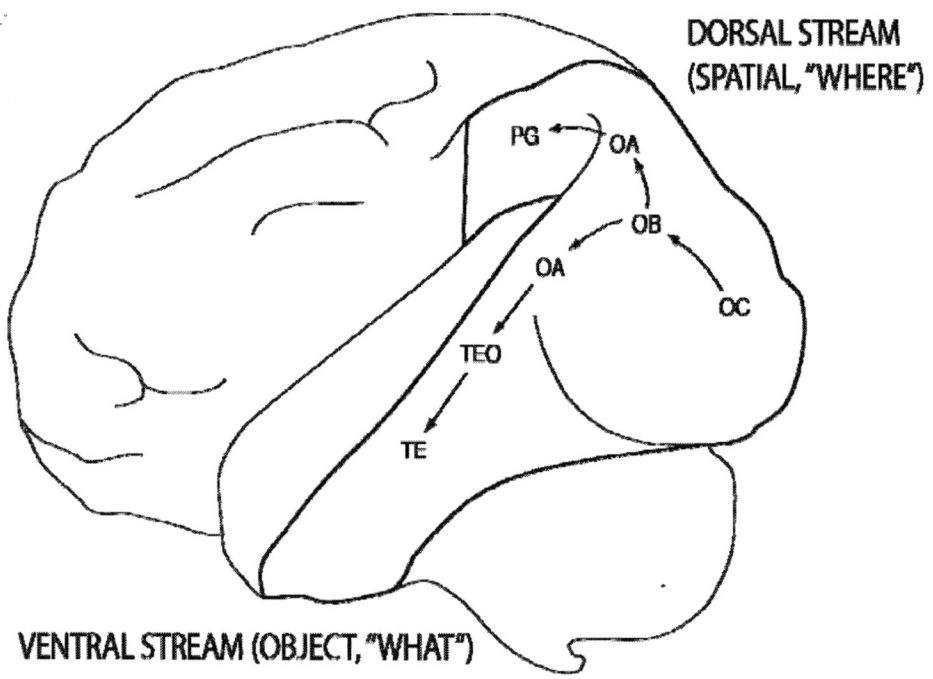

Figure 1.12. Stream segregation in the visual system in the monkey. PG: Parietal OA: OB: OC: occipital; TEO: Posterior inferior temporal cortex and TE: Anterior inferior temporal cortex. (Modified from Mishkin, M., Ungerleider, L.G., Macko, K.A. 1983. Object vision and spatial vision: Two cortical pathways. *Trends Neurosci.* 6, 415-417. Reprinted with permission of Elsevier [8]).

5. THE BRAIN

The adult brain weighs between 1,300-1,400 grams (about 3 pounds), but uses about 20% of the body's oxygen while resting. A newborn's weighs 350-400 grams. The brain is enormously intricate, and it is impossible to imagine its complexity. It is not known exactly how many nerve cells in the brain there are, but it is estimated to be in the range of 100 billion; this is 300 times the population of the US. Most of these (about 70 billion) are in the cerebellum and 12-15 billion are in the telencephalon (forebrain including the cerebral cortex). The human spinal cord has about 1 billion nerve cells [1]. Some investigators have arrived at slightly different numbers; Pakkenberg [10] for example, reported that the average number of nerve cells in the neocortex is slightly different in males and females (females 19.3 billion and males 22.8 billion, a difference of 16%).

The same investigator [10] estimated the total number of nerve cells in the human cortex to be 2,600,000,000 in a single individual (an 18 year old man). There are considerable variations, and information from single individuals must therefore be interpreted with caution. The total length of axons is about 150,000 to 180,000 kilometers (93,000 to 112,000 miles) in young people [10]. The total length of axons was shorter in older people. The number of nerve cells changes considerably during early childhood. In the cerebral cortex the number of contacts on each cell has been estimated at about 1,500 when we are born; 15,000 in early childhood; and 7,500 in adulthood on average. The total number of synapses in the human cortex has been estimated to 1500×10^{12} (1500 trillion) but these numbers have a high degree of uncertainty.

Other studies using data from many individuals have shown that the visual cortex in an unborn fetus at 20 weeks of gestation has a density of more than one million nerve cells per cubic millimeter, decreasing more than tenfold until birth when it is about 90,000 cells per cubic millimeter. It continues to decrease after birth reaching 40,000 per cubic millimeter at the age of 4 months after which it remains more or less stable at 35,000 nerve cells per cubic millimeter. The density increases slightly with age, reaching 44,000 nerve cells per cubic millimeter, as determined in five individuals at age 80 years [6]. Each one of these nerve cells makes connections to many other nerve cells.

The volume of the brain changes with age. Again, it was the visual cortex that was studied [7]. The thickness of the cerebral cortex increases about 83% between 21 gestational weeks and birth, and the volume increased about 31%. The number of nerve cells varies widely from one person to another but these investigators could not find any noticeable decrease after birth.

The difference in the total number of neocortical nerve cells over a range of 70 years (range 20–90 years) was 9.5%, providing an average "loss" of nerve cells of about 85,000 per day, or about 1 per second [10]. There is therefore no evidence of any major loss of nerve cells with, presumed healthy, aging.

The same study showed that there were several trillion connections (synapses) in the neocortex. The number of such connections between different nerve cells varies; on an average each nerve cell connects to thousands of other nerve cells. The effect of aging was only about 10%, which is less than the effect of the gender difference (16%).

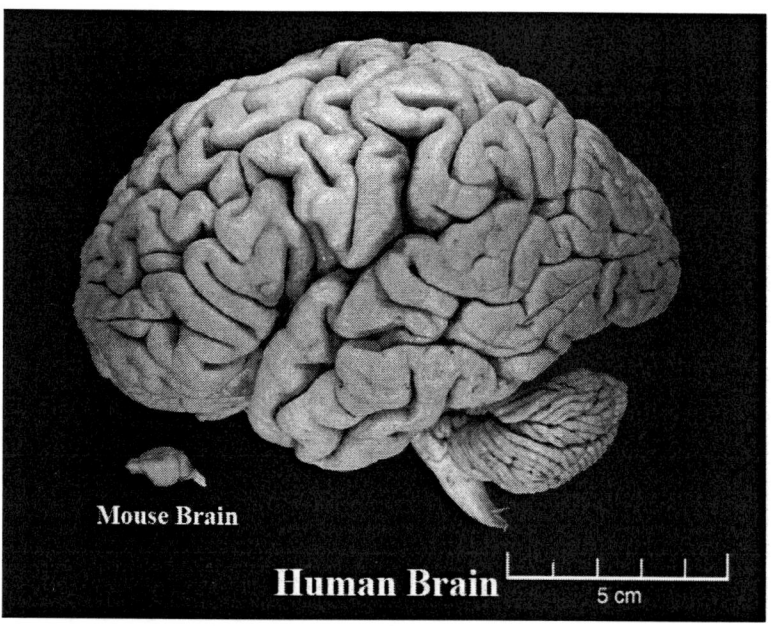

Figure 1.13. Comparison the size of the human brain and that of a mouse, often used in biomedical studies. (Courtesy Dr. Edwin Rubel).

REFERENCES

[1]   Brodal A. *The Central Nervous System Third Edition*. New York: Oxford University Press; 2004.

[2]   Conel JL. *The postnatal development of the human cerebral cortex*. Cambridge, MA: Harvard University Press; 1939.

[3]   Damasio AR. Brain and Language. *Mind and Brain: Readings from Scientific American Magazine*: W.H. Freeman and Co.; 1993.

[4]   Horng SH, Sur M. Visual activity and cortical rewiring: Activity-dependent plasticity of cortical networks. In: Møller AR, editor. *Reprogramming the brain*. Amsterdam: Elsevier; 2006. p. 3-11

[5]   Kenet T, Froemke RC, Schreiner CE, Pessah IN, Merzenich MM. Perinatal exposure to a noncoplanar polychlorinated biphenyl alters tonotopy, receptive fields, and plasticity in rat primary auditory cortex. *Proc Natl Acad Sci U S A*. 2007;104(18):7646-51.

[6]   Leuba G, Garey LJ. Evolution of neuronal numerical density in the developing and aging human visual cortex. *Hum Neurobiol* 1987;6(1):11-8.

[7]   Leuba G, Kraftsik R. Changes in volume, surface estimate, three-dimensional shape and total number of neurons of the human primary visual cortex from midgestation until old age. *Anat Embryol (Berl)*. 1994;190(4):351-66.

[8]   Mishkin M, Ungerleider LG, Macko KA. Object vision and spatial vision: Two cortical pathways. *Trends Neurosci*. 1983;6:415-7.

[9]   Møller AR. *Hearing: Anatomy, Physiology, and Disorders of the Auditory System, 2nd Ed.* Amsterdam: Academic Press; 2006.

[10] Pakkenberg B, Pelvig D, Marner L, Bundgaard MJ, Gundersen HJ, Nyengaard JR, et al. Aging and the human neocortex. *Exp Gerontol.* 2003;38(1-2):95-9.

[11] Williams R, W., Herrup K. The control of neuron number. *Ann Rev Neurosci.* 1988;11:423-53.

Chapter II

NEURAL PLASTICITY

ABSTRACT

Neural plasticity is the ability of the nervous system to change its function. It is a property of the nervous system and its presence only becomes evident when activated (turned on). Lack of sensory signals and inactivity such as lack of muscle usage are the most common factors that can induce plastic changes. However, some forms of activation of the nervous system can also activate neural plasticity. Activation of neural plasticity is necessary for normal development of the brain at birth. Sensory signals help guide the development of the brain during early childhood and neural plasticity provides a "midcourse correction" of what was laid down before birth.

The changes that are induced through activation of neural plasticity involve the way connections between nerve cells (synapses) work. The efficacy of synapses can change, new synapses can be formed and synapses can be eliminated. Other changes that can occur involve alterations in protein synthesis in nerve cells, creation of new nerve fibers and dendrites as well as elimination of existing ones. Even entire nerve cells can be eliminated as a result of activation of neural plasticity.

Activation of neural plasticity is a form of learning, but neural plasticity is different from memorizing in that the changes are always available whereas what is learned must be recalled from memory.

Throughout life, activation of neural plasticity can reorganize the nervous system by opening new routes for information. Activation of neural plasticity can enhance or suppress reflexes and change which parts of the brain are used for different tasks. Activation of neural plasticity can also close routes that are normally used by making active synapses inactive (dormant), eliminating synapses, axons or dendrites. The maps on the cerebral cortex of the surface of the body can change by activation of neural plasticity, and so can other sensory representations on the cerebral cortex and on other structures of the brain.

Neural plasticity can be turned on by absence of normal sensory signals such as occurs when sense organs are not functioning. This in turn can be caused by congenital disorders or acquired diseases and by trauma, for example amputations of limbs. Lack of sensory signals during the development prevents normal development of the affected parts of the brain, and lack of sensory signals later in life can cause symptoms such as tinnitus. Extended use of senses improves functions and extended use of muscles or muscle groups can improve manual skills.

1. INTRODUCTION

The brain does not change its shape in the way formable material can, but it can change the way it functions and how its cells are connected to each other ("wired"). The Activation of neural plasticity can change the way different parts of the brain are connected to each other.

Neural plasticity is based on synapses' ability to change the way they work (their *efficacy or strength*) and it may involve formation or elimination of synapses, nerve fibers and dendrites. Plastic changes also include sprouting and branching of nerve fibers, whereby new connections are created between nerve cells. Death of entire nerve cells (*programmed cell deaths*, PCD) may occur when neural plasticity is turned on. It may also cause changes in protein synthesis in nerve cells. Neural plasticity, when turned on, can cause reorganization or remodeling (re-wiring) of parts of the nervous system.

Activation of neural plasticity can change the relationship between inhibition and excitation and thereby change how easily nerve cells can be activated. It can also affect temporal summation, which is an important part of the normal function of the nervous system.

Change in synaptic efficacy, changes in protein synthesis and changes in the membrane potential of nerve cells can alter how easily nerve cells can be activated. Synapses provide connections between nerve cells. Synapses do not always functions, and these are said to be *dormant*. The creation of new nerve cells or opening of blocked connections (*unmasking of dormant synapses*) may cause reorganization ("*re-wiring*") of the neural network and can redirect the flow of neural traffic in pathways in the brain. Plastic changes occur more easily in young individuals but may also take place in adults.

Neural plasticity has many similarities with memory but there are also differences. Both memory and plasticity are based on changes in the brain that occur because of experience and practice. The changes in the function of the brain involved in memory and learning entail modification in both synaptic strength and in the organization of neural networks. Memory may be defined as something that can be consciously recalled, whereas neural plasticity involves changes in the function of the spinal cord and the brain that occur unconsciously and which cannot be recalled willfully. What has been learned by practice has to be retrieved actively and voluntarily. However, changes in skills acquired through activation of neural plasticity by training are there automatically every time the skills are used.

Learning and memory make it possible to recall both external (sensory) and internal events (thoughts, dreams). (Learning is different from understanding.) Learning leaves permanent traces in the brain consisting of neural circuits that are created in different places in the brain every time something is learned. These neural circuits may stay active for a lifetime. However, it may be difficult to retrieve the information. Neural plasticity involves the ability to change the function and the organization of the nervous system in a similar way as learning but the plasticity changes cannot be directly recalled as a memory.

An example of plastic changes in body functions that can be achieved through training is increasing the ease with which muscle reflexes can be elicited. Training an individual to speak uncommon words is another example that involves activation of neural plasticity. Memory is involved when a person chooses what to say.

It is now well documented that activation of neural plasticity is involved in recovery from damages to the spinal cord and the brain and its importance for normal development of the nervous system is beginning to be recognized. It is, however, not generally known that activation of neural plasticity can cause symptoms and signs of common diseases such as some forms of pain and tinnitus[5] and movement disorders such as spasm[6] and synkinesis[7] . I call all these diseases "plasticity diseases". Neural plasticity may also be involved in such diseases as Alzheimer's disease, depression, autism and dementia.

The study of neural plasticity is a rapidly growing area of neuroscience. It is poorly covered in books on medical diagnosis and treatment and is just beginning to attract the interest of neurologists and other clinicians.

In this Chapter, I will discuss the basis for neural plasticity, how it can be turned on, what changes in the function of the nervous system can occur, and the consequences these changes can have.

2. NATURE OF PLASTIC CHANGES

Activation of neural plasticity can 1) change synaptic efficacy and create or eliminate contacts (synapses) between nerve fibers and nerve cells and their dendrites, 2) create or eliminate nerve fibers and dendrites, and 3) cause programmed cell death. It is possible that new nerve cells can be created. The changes in function can develop rapidly, or it may take hours or days to develop. Plastic changes in function can last a short time (hours), or they can last long (lasting days or as long as a lifetime).

One of the first scientists to show that the function of the brain is plastic and could be changed was Goddard who showed impulses of electrical currents that were passed through the *amygdala*[8] in rats could cause the development of epileptic seizures. First there were no visible reactions from the rats, but after doing it every day for 4-6 weeks the electrical current began to evoke epileptic seizures [10]. Goddard likened it with lighting a fire and called this way of evoking epileptic seizures "*kindling*". Similar reactions have later been shown to occur in many other parts of the brain [26,28,39].

The ability of synapses to change their function is a key factor in all the different effects of neural plasticity. As mentioned in Chapter I, the synapse is the element that connects nerve fibers to nerve cells. There is also another way nerve cells can communicate with each other, known as *ephaptic* transmission [32], where the electrical field generated by nerve cells spreads to other nerve cells and activates many nerve cells at the same time. This is not regarded to be a normal way for nerve cells to communicate with each other, but rather as a cause of harmful neural activity such as epileptic seizures [19].

---

[5]   Tinnitus: ringing in the ears and hearing sounds that does not come from outside the body.
[6]   Spasm: *A sudden involuntary contraction of one or more muscles; includes cramps, and contractures.* (Stedman's Electronic Medical Dictionary, Version 7.0).
[7]   Synkinesis: *Involuntary movement accompanying a voluntary one, as the movement of a closed eye following that of the uncovered one, or the movement occurring in a paralyzed muscle accompanying motion in another part.* (Stedman's Electronic Medical Dictionary, Version 7.0).
[8]   The amygdala is a group of nuclei (which are clusters of nerve cells) that is part of the limbic system (the "emotional brain").

The amygdala consists of several groups of nerve cells in the limbic system. The amygdala is involved in emotions such as fear and mood and it is also known as the visceral brain, and often called the emotional brain. The limbic system consists of several other brain structures; the hippocampus, which makes long term memory possible, and the cingulate gyrus that concerns autonomic functions and also processes cognitive information. An additional structure of the "old" brain is the hypothalamus which regulates the autonomic nervous system by the hormones it produces; it controls sleep/wake cycles, hunger and thirst, and sexual arousal. A similar structure located in the forebrain, the nucleus accumbens, is involved in reward, pleasure, and addiction. These structures are all interconnected and regarded as parts of the "old" brain because they are found in animals that have evolved a long time ago.

2.1. Plastic Changes in the Way Synapses Function

Synapses have an important role in neural plasticity. Activation of neural plasticity can change in the efficacy of synapses, creation and elimination of synapses. The function of synapses was briefly discussed in Chapter I. Here it will be discussed in more detail. The transmission of signals in a nerve fiber to a nerve cell depends on the efficacy of the synapse that connects the nerve fiber to the nerve cells. Since activation of neural plasticity can change the efficacy of synapses, it can control connections in the nervous systems.

2.1.1. Synaptic Transmission between Nerve Cells

Let's for a moment discuss how synapses work. The basics of the processes that take place in synapses were described in Chapter I. These processes make it possible for a nerve impulse that arrives at a nerve cell to affect the electrical potential inside the cell (the membrane potential). There are mainly two kinds of synapses: excitatory and inhibitory synapses. Activation of synapses changes the electrical potentials inside the receiving cell (the *membrane potential*). The change in the membrane potentials is known as an *excitatory postsynaptic potential (EPSP)* if caused by an excitatory synapse. The inside of a nerve cell normally has a negative potential, and the EPSP makes the inside of a cell less negative known as *depolarizing* the cell. The potentials that are generated by an inhibitory synapse have the opposite polarity of that generated by an excitatory synapse and is known as an *inhibitory post synaptic potential (IPSP)*; it makes the potential inside the cell more negative, known as *hyperpolarizing* the cell. If excitation is dominating and the cell's membrane becomes sufficiently depolarized, the cell will fire an action potential in its nerve fiber (axon).

Most nerve cells in the brain receive both the excitatory signals causing increased activation and inhibitory signals that decrease activation. Nerve cells thereby work in a similar manner as driving an automobile by constantly holding one foot on the brake and the other on the accelerator, controlling the car's speed by varying the relation of pressure on each pedal.

2.1.2. Temporal Summation

The EPSPs caused by single nerve impulses that arrives at a synapse cause very small changes in the membrane potential and a single EPSP is rarely able to get the membrane potential to reach the threshold for firing a nerve impulse in its axon. In most situations, summation of many EPSPs is necessary. The EPSP caused by a nerve impulse that arrives at a synapse a short time after another nerve impulse will add to the EPSP of the first nerve impulse. This is called temporal summation. Because an EPSP decays with time, the addition of two EPSPs depends on the time between the two nerve impulses. Normally, many EPSPs must be added in order for the membrane potential to reach the threshold for the cell firing a nerve impulse. The impulses have to appear with a certain short interval in order for temporal summation to cause the generated EPSP to reach the threshold of the cell. The interval between the impulses in the axon that leads to a synapse will therefore affect the way that EPSPs are added (see Figure 2.1). In the situation shown in this figure, the period of rapid firing of the axon (burst firing) is what caused the membrane potential to reach threshold.

The membrane potentials are affected by inhibitory synapses that generate IPSPs that counteract EPSPs in raising the membrane potential towards the threshold. The ability to exceed a cell's threshold for firing a nerve impulse in its axon therefore depends on the relationship between activation of inhibitory and excitatory synapses.

One reason the signals that reach a synapse do not activate a target nerve cell may be that the nerve impulses do not have a sufficiently high frequency, or rather the intervals between the impulses are too long (see Figure 2.1).

Since the size of the EPSPs (and IPSPs) can be altered by change in synaptic efficacy, activation of neural plasticity may make it possible for signals that arrive at a nerve cell to generate a sufficiently large EPSP to reach the threshold in cells where it was not possible before neural plasticity was activated.

If the signals that normally reach a synapse cannot activate the cell the synapse is said to be dormant. Change in synaptic efficacy can activate a cell that would normally remain dormant.

Dormant synapses may be able to activate the cell they make contact with if 1) the firing rate of the nerve fiber is increased, 2) the firing changes from a continuous stream of impulses to bursts of impulses (burst firing) (Figure 2.1), 3) synaptic efficacy is increased, and 4) if the cell's threshold is lowered. Activation of dormant synapses can re-route information because it can open routes that are normally blocked.

2.1.3. Spatial Summation

In textbooks neural connections are often shown as a single synapse attached to a nerve cell. This is naturally an extreme simplification. Nerve cells in the spinal cord and the brain have many, hundreds and sometime thousands, of synapses that receive signals through as many axons.

This means nerve cells can add signals they receive from many sources. Such *spatial summation* is another important function of the nervous system that can be altered by activation of neural plasticity.

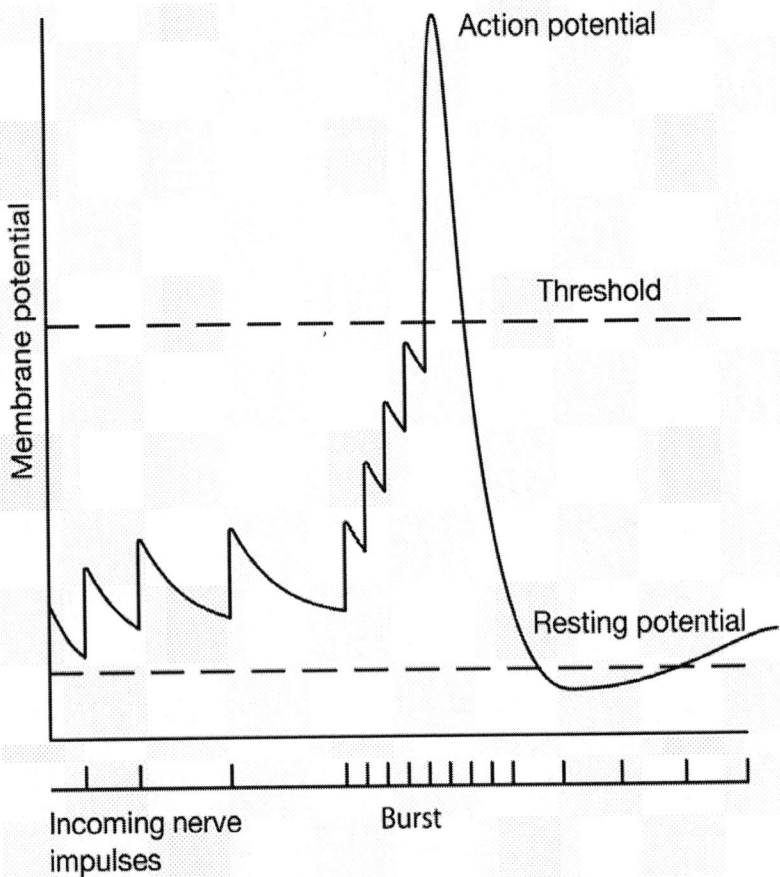

Figure 2.1. Illustration of how temporal summation of impulses is necessary for activating a nerve cell. Only because of a burst of high frequency nerve impulses did the EPSP exceed the threshold and an action potential in the outgoing axon is generated (From Møller, A.R. 2006. *Neural plasticity and disorders of the nervous system* Cambridge University Press Cambridge, Copyright © 2006. Cambridge University Press. Reprinted with the permission of Cambridge University Press.)

Figure 2.2 shows four nerve fibers come together on a nerve cell by excitatory synapses. When the nerve impulses arrive at exactly the same time the resulting EPSP is a brief change in the membrane potential (A in Figure 2.2). As the EPSP exceeds the threshold, the cell fires a nerve impulse. It only fires one nerve impulse because the EPSP is over before the end of the cell's *refractory period*.

The situation becomes more complicated when the nerve impulses do not arrive at the same time (Figure 2.2B&C). This may occur because of injury to a nerve or a fiber tract in the spinal cord or brain. Such injuries generally slow neural transmission and because different fibers are affected equally, nerve impulses will arrive at their target at different times. This increased "*temporal dispersion*" of nerve impulses causes the sum of the EPSPs in a cell on which many nerve fibers converge to be broader and of a lower amplitude (Figure 2.2B&C) than what would occur when the nerve impulses arrived at the same time (Figure 2.2A). When the EPSP does not reach the threshold of the cell (Figure 2.2B) it does not deliver a nerve impulse in its axon.

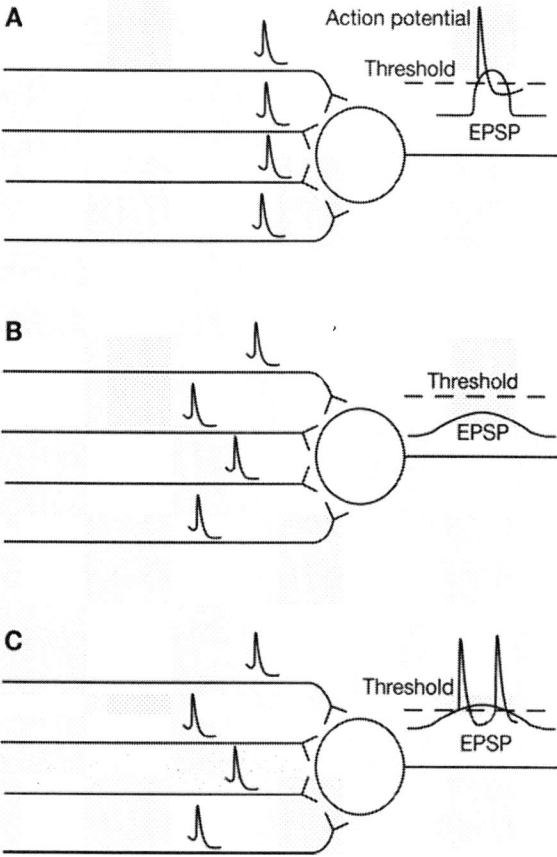

Figure 2.2. Hypothetical illustration of the effect of spatial integration by a cell on which many axons converge. A: All nerve impulses occur at the same time (little spatial dispersion). B: Nerve impulses in the axons do not occur at the same time (large spatial dispersion). The EPSP does not reach the threshold of the cell preventing it from firing. C. Same degree of spatial dispersion as in B but the threshold of the cell is lower and the EPSP makes the nerve cell fire twice. (From Møller, A.R. 2006. *Neural plasticity and disorders of the nervous system* Cambridge University Press Cambridge, Copyright © Cambridge University Press 2006. Reprinted with the permission of Cambridge University Press).

If, on the other hand, the sum of EPSPs exceeds the cell's threshold the cell may fire two nerve impulses because the EPSP lasts longer than the cell's refractory period. This means that when the nerve impulses are spread out in time the result can be either less activation of the target cell or more activation because it allows two nerve impulses to be generated.

2.2. Neural Plasticity and Memory

Activation of neural plasticity can both increase and decrease synaptic efficacy. These changes are similar to those that occur in memory. In studies of memory, these two kinds of changes in efficacy of synapses are known as *long term potentiation (LTP)* and *long term depression (LTD)*. Both learning and plasticity also involve creation and elimination of synapses.

LTP and LTD have been studied extensively in the hippocampus but are not limited to this area of the brain. Both LTP and LTD occur commonly in synapses in many other parts of the brain and the spinal cord. LTP and LTD are induced by neural activity and the changes are therefore *use-dependent*. The use-dependent LTP and LTD are caused by changes in the synapses that use the neural transmitter glutamate, which is the most common neural transmitter in the brain and spinal cord.

The most effective way of experimentally inducing LTP is by electrical stimulation of the nerve fiber that leads to a synapse on the dendrites or cell membrane of a nerve cell. High frequency electrical impulses (such as 200 pulses per second) are most effective. LTD can be induced by low frequency stimulation (1-2 pulses per seconds) of its nerve fiber and that can reverse LTP.

2.3. Reorganization of the Central Nervous System

Reorganization of the nervous system can occur in two ways, 1) by creation of new connections (nerve fibers) and 2) by opening existing pathways that are inactive because of dormant synapses. Unmasking dormant synapses can occur through activation of neural plasticity.

2.3.1. Creation of New Connections

Neural activity that occurs at the same time in many nerve cells can increase synaptic efficacy and cause creation of new connections between nerve cells. This is known as *Hebb's principle*: "Nerve cells that fire together wire together". In that way, plastic changes can become permanent. This suggestion by Hebb [12] has been confirmed by many later studies [36] showing that branching and sprouting of nerve fibers can occur after nerve cells have been firing together. This means that neural activity has control over not only the functional organization of neural network but also the anatomical organization of the brain and spinal cord, how it can develop, and how its organization can be changed.

2.3.1.1. Sprouting of Nerve Fibers

Some studies suggest that large diameter myelinated nerve fibers, Aβ fibers, that arrive to the spinal cord from receptors such as touch receptors in the skin can sprout from a location deep in the dorsal horn of the spinal cord into parts where small unmyelinated fibers (C-fibers) normally terminate (lamina II of the dorsal horn, [see Figure 2.3]) and there make synaptic contacts with nerve cells that are normally activated by painful stimuli [8,15,16,45]. Sprouting in other places may explain *allodynia*[9] after peripheral nerve injuries but allodynia may also be explained by changes in synaptic efficacy.

---

[9] The term "allodynia" means pain from a light touch on the skin. It is caused by redirection of the signals from receptors that normally signal touch to neural circuits that conduct pain signals. Sensitization, as often occurs in chronic pain, may also be involved (sensitization is discussed on page 120).

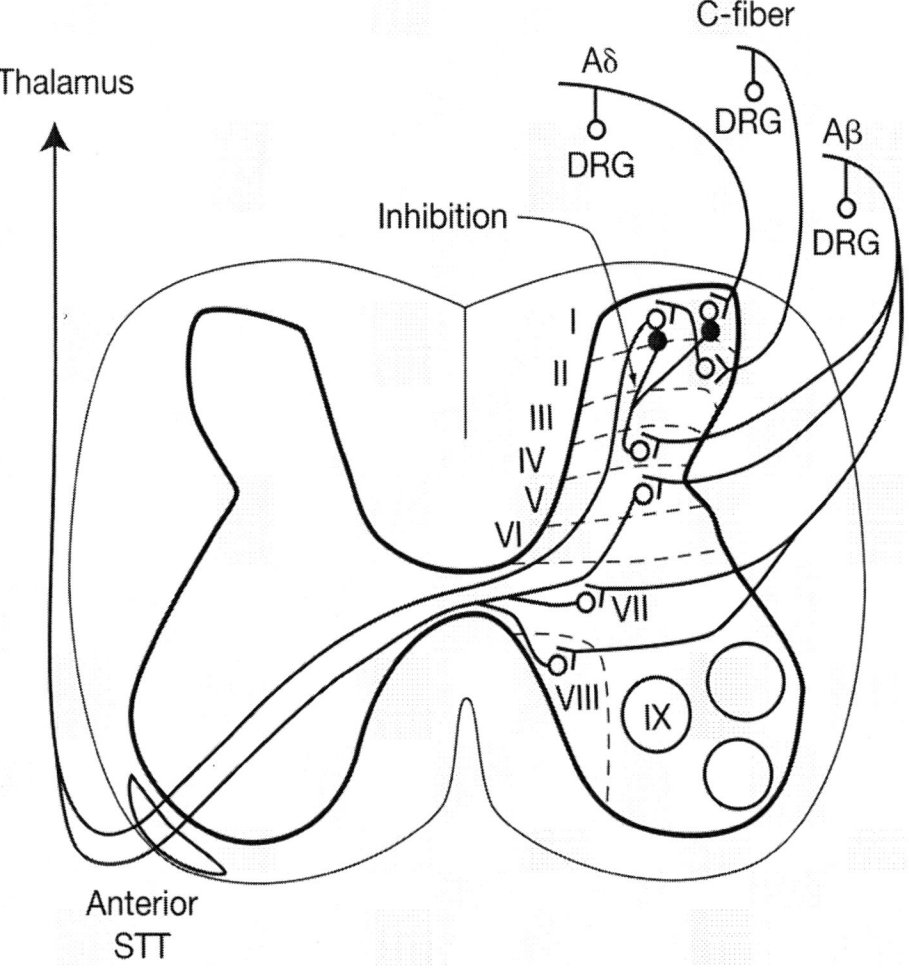

Figure 2.3. Schematic drawing of connections to nerve cells in the dorsal horn showing how signals from Aβ fibers can inhibit activity in nerve cells that are innervated by Aδ and C fibers and involved in acute pain. (Modified from Møller, A.R. 2006. *Neural plasticity and disorders of the nervous system*, Cambridge University Press, Copyright © Cambridge University Press 2006. Reprinted with the permission of Cambridge University Press).

2.3.1.2. Unmasking of Dormant Synapses

Expression of neural plasticity may cause changes in the organization ("wiring") of neural networks because it changes the efficacy of synapses that connect nerve cells to each other and thereby change how efficient incoming trains of nerve impulses are in activating a target nerve cell.

Many synapses cannot activate the nerve cells on which they are located in the spinal cord and brain. Dr. Patrick Wall, a neurologist at Oxford University who performed fundamental research on pain, called such synapses "*dormant synapses*" [40]. Dr. Wall showed that turning on neural plasticity can change the property of synapses so those previously dormant can activate their target cell (unmasking dormant synapses). Also, the opposite can occur where synapses that normally can activate the cell to which they connect can become "masked" through activation of neural plasticity. The result can be that the normal traffic flow between nerve cells is interrupted.

> Nerve fibers that enter a segment of the spinal cord as dorsal root fibers branches many other segments but activation of dorsal root fibers can only activate nerve cells in the segment where the fibers enter the spinal cord and cells in a few adjacent segments. This is because the synapses of these branches in distant segments are dormant (see Figure 2.4). Dr. Wall showed that cutting a dorsal root to a segment of the spinal cord unmasks inactive synapses in that segment so it became possible for branches of dorsal root fibers to activate the cells in more distant segments of the spinal cord [40] (see Figure 2.4).
>
> These studies of pain gave one of the first strong signs of how dormant synapses can be unmasked by turning on neural plasticity and how this can change the function of neural circuits in the spinal cord.

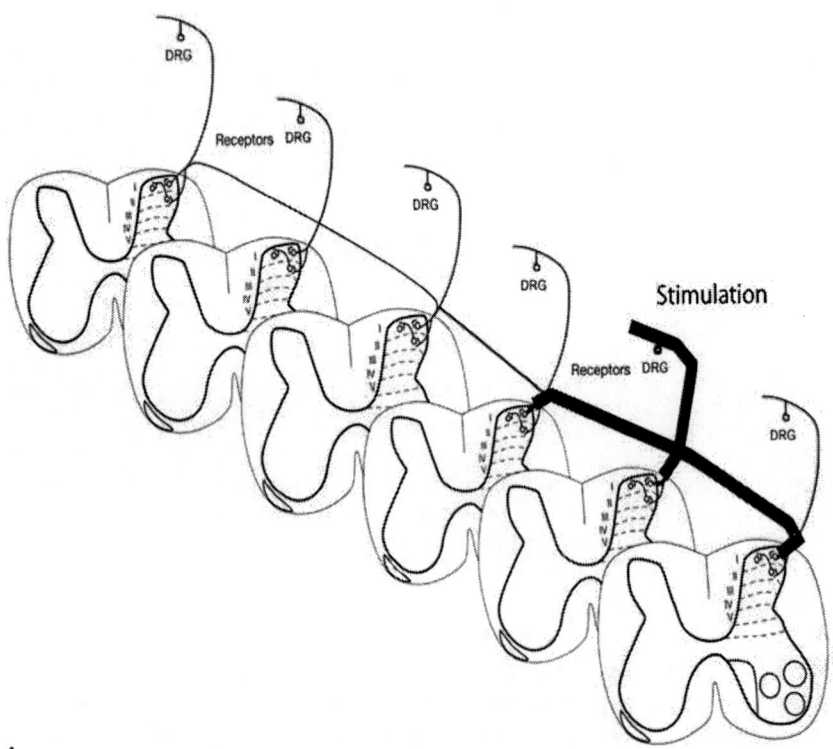

Figure 2.4A. Connections between nerve fibers from the body to cells in different segments of the spinal cord. Heavy lines show connections that are active.

Other investigators at about the same time [11] also showed the existence of ineffective connections in the spinal cord. The publication of these studies was followed by many others that showed different ways in which activation of neural plasticity could change the function of the spinal cord and brain.

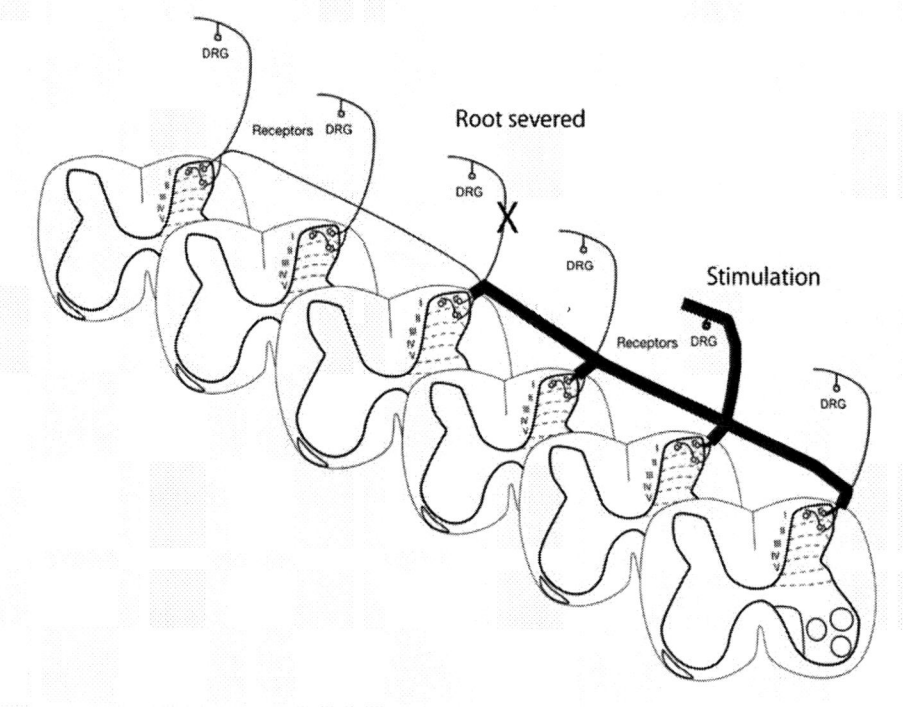

Figure 2.4B. Effect of cutting a dorsal root to a segment of the spinal cord (at X on the third segment from top) makes it possible to activate cells in that segment from a dorsal root that enter a segment of the spinal cord that is far away. Heavy lines show connections that are active. Before the dorsal root was cut, this segment could not be activated (see Figure 2.4A)

2.4. Redirection of Information through Neural Plasticity

Studies as those illustrated in Figure 2.4 show that activation of neural plasticity can change the arrangement ("wiring") of neural circuits by opening pathways that have been blocked because of inactive synapses.

Similar changes in synaptic efficacy in other places in the brain and spinal cord may re-route information to regions that are not normally receiving such signals. For example, activation of neural plasticity may cause hearing information to reach the amygdala (a part of the emotional brain) directly from the thalamus in connection with some forms of tinnitus [30].

A very simplified illustration of how the efficacy of synapses can control where signals are going in the brain or spinal cord is shown in Figure 2.5. In this example, an axon branches and each branch ends in a synapse on a nerve cell. One of the two synapses is masked and therefore, only signals flow in the other branch. If the masked synapse is unmasked, signals can flow to both target cells. This example shows how nerve cells can act as switching devices where change in synaptic efficacy operates the switch. No structural changes need to occur for such switching to take place.

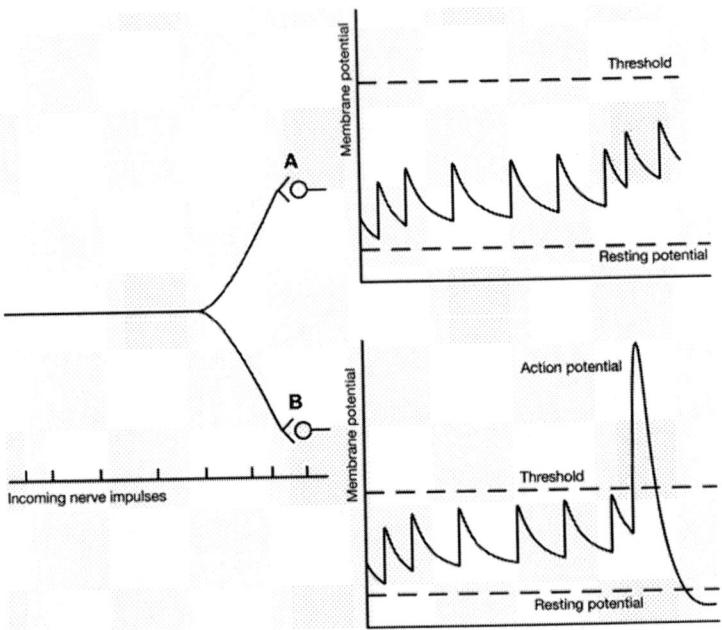

Figure 2.5. A nerve fiber branches into two axons (bifurcate), each of which ends in a synapse on two different nerve cells. Only one (B) of these two nerve cells can be activated by the nerve impulses in the axon because the synapse in the other branch (A) is not strong enough to activate the cell (the excitatory postsynaptic potential, EPSP, does not reach the cell's threshold). (From Møller, A.R. 2006. *Neural plasticity and disorders of the nervous system*, Cambridge University Press Cambridge, Copyright © Cambridge University Press 2006. Reprinted with the permission of Cambridge University Press.

Changing synaptic efficacy, the threshold of a nerve cell, or altering the interplay between inhibition and excitation can therefore change the selection of pathways for motor instructions or for sensory information.

Pathways that end in dormant synapses can be viewed as redundant systems that can be brought into use through activation of neural plasticity which unmask synapses. The pathways that are normally unresponsive can thereby be made available to the organism and be brought into use when neural plasticity is turned on. As we will see later in this book, such activation of neural plasticity can either be beneficial (see Chapter III) or cause symptoms of disease (see Chapter IV).

Other examples of re-direction of the flow of impulse traffic in the brain's fiber tracts come from the balance system. Diseases and ingestion of certain substances can change the way the balance system connects to other parts of the brain and cause awareness of moving the head. Ingestion of too much alcohol is a typical action that can cause such changes. After having too much alcohol, signals from the balance organs may be re-directed to reach the part of the brain that produces conscious reactions. The change is reversed when the ingested alcohol and its metabolites have left the body.

Since the redirection can occur within a short time, it cannot involve structural changes that entail outgrowth of nerve fibers or dendrites. It must, however, be caused by rapid action such as opening of dormant connections [40] or change of RNA (ribonucleic acid) causing a change in the synthesis of proteins [35].

2.5. Cross-modal Interaction

An example of re-direction of information in the brain through activation of neural plasticity regards the connections between different sensory systems. The different sensory systems have anatomical connections to each other, but many times the nerve fibers that come from one sensory system to another end in dormant synapses. Activation of neural plasticity can also open such connections, possibly causing one sense to affect another as can occur in non-classical pathways [1]. For example, such *"cross modal interaction"* in sensory systems can cause the perception of sounds to change when rubbing the skin and it can even make rubbing the skin give a sensation of sounds [24]. This means that signals from receptors in the skin have been re-directed to the hearing nervous system where they interfere with processing of signals in the hearing pathways, causing changes in hearing sounds [4,5,18,30]. Changes in the efficacy of connections between nerve cells (unmasking of dormant connections, or masking of functional connections) can also explain such changes in the function of sensory systems. Interaction between sensory modalities does not normally occur in adults [30]. It does, however, occur normally in young children [31]. There is also evidence that cross-modal interaction occurs in some individuals with autism [27,29] (see Chapter IV).

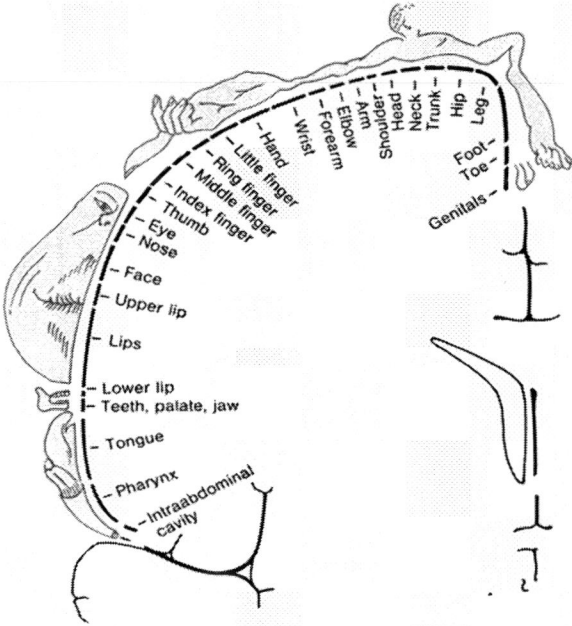

Figure 2.6. Representation of the body surface on the primary cortex. The studies behind this illustration were made by Wilder Penfield and his co-workers in the early 1930s. Results from duplications of these studies have never been published. (Reproduced from Everett, N.B. *Functional Neuroanatomy*, Lea & Fibiger, Philadelphia 1971 after Penfield and Rasmussen).

Topographic maps can best be described as a projection of a receptor surface onto the surface of a part of the brain, such as the cerebral cortex. Examples are the organization of the somatosensory cortex where body surface is projected on the surface of the cerebral cortex often illustrated by a homunculus (little man) (Figure 2.6). The functional importance of this orderly organization of nerve cells is not known.

2.6. Topographic and Computational Maps

Nerve cells in many parts of the brain are arranged anatomically in relation to what they respond to nerve cells with similar characteristics are anatomically located close to each other. Maps of the allocation of nerve cells in sensory nuclei and cerebral cortices according to what the cells respond to are of two kinds: *topographic* and *computational*.

Other senses, such as hearing, also have topographical maps known as *tonotopic* maps. Here it is the surface of the basilar membrane, which separate sounds according to their frequency that is projected onto the surface of brain structures such as the cerebral cortex. These maps show how nerve cells that respond best to different frequencies are distributed over the surface of a structure of the brain such as the cerebral cortex.

Maps showing how the surface of the body is projected onto the cerebral cortex which receives signals from receptors in the skin (somatosensory cortex) are two-dimensional representing a surface, as do maps in the visual cortex whereas tonotopic maps are one-dimensional showing how cells are located according to the frequency to which they respond best. Examples of computational maps are the distribution of nerve cells that respond to sound that comes from different directions [25].

2.6.1. Plastic Changes in Cortical Maps

Dr. Merzenich and his colleagues were some of the first to show that activation of neural plasticity can change how cells in the cerebral cortex respond and how the representation of the surface of the body (topographical map) on the cerebral cortex can be altered by eliminating sensory signals from receptors in a small path of skin [20,21].

In their experiments, interruption of signals from the skin to nerve cells in the dorsal column nuclei due to amputation turned on neural plasticity. This changed the synaptic efficacy of some of the nerve cells in the cerebral cortex that responded to touch. The result was cells in the cerebral cortex that had received signals from receptors in the skin of the amputated finger became taken over by receptors in the skin adjacent to the skin that was removed [13].

This can be explained by a shift in the tonotopic map on the cerebral cortex caused by changes in the efficacy of the synapses that connect the nerve fibers from the receptors to the cells in the cortex. This change was therefore not caused by alterations in the anatomy of the connections ("wiring") but by changes in the efficacy of synapses.

Since Dr. Merzenich and his colleagues' studies were first published many other studies showed that the maps of the body's surface on the cerebral cortex can be altered through activation of neural plasticity. In one such study, Edward Taub and his colleagues [3,17,42] showed that the receptive fields of nerve cells in a human's somatosensory cortex change when the demand changes.

Several different studies have shown that the representation of different parts of the body on the (primary) somatosensory cortex depends on how much the parts are used. The changes are opposite to those described above that occur when a patch of skin is removed. For example, extensive activation of a part of the body can change cortical maps. Instead of giving away a groups of nerve cells in the cerebral cortex that lost their signals, regions of the cerebral cortex that represented areas of the skin that were used more expanded. This has been demonstrated in studies of a musician (a string player) who uses the fingers of one hand repeatedly. The representation of these fingers on the somatosensory cortex was enlarged compared with that of fingers that were used to a normal extent [9].

Other studies showed that such increased representation was more pronounced for people who began to play early in life than people who began later in life. Braille users also develop changes in the organization of their somatosensory cortex [37].

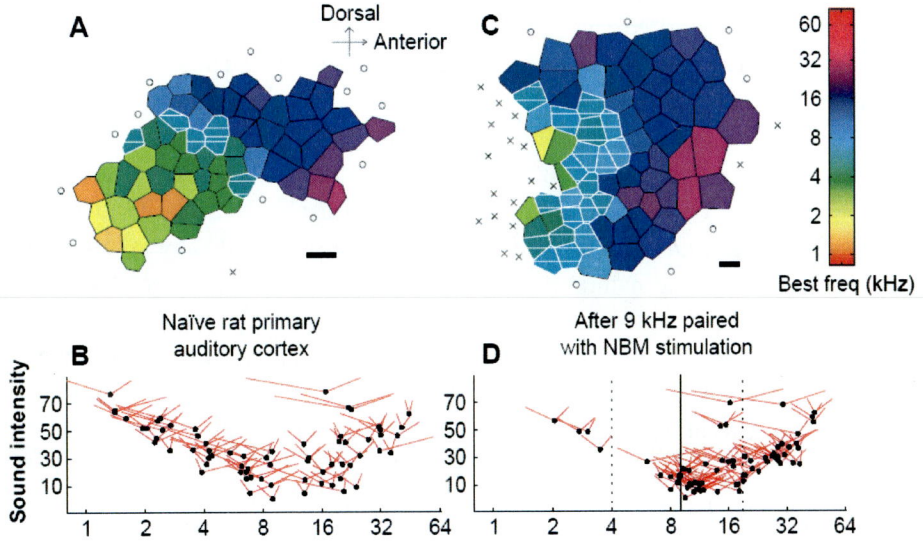

Figure 2.7. Illustration of how cortical maps depend on previous sound exposures. The results were obtained in rats in recordings from the primary hearing cortex (A1). A and B: No previous sound exposure. C and D: After exposure to 9 kHz tones simultaneously with electrical stimulation of nucleus basalis (which promote expression of neural plasticity). Penetrations that were either not responsive to tones (O) or did not meet the criteria of A1 responses (X) were used to determine the borders of A1. Each polygon in A and C represents one electrode penetration. B and D: Tuning curve tips at every A1 penetration indicating the BF, threshold, and receptive field width 10 dB above the threshold for nerve cells recorded at each penetration. Scale bar, 200 μm. (Modified from: Kilgard MP and Merzenich MM. Cortical map reorganization enabled by nucleus basalis activity. *Science* 279: 1714-1718, 1998, with permission from the American Association for the Advancement of Science) [14].

Tonotopic maps on the hearing cortex are also subject to plastic changes in a similar way as the topographical maps on the somatosensory cortex. The way sound is represented on the hearing cortex has been shown to depend on the exposure to sounds of different kinds. When the same sound, such as a tone, is presented to an animal many times the tonotopic maps change [14,41], as shown in Figure 2.7. These investigators also showed the importance of neuromodulators such as acetylcholine secreted from a nucleus deep in the forebrain (nucleus basalis) in making plastic changes possible [2,14].

The response area of regions of the brain where nerve cells respond to pain can also be modified by stimulation [6,8,44].

3. How may Neural Plasticity be Turned on?

The examples given above show that neural plasticity can be turned on by decrease or by increase in sensory signals to the brain. This occurs in general when the flow of signals from receptors in the skin, muscles and tendons, as well as from receptors in the four other sense organs (the ears, eyes, tongue and nose) is interrupted [26]. Lack of or reduced signals that typically occur after traumatic injuries, including amputations, can change synaptic efficacy that may re-organize neural circuits in the spinal cord and the brain and it can lead to pain. This may explain why injury and amputations often are followed by pain long after the wounds have healed.

These observations emphasize that correct arrangement of nerve cells in sensory nervous systems depends on sensory activation. These findings are clear signs that one should not damage or cut nerves or perhaps not even do long term nerve blocks in attempts to treat disorders such as pain, tinnitus and spasticity. Neural plasticity is already involved in most of these diseases and reducing natural signals to reach the spinal cord by cutting or blocking nerves may, over time, make the problems worse by inducing additional neural plasticity.

Deprivation of sensory signals has been shown to change in cells' RNA in the cochlear nucleus, resulting in changes in synthesis of protein [35]. The effect of such abnormalities propagates up the ascending hearing pathways and reaches the structures in the brain that cause symptoms and signs. Stronger than normal stimulation of receptors, such as from exposure to very loud sounds, can also turn on neural plasticity [22,23,38,43]. This is probably one of the ways in which exposure to loud sounds can cause tinnitus.

It is not only loss of sensory signals that can turn on neural plasticity. Also, loss of muscle function and changes in the use of muscles can turn on neural plasticity and cause hyperactivity (spasm, tremor etc.) and abnormal functions such as synkinesis (involuntary contraction of other muscles than those intended to be activated).

Neural plasticity can also be turned on from inside the body, for example, by inflammation and injuries to nerves, the spinal cord, or the brain. Diseases that upset the normal regulation of many bodily functions can also turn neural plasticity on. Internal signals from the brain and spinal cord or from internal organs (viscera) are also powerful initiators of neural plasticity.

3.1. Neural Plasticity Turned on by Artificial Means

Neural plasticity can be activated by artificial means such as electrical stimulation of ▯al nerves causing change in the function of the spinal cord, which is effective in ▯ pain conditions (transderm electric nerve stimulation, TENS, see p 122). Electrical stimulation of the facial nerve can create hemifacial spasm-like signs, by turning on neural plasticity in the facial motonucleus in the brainstem as shown in animal studies [33]. Electrical stimulation of various parts of the brain (deep brain stimulation) [34] using stereotaxically techniques and electrical stimulation of the cerebral cortex [7] is becoming in increasing use to treat plasticity diseases by reversing harmful plasticity.

4. Changes in Early Childhood

Neural plasticity plays extensive and very important roles in childhood development and childhood development depends on plastic changes in several ways. Activation of neural plasticity provides a "midcourse correction" that occurs during the first few years of life and it supplements the development of the nervous system that occurred before birth. Neural plasticity also plays a role in shaping sensory systems later in life based on exposure to sensory signals. Little is known about how this kind of plasticity is activated but it is necessary for normal development of the nervous system and for maintenance of the normal abilities of sensory and motor functions throughout life.

Childhood development of the brain and the spinal cord involves plastic changes that may be directed by *programs (rules)* that may have been laid down before birth and activated by environmental (external) factors or controlled internally. We know very little about the programs (or rules) that control childhood development and it is not known what turns on the neural plasticity that makes childhood development possible. It is believed that some developmental disorders may be caused by the "midcourse correction" not occurring correctly (see p 196).

Study of neural plasticity is still in its infancy and there are most likely many unknown ways it can be turned on. Many of the signs of activation of neural plasticity are so far unknown.

I will discuss neural plasticity in more detail in the following two Chapters. Chapter III deals with neural plasticity that is beneficial to the individual, and Chapter IV will discuss neural plasticity that causes signs and symptoms of what I will call "plasticity diseases". A developmental disorder, autism, is discussed in Appendix C.

References

[1]   Aitkin LM. *The auditory midbrain, structure and function in the central auditory pathway.* Clifton, NJ: Humana Press; 1986.
[2]   Bakin JS, Weinberger NM. Induction of a physiological memory in the cerebral cortex by stimulation of the nucleus basalis. *Proc Natl Acad Sci USA.* 1996;93(20):11219-24.
[3]   Braun C, Schweizer R, Elbert T, Birbaumer N, Taub E. Differential activation in somatosensory cortex for different discrimination tasks. *J Neurosci.* 2000;20 ' '·446-50.
[4]   Cacace AT. Expanding the biological basis of tinnitus: crossmodal origins of neuroplasticity. *Hear Res.* 2003;175:112-32.

[5] Cacace AT, Lovely TJ, McFarland DJ, Parnes SM, Winter DF. Anomalous cross-modal plasticity following posterior fossa surgery: Some speculations on gaze-evoked tinnitus. *Hear Res*. 1994;81:22-32.

[6] Coderre TJ, Katz J, Vaccarino AL, Melzack R. Contribution of central neuroplasticity to pathological pain: Review of clinical and experimental evidence. *Pain*. 1993;52:259-85.

[7] De Ridder D, De Mulder G, Menovsky T, Sunaert S, Kovacs S. Electrical stimulation of auditory and somatosensory cortices for treatment of tinnitus and pain. In: Langguth B, Hajak G, Kleinjung T, Cacace AT, Møller AR, editors. *Tinnitus, Pathophysiology and Treatment*. Amsterdam: Elsevier; 2007. p. 377-88.

[8] Doubell TP, Mannion RJ, Woolf CJ. The dorsal horn: state-dependent sensory processing, plasticity and the generation of pain. In: Wall PD, Melzack R, editors. *Handbook of Pain*. 4 ed. Edinburgh: Churchill Livingstone; 1999. p. 165-81.

[9] Elbert T, Pantev C, Wienbruch C, Rockstroh B, Taub E. Increased cortical representation of the fingers of the left hand in string players. *Science*. 1995;270(5234):305-7.

[10] Goddard GV. Amygdaloid stimulation and learning in the rat. *J Comp Physiol Psychol*. 1964; 58:23-30.

[11] Goshgarian HG, Guth L. Demonstration of functionally ineffective synapses in the guinea pig spinal cord. *Exp Neurol*. 1977;57:613-21.

[12] Hebb DO. *The organization of behavior*. New York: Wiley; 1949.

[13] Jenkins WM, Merzenich MM, Ochs MT, Allard T, Guic-Robles E. Functional reorganization of primary somatosensory cortex in adult owl monkeys after behaviorally controlled tactile stimulation. *J Neurophysiol*. 1990;63(1):82-104.

[14] Kilgard MP, Merzenich MM. Cortical map reorganization enabled by nucleus basalis activity. *Science*. 1998;279:1714-8.

[15] Koerber HR, Mirnics K, Kavookjian AM, Light AR. Ultrastructural analysis of ectopic synaptic boutons arising from peripherally regenerated primary afferent fibers. *J Neurophysiol*. 1999;81:1636.

[16] Kohama I, Ishikawa K, Kocsis JD. Synaptic reorganization in the substantia gelatinosa after peripheral nerve neuroma formation: aberrant innervation of lamina II neurons by beta afferents. *J Neurosci*. 2000;20:1538-49.

[17] Lenz FA, Lee JI, Garonzik IM, Rowland LH, Dougherty PM, Hua SE. Plasticity of pain-related neuronal activity in the human thalamus. *Progr Brain Res*. 2000;129:253-73.

[18] Lockwood A, Salvi R, Coad M, Towsley M; Wack D, Murphy B. The functional neuroanatomy of tinnitus. Evidence for limbic system links and neural plasticity. *Neurology*. 1998;50:114-20.

[19] McCormick DA, Contreras D. On the cellular and network bases of epileptic seizures. *Ann Rev Physiol*. 2001;63:815-46.

[20] Merzenich MM, Kaas JH, Wall J, Nelson RJ, Sur M, Felleman D. Topographic reorganization of somatosensory cortical areas 3b and 1 in adult monkeys following restricted deafferentation. *Neuroscience*. 1983; 8(1):3-55.

[21] Merzenich MM, Nelson RJ, Stryker MP, Cynader MS, Schoppmann A, Zook JM. Somatosensory cortical map changes following digit amputation in adult monkeys. *J Comp Neurol*. 1984;224(4):591-605.

[22] Morest DK, Ard MD, Yurgelun-Todd D. Degeneration in the central auditory pathways after acoustic deprivation or over-stimulation in the cat. *Anat Rec*. 1979;193:750.

[23] Morest DK, Bohne BA. Noise-induced degeneration in the brain and representation of inner and outer hair cells. *Hear Res*. 1983;9:145-52.

[24] Møller AR. Pathophysiology of Tinnitus. In: Sismanis A, editor. *Otolaryngol Clin N Am*. Amsterdam: W.B.Saunders; 2003. p. 249-66.

[25] Møller AR. *Hearing: Anatomy, Physiology, and Disorders of the Auditory System, 2nd Ed*. Amsterdam: Academic Press; 2006.

[26] Møller AR. *Neural plasticity and disorders of the nervous system*. Cambridge: Cambridge University Press 2006.

[27] Møller AR. Neurophysiologic abnormalities in autism. In: Mesmere BS, editor. *New Autism Research Developments*. New York: Nova Science Publishers; 2007.

[28] Møller AR, Jannetta PJ. On the origin of synkinesis in hemifacial spasm: Results of intracranial recordings. *J Neurosurg*. 1984;61:569-76.

[29] Møller AR, Kern JK, Grannemann B. Are the non-classical auditory pathways involved in autism and PDD? *Neurol Res*. 2005;27:625-9.

[30] Møller AR, Møller MB, Yokota M. Some forms of tinnitus may involve the extralemniscal auditory pathway. *Laryngoscope*. 1992; 102: 1165-71.

[31] Møller AR, Rollins P. The non-classical auditory system is active in children but not in adults. *Neurosci Lett*. 2002;319:41-4.

[32] Rasminsky M. Ephaptic transmission between single nerve fibers in the spinal nerve roots of dystrophic mice. *J Physiol (Lond)*. 1980;305:151-69.

[33] Sen CN, Møller AR. Signs of hemifacial spasm created by chronic periodic stimulation of the facial nerve in the rat. *Exp Neurol*. 1987;98:336-49.

[34] Shils JL, Tagliati M, Alterman RL. Neurophysiological monitoring during neurosurgery for movement disorders. In: Deletis V, Shils JL, editors. *Neurophysiology in Neurosurgery*. Amsterdam: Academic Press; 2002. p. 405-48.

[35] Sie KCY, Rubel EW. Rapid Changes in Protein Synthesis and Cell Size in the Cochlear Nucleus following Eighth Nerve Activity Blockade and Cochlea Ablation. *J Comp Neurol*. 1992;320:501-8.

[36] Stent GS. A physiological mechanism for Hebb's postulate of learning. *Proc Nat Acad Sci*. 1973;70(4):997-1001.

[37] Sterr A, Muller MM, Elbert T, Rockstroh B, Pantev C, Taub E. Perceptual correlates of changes in cortical representation of fingers in blind multifinger Braille readers. *J Neurosci*. 1998;18(11):4417-23.

[38] Szczepaniak WS, Møller AR. Evidence of neuronal plasticity within the inferior colliculus after noise exposure: A study of evoked potentials in the rat. *Electroenceph Clin Neurophysiol*. 1996;100:158-64.

[39] Wada JA. *Kindling 2*. New York: Raven Press; 1981.

[40] Wall PD. The presence of ineffective synapses and circumstances which unmask them. *Phil Trans Royal Soc (Lond)*. 1977;278:361-72.

[41] Weinberger NM. Learning-induced physiological memory in adult primary auditory cortex: Receptive field plasticity, model, and mechanisms. *Audiol Neuro-Otol.* 1998;3:145-67.

[42] Weiss T, Miltner WH, Huonker R, Friedel R, Schmidt I, Taub E. Rapid functional plasticity of the somatosensory cortex after finger amputation. *Exp Brain Res.* 2000;134(2):199-203.

[43] Willott JF, Lu SM. Noise induced hearing loss can alter neural coding and increase excitability in the central nervous system. *Science.* 1981;16:1331-2.

[44] Woolf CJ, Salter MW. Neural plasticity: Increasing the gain in pain. *Science.* 2000;288:1765-8.

[45] Woolf CJ, Shortland P, Cogershall RE. Peripheral nerve injury triggers central sprouting of myelinated afferents. *Nature.* 1992;355:75-8.

,

Chapter III

BENEFICIAL NEURAL PLASTICITY

ABSTRACT

There are numerous ways our bodies benefit from activation of neural plasticity. For example, the recovery that occurs a long time after a stroke is a result of activation of neural plasticity. The aim of therapy after strokes is mainly to induce neural plasticity that can reorganize (re-wire) parts of the brain to take over the functions that were lost to damage. The benefit from this kind of activation of neural plasticity requires that there is sufficient additional capacity (redundancy) in the brain that can do the same functions as are lost. Adaptation to changing demands, such as in use of prostheses, depends on activation of neural plasticity. The training that is done in connection with prostheses such as leg and arm prostheses and, perhaps most prominent, regarding the use of cochlear and brainstem implants are examples of how activation of neural plasticity can benefit adaptation to using various kinds of prostheses.

Exposure to sensory stimulation and normal use of muscles activate neural plasticity to guide development of the brain and spinal cord and it is necessary to maintain both cognitive and physical skills. Prostheses such as cochlear and auditory brainstem implants do not deliver the same code as the ear. The brain must therefore be re-programmed through training to activate neural plasticity. In children who are born deaf the situation is different in that the hearing nervous system needs signals to develop normally. These hearing prostheses can deliver such signals. There are limitations in the benefit that can be achieved from activation of neural plasticity. Redundancy (duplication of functions) is necessary for successfully replacing functions that have been lost to damage to the brain and spinal cord.

Activation of neural plasticity is necessary for normal childhood development of the brain. The nervous system must be activated early in life in order to not miss the "critical period" in which normal organization of the nervous system can be established. Without signals from sense organs or other forms of activation (by prostheses) of sensory systems cognitive and other deficits occur. Lack of sensory stimulation, such as occurs from deafness at birth, prevents normal development of the auditory system. Sensory activation by cochlear and cochlear nucleus implants can substitute normal sensory input in guiding the development of the nervous system during a few early critical years of life.

The balance system is one of the most plastic systems, as shown by the reflex that moves the eyes in the opposite direction of head movements so an image on the retina is steady (the vestibular ocular reflex). Exercise that activates plasticity can ameliorate some forms of dizziness such as those that results from changing spectacles.

Training can ameliorate symptoms such as synkinesis through activation of neural plasticity. Training that activates neural plasticity can make it possible to do separate movements such as using only one finger at a time. It is also possible to suppress reflexes through training, which activates neural plasticity. It is also possible to strengthen reflexes by activating neural plasticity.

1. INTRODUCTION

The recovery that normally occurs after ischemic strokes is a typical example of the beneficial effect from activation of neural plasticity. It is not usually possible to repair damage to the spinal cord and brain, but functions that have been lost can often be regained (partly) by shifting the function to another part of the brain. This is possible because the brain is malleable and because some functions can be done in more than one part of the brain as was discussed in Chapter II. Re-organization of the brain through activation of neural plasticity makes it possible for a person to recover some of the functions that are lost because of injury to the brain. Activation of neural plasticity can shift functions from a damaged part of the brain to parts of the brain that function. When people learn to speak after a stroke, the speech therapy promotes rewiring of the brain to use other parts than those that are destroyed by the stroke. Shifting functions from damaged parts of the brain to those that are functioning is an important feature of neural plasticity, and it is perhaps the best-known benefit. The training that is used for rehabilitation may activate neural plasticity and cause recovery of lost functions. This recovery (totally or partially) requires sufficient *redundancy* of the brain function that has been lost so that the lost function can be taken over by other parts of the brain. This means that the lost function can be performed by more than one part of the brain. This is not always the case. For example, the control of movements of limbs can only be controlled by one part of the brain and if that is lost it cannot be taken over by other parts. Speech depends on several parts of the brain and speech therapy is very effective in restoring the ability to speak after a stroke for some forms of speech deficits (aphasia), depending on which parts of the brain that has been damaged.

Turning on neural plasticity does not repair damaged parts of the brain, but it makes other parts take over some functions that were lost from the destruction of neural tissue. Perhaps these parts of the brain must be adapted to their altered tasks to be able to replace lost functions, and that requires other forms of plastic changes to be activated.

Activating neural plasticity has other kinds of benefits as well. For instance, the ability to adapt to use a cochlear or brainstem implant which could restore hearing when the cochlea or hearing nerve is damaged depends on the brain being malleable. Also, the use of leg and arm prostheses is only possible by the benefit from activation of neural plasticity. It was earlier believed that neural plasticity could not be activated after a certain age, but it is now known that neural plasticity can be induced also after childhood, although to a lesser degree (see page 67 regarding critical period) [23,25,26]. These discoveries have opened new possibilities for rehabilitation after strokes and other forms of brain injury and it has changed our view on diseases such as tinnitus, pain, and some forms of muscle spasm.

Recently, we have learned the mature brain can even grow new nerve cells – something we did not know just a few years ago. Understanding neural plasticity and how it can be turned on is important for obtaining the best effect of rehabilitation and for adaptation to changes it demands. This Chapter provides such information.

Last, but not least, it is worth mentioning that neural plasticity becomes turned on during early childhood and extends the brain's development that occurred before birth. It has been known for many years that the development of the brain is not finished at birth but needs to develop further in order to reach its normal function. This *"midcourse correction"* that normally occurs in early childhood is absolutely necessary to achieve normal functions of many parts of the brain. The development that occurs after birth is accomplished by activation of neural plasticity, but it is not known how this form of neural plasticity is being turned on. When this early childhood development does not proceed normally, the results are severe developmental diseases (discussed in Chapter IV).

Experience from exposure to sensory stimulations is also necessary for the normal development of our senses. Even the ability to perceive pain requires experience of pain in early childhood. Also muscle functions are not fully developed at birth, and the use of muscle functions during early childhood is necessary for their normal development. In fact, the brain's development is not finished before the approximate age of 20. In this Chapter, I will discuss beneficial effects of neural plasticity in more detail.

2. REHABILITATION AFTER INJURY TO THE BRAIN AND SPINAL CORD

Strokes and trauma are the most common causes of injury to the brain and the spinal cord. In the US, about 700,000 people experience a stroke, of which 500,000 for the first time, while the remaining have their second stroke. Of the individuals who had a stroke, about 275,000 die. About one in every sixteen deaths in the United States are from strokes. Ischemic strokes are caused by occlusion of a blood vessel and are the most frequent form of strokes. They cause damage to the parts of the brain that get deprived of blood supply. Nerve cells in the affected part of the brain die if blood supply is not restored within a short time after the occurrence of the stroke. If an ischemic stroke is not treated promptly (within one hour) the damage is permanent because it is causing brain tissue to die from deprivation of oxygen and nutrients. This can cause death or result in deficits of various kinds in those who survive. The kind of deficits depends on which parts of the brain are affected. Ischemic strokes also affect other parts of the brain than the region that was damaged immediately after blood supply was interrupted.

Hemorrhagic strokes can cause widespread damage because blood may spread over large parts of the brain. Blood that is in contact with the surface of the brain acts as a toxic substance to brain cells and when it takes up space around the brain it may cause damage by compressing the brain.

Traumatic brain injuries have many degrees of severity, from deadly injuries to those that cause headache and memory loss and often tinnitus (ringing in the ears). Concussions, which are often regarded as a minor injury, can cause severe symptoms such as tinnitus, memory loss and personality changes.

2.1. Replacement of the Functions of Damaged Parts of the Brain

Nerves can repair themselves but the brain and the spinal cord have less ability to do so after injury. However, shifting functions that are normally done by injured parts to other parts of the brain through activation of neural plasticity can make it possible to regain some lost functions. When people learn to speak after a stroke, the speech therapy promotes activation of neural plasticity that can reorganize (re-wire) affected parts of the brain to use other parts than those that have been destroyed by the stroke.

Plastic changes causing re-organization normally start as a natural reaction to the loss of functions. Reorganization can be helped by training, and more recently it has been shown that impulses of electrical current applied to the brain can help the process of reorganizing so that other parts can take over functions that were done by the brain tissue that has been destroyed [1,4].

The success of neural plasticity in rehabilitation depends on the ability of the brain to reorganize. This requires that there are spare, or "redundant", systems in the brain that can take over from regions with damaged functions.

Not all functions can be performed by more than one part of the brain. Such lack of redundancy is apparent in connection with injuries to the parts of the nervous system that are important for speech. The parts of the brain that control movements of arms, hands, and legs also have very little redundancy, and that is why paralysis from strokes does not recover to any great extent. Some kinds of aphasia are caused by injury to parts of the brain, the function of which cannot be replaced by other parts of the brain.

There are a few regions of the brain that are completely duplicated and thereby capable of taking on lost functions directly without much help from neural plasticity. One example is the hearing cortex. The hearing cortex on one side receives signals from both ears, and impairment of the function of the cortex on one side has little practical influence on everyday hearing. Only when hearing is attempted in difficult environments and the sounds are distorted does hearing from the opposite side of the lesion become noticeably impaired (the hearing pathways are crossed, see Appendix A) [37].

In strokes, the focus is on the area of the brain where the primary damage has been done by the lack of oxygen caused by the occlusion of a blood vessel. This is what can be seen on imaging studies such as MRI. However, there are also changes in the regions around this area, and there can be changes in brain regions far from where the occluded vessel did its initial damage. For example, injury from lack of oxygen to the motor cortex on the left side of the brain that causes paralysis of the right hand may be followed by impairment of controls of the left hand because of changes in the function of the motor cortex on the left side [8]. These far away changes occur after the initial damage (discussed in Chapter IV), and they are likely caused by activation of neural plasticity and rehabilitation must include reversal of these plastic changes.

Such weakness in the opposite limb after a stroke can often be decreased by restricting the movement of the same limb on the other side (constraint-induced movement therapy) [50]. This is an example of how the two sides of the brain interact with each other in many ways.

Two regions of the brain, known as Wernicke's area and Broca's area, control speech. Wernicke's area controls what to say (the content of speech) and it is also involved in understanding speech. Broca's area controls the muscles that move the tongue and the lips and it controls the voice box (larynx), all of which are necessary for producing speech. When Broca's area on the left side is damaged the same area of the brain on the other side cannot replace the function of the damaged area because Broca's area is only found on one (normally the left) side of the brain and when that part it is damaged it is difficult or impossible to regain the ability to speak. Damage from strokes or other forms of injury to Broca's area causes what is known as expressive aphasia (motor aphasia, non-fluent aphasia), while damage to Wernicke's area of the brain causes what is known as receptive aphasia. Injuries of Wernicke's area also inflict on understanding speech.

3. ADAPTATION TO ALTERED DEMANDS

There are many examples that can illustrate how the brain can adapt or accommodate to altered demands. Use of prostheses is an example of changing demands that require the nervous system to alter its function and organization.

Activation of neural plasticity can make it possible to effectively use many different kinds of prostheses. One such kind of prostheses that requires extensive changes in the way the nervous system functions is cochlear and brainstem implants, which are (neuro) prostheses that make it possible for deaf people to hear and understand speech and enjoy many other sounds. These devices do not produce the same neural code (language) as the normal ear. The success of cochlear or brainstem implants is achieved only after appropriate re-programming of the hearing nervous system has occurred. The brain can interpret the signals from these prostheses despite they are different from the messages the ear normally sends to the brain. When a person learns to use prostheses of legs the same happens: the brain is reprogrammed to send different kinds of commands to muscles that make it possible to stand and to walk on an artificial limb.

3.1. Adapting to the Use of Prostheses

The most successful kinds of prostheses of the nervous system are those that can provide hearing in totally deaf people, known as cochlear and cochlear nucleus implants (or auditory brainstem implants, ABIs) [6,34]. Their success depends on proper activation of neural plasticity.

Also adapting to the use of other prostheses, such as leg or arm prostheses, requires activation of neural plasticity. The use of cochlear and brainstem implants to treat deafness requires reprogramming of the hearing nervous system, and leg and arm prostheses require re-programming of the systems in the brain and spinal cord that control muscles.

I will discuss cochlear and cochlear nucleus implants in more detail below because these implants are excellent examples of the importance of neural plasticity in adaptation to changing demands. These prostheses are, first of all, the most successful of prostheses of the nervous system, and that is to a great extent a result of the ability of the hearing nervous system to be re-programmed through activation of neural plasticity. Much research has been done regarding the role of neural plasticity in adaptation in connection with cochlear and brainstem implants. The knowledge that has been gained through such research has helped understand many features of neural plasticity [20,22], and it has helped to understand how the ear and the hearing nervous system normally work [11]. Such research has particularly contributed to our understanding of how the ear and the hearing nervous system make it possible to understand speech.

3.1.1. Cochlear Implants

Cochlear implants are devices that activate the hearing nerve by applying impulses of electrical current to the part of the hearing nerve where it is located in the cochlea. The earliest implants had only one electrode placed in the cochlea [16,29]. It was a major improvement when it became possible to implant several electrodes and apply impulses that were controlled by the energy in different bands of the sound spectrum (distribution of sound energy over frequencies) to the different electrodes [34].

Modern cochlear implants consist of an array of electrodes that are implanted in the cochlea. These electrodes are connected to a device placed somewhere under the skin which makes it possible to activate the implants from outside the body [32]. A small computer worn by the individual converts the sound signals that are picked up by the microphone worn by the person. The computer turns the signals from the microphone into a code of electrical impulses that are applied to the hearing nerve through the implanted electrodes.

From the beginning, the focus for these devices was to make it possible to understand speech, but as cochlear implants became more and more sophisticated it also became possible to enjoy and understand the meaning of other sounds such as environmental sounds and music.

3.1.1.1. History of Cochlear Implants

Cochlear implants were introduced by the ear nose and throat surgeon, William House [16] in Los Angeles. He worked with Robin Michelson and Blair Simmons who both had done pioneering work on electrical stimulation of the cochlea [29,49] (for a historical overview of cochlear and brainstem implants, see [34]). It was known many years ago that electrical current that passed through the hearing nerve could give a sensation of sound in people [9,49], but these discoveries had not resulted in any practical solutions that could help deaf individuals (see also [32]) until House and Michelson developed cochlear implants.

These early cochlear implants were very different from those we have now – they consisted of a single electrode placed bluntly in the cochlea and the conversion of sounds into electrical signals that were applied through this electrode was primitive with today's

> *measures. The individuals who had these first implants did not get actual speech comprehension, but they got sound awareness and that was useful as an addition to lip-reading.*

The undertakings of developing cochlear implants were met with great skepticism from researchers and physicians. Nobody would believe that such a primitive device could replace the function of the complex organ of the ear. Further development of cochlear implants proved these skeptics wrong. It was indeed possible to get speech comprehension by cochlear implants, and there are now many people whose lives were changed for the better by these devices [11,47]; see also [32].

This lesson tells us that researchers as well as physicians, and other health care professionals are often very conservative and have difficulty thinking in nontraditional paths. Such "thinking outside the box" as Dr. House did has often produced revolutionary results. The grant system for supporting research does not usually appreciate novel research ideas, because so many people need to agree upon a research project to get it funded, and that impedes innovations that are outside the mainstream of thinking. It would have been unlikely that Dr. House would have been able to obtain a grant for carrying out the project of developing cochlear implants. Dr. House undertook it on his own and carried it to a successful completion without monetary support and against his colleagues' resistance. If such brave individuals as Dr House had not taken this bold step to try to provide some form of hearing to deaf people, we would probably not have had the cochlear implants we have today.

> Cochlear implants activate hearing nerve fibers directly and thereby bypass several normal functions of the cochlea. One such function is the frequency selectivity that separates sounds in the normal cochlea according to their frequencies before the sensory cells (these receptors are known as "hair cells" because of the hair-like structures on their top) are activated.
>
> The frequency selectivity of the cochlea is accomplished by a structure known as the basilar membrane, which is set into vibrations by sound (see Chapter I). The sensory receptors (hair cells) are located along the basilar membrane. The vibrations of the basilar membranes depend on the frequency of the sound in such a way that low frequency sounds produce their largest vibrations in the far end of the membrane while high frequencies give rise to the largest amplitude at the beginning of the membrane (see Figure 3.1). The result is that hair cells along the membrane are activated according to the frequency of the sounds, and naturally, according to how strong the sounds are.
>
> The hair cells in the normal cochlea transform the vibration of the basilar membrane into electrical signals that control the activity in the hearing nerve fibers. In cochlear implants, electrical impulses from the implanted electrodes activate the hearing nerve fibers directly. This means that cochlear implants bypass the frequency selectivity of the basilar membrane and the properties of the neural transduction in the hair cells. The complex functions of the basilar membrane and the hair cells are simulated in a small computer that is a part of the cochlear implant system. The computer processes the sounds that reach a microphone worn by the person who has a cochlear implant. The ability of the

basilar membrane to separate sounds according to frequency is imitated by the computer, which separates sounds in a few frequency bands, each band controlling the electrical impulses that are applied to each electrode pair in the cochlea. The number of frequency bands used varies from 8-20 in different commercially available cochlear implants devices.

The basilar membrane is a highly nonlinear structure that in addition to its frequency selectivity also compresses the vibrations of the basilar membrane before the hair cells are activated. This feature of the normal cochlea is also implemented in the processing done by the computer of cochlear implants systems.

The computer in the cochlear implant performs only some of the functions that normally are carried out by the basilar membrane and the hair cells. For example, what is known as "two-tone inhibition"[10] is not provided by cochlear implants.

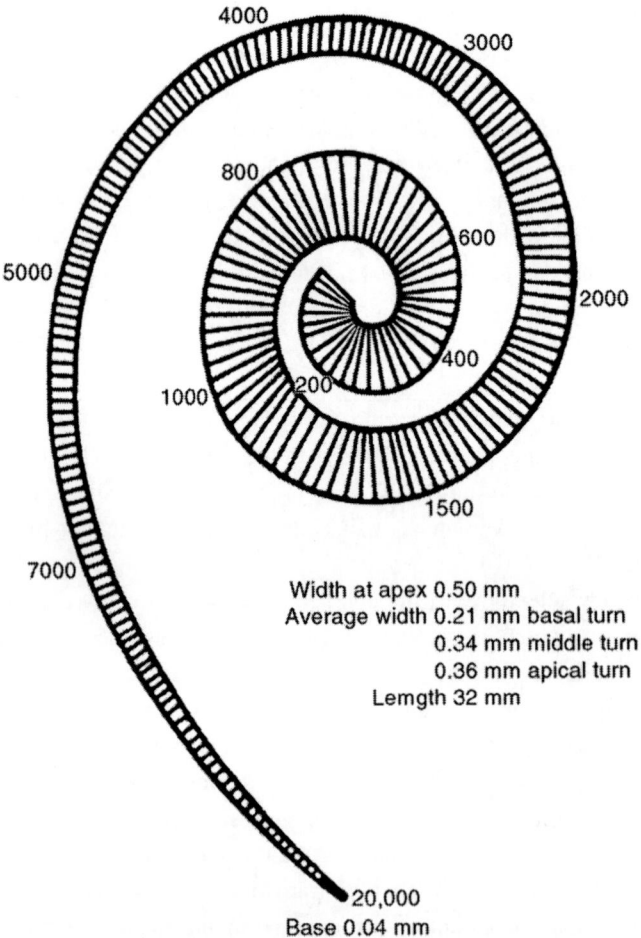

Width at apex 0.50 mm
Average width 0.21 mm basal turn
0.34 mm middle turn
0.36 mm apical turn
Lemgth 32 mm

Figure 3.1. The cochlea separates sounds according to their frequency. (From Stuhlman, 1943 *An Introduction to Biophysics*, Wiley, New York)

---

[10] Two-tone inhibition is a property of the ear that makes it possible for one tone to suppress the response to a tone with a different frequency. It is assumed to help separate sounds on the basis of their frequencies.

Since the most important function of cochlear implants is to provide speech comprehension, the design of their processors is aimed at extracting important features of speech sounds and code them in trains of electrical impulses for activating the hearing nerve fibers in the cochlea.

The coding of sounds in the hearing nerve that cochlear implants produce is different from that of the normal ear. Modern cochlear implant processors perform only two of the main functions of the ear, namely separation of the sounds according to their frequency and how the strength of sounds varies. The use of implants therefore must rely on reprogramming of the hearing nervous system through activation of neural plasticity. The fact that speech sounds have a considerable degree of spare (redundant) information is a great help because it means it is not necessary to provide the same amount of information about the speech signals to the brain as the normal ear does. Processing of sounds in the normal ear and nervous system also has a large degree of redundancy.

Cochlear implants activate groups of hearing nerve fibers in an identical way, which is much different from the normal situation where each nerve fiber is activated independently. This is one of the reasons why activation of neural plasticity is necessary to make it possible to understand speech through cochlear implants.

Earlier cochlear implants provided information to the hearing nerve about the time pattern of the signals in the different frequency bands [28]. It was shown that spectral information alone could provide good speech discrimination when processed using a small number of frequency bands [10]. Modern cochlear implants therefore only make use of information about the energy in a few (8-20) frequency bands, and information about the time pattern of sounds is discarded. (The function of the ear and the hearing nervous system is discussed in Appendix A). It was earlier believed that the waveform of the speech signals was important for understanding speech, but it was recognized later that good speech discrimination could be achieved on the basis of the spectrum of sounds.

3.1.1.2. The basis for Modern Cochlear Implants is the Channel Vocoder

During the 1950s, much effort was devoted to compress the information in speech signals to save bandwidth for telephone signals sent over long telephone lines so that many telephone conversations could be transmitted with limited bandwidth. One of the systems developed for that purpose was known as the "vocoder" [44]. These systems determined the energy of speech sounds in a few (up to 14) frequency bands and then sent the information about the energy in these bands to the receiver far away, where the signals were interpreted and used to synthesize speech. These slowly varying signals that provided information about the spectrum of the sounds required much less bandwidth for transmission than the speech signals, and therefore many more speech conversations could be transmitted over the low-bandwidth lines that were available at the time.

The development of other technologies, first of satellites and later of fiber optic lines, made these endeavors unnecessary. The research results that led to the development of these "analysis-synthesis" telephony systems became forgotten. It was not until relatively recently that it become apparent that research results on the *"channel vocoder"* were applicable to cochlear implants.

Cochlear implants that use the vocoder principle also extract the energy of sounds in a few (8-20) frequency bands [28]. The energy in each of these bands controls the electrical impulses that are applied to each pair of electrodes implanted in the cochlea for activating hearing nerve fibers. The processor in such implants discards information about the fine pattern of the speech waves.

The studies on the channel vocoder have shown that the spectrum of sounds (known as place coding, see Chapter I) alone is therefore sufficient for speech discrimination, and coding of the waveform of the speech wave alone is equally sufficient for speech discrimination. Often studies of which parts of the speech signals are necessary for speech comprehension have shown that information about the speech wave (temporal information) alone could provide good speech discrimination [45]. This is again a sign of the redundancy of the speech signal, making it possible to achieve good speech discrimination using only some parts of the properties of the speech signal.

Studies of the success of cochlear implants confirm that the speech signal has considerable redundancy and that also the normal hearing system has considerable redundancy and flexibility in the way it processes sound such as speech sounds [11]. The hearing system can be trained to discriminate speech signals from cochlear implants processors showing the power of neural plasticity.

3.1.1.3. Adding more Channels to Cochlear Implants was a Major Improvement over Early Cochlear Implants for Speech Discrimination

When it became technically possible to implant many electrodes in the cochlea, the question arose about how many channels (frequency bands) were needed for good speech discrimination. This has been studied in individuals with normal hearing by computer simulation of cochlear implants with different number of frequency bands (Figure 3.2 [11]). The obtained results were compared with results from real cochlear implants of different kinds by many actual cochlear implant wearers.

The success regarding achieving speech comprehension depends on the principles used for processing speech sounds in cochlear implants and on how many channels (frequency bands) are used (Figure 3.2). Computer simulations [11] have shown that speech comprehension improves when the number of frequency bands is increased, but only up to about 8 bands-- above that the gain is small (solid lines in the graphs in Figure 3.2).

The degree of speech comprehension obtained by a cochlear implant wearer varies considerably as seen from the results obtained in the study of actual cochlear implant wearers (open circles in Figure 3.2). Great individual variation in success is often seen when systems are challenged, such as when the redundancy in the information is reduced. Normal hearing individuals rely not only on the energy in different frequency bands but also the waveform of speech sounds, and that provides redundancy that increases the "safety with respect to transmission faults" as communication engineers calls it.

3.1.2. Cochlear Nucleus Implants

Signals from the ear normally reach the first relay nerve cells of the ascending hearing pathways, the cochlear nucleus (see Appendix A). When the hearing nerve is damaged this cannot occur and the person is deaf even if the cochlea may be intact. Cochlear implants are therefore not of any benefit for such individuals. Instead, electrical impulses are applied directly to the cochlear nucleus (known as cochlear nucleus implants or brain stem implants) can provide hearing sensations in such individuals. These devices activate the cells in the cochlear nucleus directly and therefore bypass not only the cochlea but also the hearing nerve. In cochlear nucleus implants, electrical impulses are applied to the surface of the nucleus by electrodes placed on a plastic sheet.

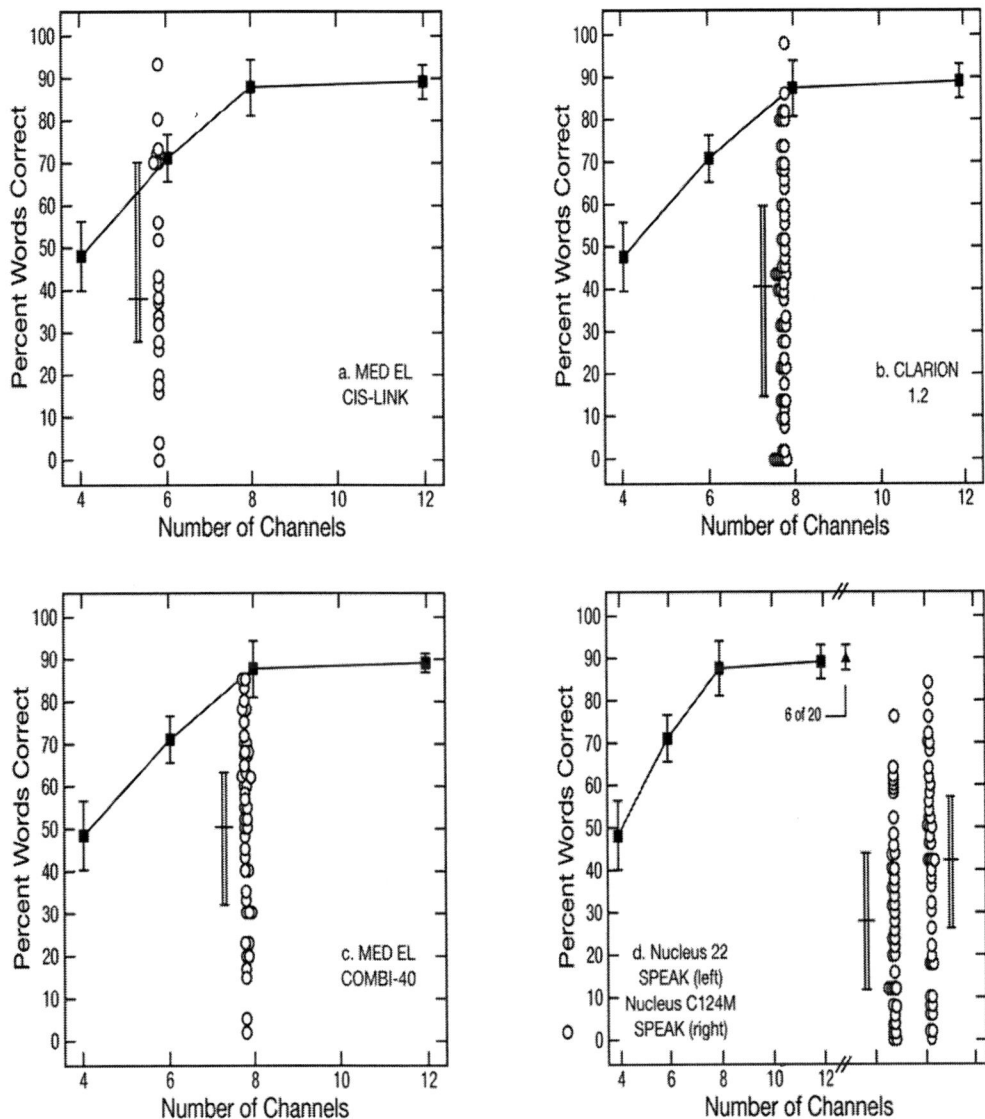

Figure 3.2. Improvement of speech comprehension by increasing the number of frequency bands. Solid lines and squares: Simulation of cochlear implants with 4, 6, 8 and 12 channels on people with normal hearing. Open circles: Actual cochlear implant wearer using 6, 8 and 22-channel cochlear implants. The two columns in the graph showing results from Nucleus 22 represent 22 channels. (Reproduced from: Møller, A.R. 2006. *Hearing: Anatomy, Physiology, and Disorders of the Auditory System*, 2nd Ed. Academic Press, Amsterdam, after Dorman, 2000 [11] with permission from Elsevier.

Bypassing the hearing nerve would not seem to have any noticeable importance because it does not process signals; only transmit the signals from the cochlea to the cochlear nucleus. It could therefore be expected that cochlear nucleus implants would work as well as cochlear implants do. However, when cochlear nucleus implants were first introduced, the results were disappointing. The best these devices could provide was sound awareness, but no actual speech comprehension. Cochlear nucleus implants were originally used exclusively in individuals whose hearing nerves were severed on both sides because they had tumors (vestibular schwannoma) caused by a genetic defect known as neurofibromatosis type 2. When an otologic surgeon, Dr. Vittorio Colletti [5], began to use the implants in people who had their hearing nerve severed for other reasons, such as head injury and in children who had a malformation that strangled the hearing nerve, he found that equally good speech discrimination could be achieved with cochlear nucleus implants as with cochlear implants used in people with intact hearing nerves. Naturally, training and activation of neural plasticity was necessary in order to obtain these results. Children with a faulty hearing nerve (such as in internal auditory canal (IAC) atresia[11]) must be given the benefit from a cochlear nucleus (brainstem) implant [6].

This means that individuals with vestibular schwannoma on both sides may have had some defects of the cochlear nucleus in addition to the defects that caused the tumors.

3.1.3. The Role of Neural Plasticity

Cochlear implants only have a few electrodes (channels). They provide information only about the energy of sounds in a few frequency bands and activate large groups of nerve fibers in exactly the same way. This means the brain has to do with less and different information than the cochlea normally provides.

The patterns of electrical impulses the cochlear implants induce in the hearing nerve are different from that produced by the normal cochlea, but that is not the only difference. The brain must therefore learn to interpret this new neural code so the person who wears a cochlear implant can understand speech and the meaning of other sounds [25]. This is accomplished through neural plasticity turned on through training. Activation of neural plasticity changes the processing of the nerve signals produced by cochlear implants and cochlear nucleus making it possible to understand speech using these prostheses.

3.1.3.1. Critical Period

For many years it was assumed that plastic changes could only occur in young children and that only the developing nervous system could be changed (was plastic). However, many recent studies have confirmed that the adult brain is plastic as well. It is easier to activate neural plasticity in children than in adults, and the changes in function that can be achieved through activation of neural plasticity are more extensive in children. The period where it is easy to change the function of the nervous system is known as the *"critical period"* [21]. The correct organization of the brain depends on receiving sensory signals within this short period

---

[11] Atresia: means that a bony orifice is either not formed correctly of totally absent. Regarding the ear, atresia of the ear canal and of the bony canal where the hearing nerve travels, the "internal auditory canal" (IAC) are known birth defects.

after birth. The critical period has been most extensively studied in vision, [51,52], but it is also apparent in other senses, particularly hearing [23,26].

The basic discovery regarding critical periods was done in studies of the visual system [53], and still most of the research so far has been done in the visual system. Recent results of research in the hearing field have been published [23], especially in connection with cochlear implants, where knowledge about critical periods has directly influenced clinical work and planning of intervention [26,46].

The importance of sensory stimulation early in life was first shown in studies of the visual system. Kittens that were deprived of stimulation of the visual system had abnormalities in their visual nervous system [17,51] because sensory signals are necessary for the normal development of the brain. Without sensory signals, the wiring of the brain becomes different from what it is normally, and the cortical regions that do not get any signals may become invaded by nerve fibers (axons) from nerve cells of other senses that receive signals (see page 91). The structure of the thalamic nucleus (lateral geniculate nucleus) is different in animals that have not received any sensory signals early in life from that of normal animals that have received sensory signals. The critical period for vision in humans is probably 2-3 years, with different aspects of vision having different critical periods.

Children who are totally deaf because of a faulty cochlea but who have an intact hearing nerve must be given a cochlear implant so that the nervous system can develop normally [25,32]. Those who do not have an intact hearing nerve should have a cochlear nucleus implant [7]. Cochlear implants have been shown to facilitate childhood development. The result may not be exactly identical to the normal nervous system, but similar (see page 90). To achieve the best possible results, cochlear implants or brainstem (cochlear nucleus) implants should be given to deaf children as soon as possible after birth. (The cochlea does not grow after birth).

Children who have hearing loss must be given amplification (hearing aids or cochlear implants if adequate hearing cannot be established by hearing aids) so their hearing nervous system can be activated in a normal way. Adequate stimulation of the hearing nervous system during childhood is necessary for its normal development. This stimulation by meaningful sounds must occur early in life to make it possible for the hearing nervous system to develop in a normal way. Not all hearing children receive adequate exposure to sounds. It is important that the exposure to sounds occurs during the "critical period" where the brain is most malleable. During the critical period, the brain has its greatest ability to change its function. It is important that training of functions such as the spoken language is done during this period. There is evidence that missing the critical period cannot be compensated for totally by exposure to sensory signals later, although plastic changes can occur after the critical period and during the entire adult life. However, this happens to a lesser extent and it takes a longer time to achieve adaptation after the critical period.

The fact that the young brain is more malleable than the adult brain has been confirmed by studies of children and adults who have received their cochlear implants at different ages. The main proof of success is naturally the obtained speech discrimination, but there are also physiologic correlates that can help assessing the success of cochlear implants (See figure 3.3). In a study of the effect of the time of the implantation on the success of cochlear implants, such physiological methods were used. Electrophysiological potentials (evoked potentials[12]) such as those known as event related potentials (ERPs)[13] could be used for evaluation of adaptation to a cochlear implant [48]. These potentials occur in response to sounds and they can be recorded from electrodes placed on the scalp.

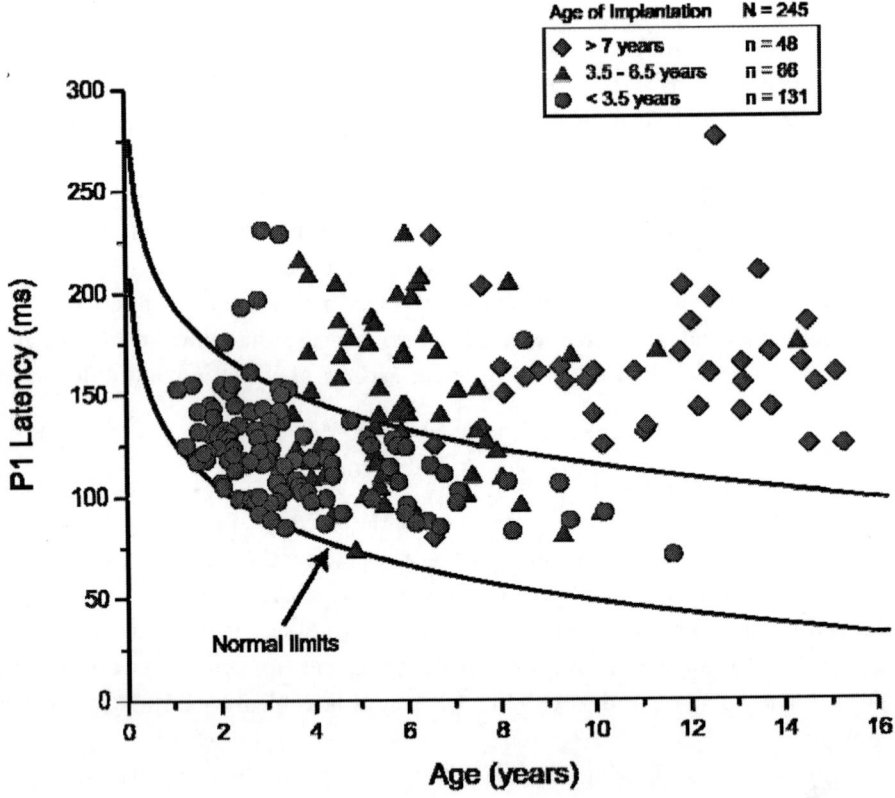

Figure 3.3. Maturation of evoked potentials in children who have normal hearing at birth and deaf children after receiving cochlear implants at different ages. Reproduced from Sharma, A., Dorman, M.F. 2006. Central Auditory Development in Children with Cochlear Implants: Clinical Implications. In: Møller, A.R., (Ed.), *Cochlear and Brainstem Implants,* Adv Oto Rhino Laryngol, Vol. 64. Karger, Basel. pp. 66-88 [46]).

The studies using recordings of ERPs have clearly shown that there is a "critical period" (see page 78, 92) during which the best results of cochlear implants are obtained [46]. Those who got their cochlear implants at a young age (within the critical period) are performing much better than those who got implants as adults (Figure 3.3). The experience with cochlear implants shows that the critical period for hearing is probably 3-4 years.

---

[12] Evoked potentials: Electrical activity in the brain that is caused by stimulation of senses such hearing, vision and body senses and which can be recorded by placing electrodes on the scalp.

[13] ERP: This term is used for evoked potential that occur a long time (100 or more milliseconds) after the activating sound.

When cochlear implants were developed, doctors were not allowed to implant such devices in young children - no FDA approval - which displays ignorance about neural plasticity in general and critical periods in particular by the FDA.

The sensory nervous system can change its function even after the critical period. The nervous system in older children and adults can adapt to changing demands [25,46] but it takes longer time to achieve the changes and they are less extensive than those that can occur during the critical period. This is why adults or older children have more difficulties adapting to the use of cochlear and brainstem implants than young children (Figure 3.3 [25,46]).

3.1.4. Prostheses of Limbs

Amputation of a limb causes re-organization of the motor cortex because of loss of connection between the motonuclei [5] and the muscles [13,40]. When a person who has lost a limb is fitted with prosthesis the motor cortex has to be re-organized in order to be able to use the limb.

Training in the use of limb prostheses is necessary for activation of neural plasticity of the motor system so that the commands that are issued by the brain can properly adapt to the changed situation. Training makes it possible to use prostheses for amputated limbs because training activates plasticity in neural circuits in the spinal cord and the brain adapting the motor system to the changed demands from the use of prostheses.

3.2. Change in Sensory or Motor Functions Function through Training

3.2.1. Ameliorating Synkinesis

Activation of neural plasticity can reduce synkinesis (involuntary contraction of other muscles than those intended). Synkinesis of muscles in the face (the mimic muscles) often occurs after recovery after injuries where the facial nerve has been damaged. Peter Johnson and his colleagues have shown that training [3] can ameliorate such synkinesis. That training can reduce synkinesis suggests that the synkinesis that occurs after completion of the outgrow of nerves from an injury is not caused by misdirection of outgrowing nerve fibers as was believed earlier. It is more likely caused by changes in the organization of the facial motonucleus[14].

Further evidence that re-organization of the facial motor nucleus can cause synkinesis and spasm[15] comes from studies of patients with hemifacial spasm[16] [31] undergoing microvascular decompression operations[17] to relieve the spasm and synkinesis (discussed in Chapter IV).

---

[14] Motonucleus: Cluster of nerve cells that send signals to muscles through motor nerves. Motonuclei are located in the front part of the spinal cord, and for the head, motonuclei are located in the brainstem.

[15] Spasm: *Involuntary movement accompanying a voluntary one, as the movement of a closed eye following that of the uncovered one, or the movement occurring in a paralyzed muscle accompanying motion in another part.* (Stedman's Electronic Medical Dictionary, Version 7.0).

[16] Hemifacial spasm: A rare disease that is characterized by episodic spasm of mimic muscles in on side of the face, and synkinesis.

[17] Microvascular decompression operations: Operations where a blood vessel is moved off a cranial nerve root, most often that of the facial, trigeminal or glossopharyngeal nerves.

3.2.2. The Balance System

When the head is turned, the balance system, also known as the vestibular system, is activated and causes the eyes to move in the opposite direction as the head to keep an image on the retina (the backside of the eye containing the receptors) from moving. This is accomplished by the *vestibular-ocular reflex (VOR)* that controls the muscles that move the eye (see Chapter II). The balance system also helps maintain posture and assists keeping in normal gait (the manner of walking).

3.2.2.1 The Vestibular Ocular Reflex

The balance organ in the inner ear reports to the brain how much the head is moved and commands are sent to the five eye muscles that control the position of the eye. Normally the eyes move in the opposite direction the head is turned and that makes an image stay still on the retina. This normally occurs without us knowing, but diseases of the hearing-vestibular nerve may cause information about movements of the head to reach consciousness and produce the sensation of dizziness and vertigo. Head motion may cause vomiting under certain conditions such as violent movements (motion sickness) or during viral infections that affect the vestibular nerve (see Chapter IV). The eyes must move exactly the same amount as the head but in the opposite direction [2]. This means the gain (the ratio between movement of the eyes and the movement of the head) of the vestibular ocular reflex must be exactly -1.0 in order to keep the image on the retina from moving. The value of the gain is set in the brain.

When a person wears spectacles the amount that the eyes must move to avoid the image on the retina moving depends on the strength of the lenses in the spectacles. A person who changes eyeglasses, or just begins to wear eyeglasses, will see objects move while moving the head. This occurs because the amount the eyes need to move when the head is turned becomes slightly different with new glasses and turning the head will cause an image on the retina to move, which is perceived as the surroundings move when turning the head. This unpleasant effect of changing spectacles will normally only last a short time because this discrepancy between head movement and eye movement will turn neural plasticity on and that will adjust the gain of the vestibular ocular reflex. When this happens, the eyes again move an appropriate amount when the head is turned so that it again can hold an image steady on the retina (vestibular ocular reflex gain of -1.0, negative sign indicating movement in the opposite direction).

3.2.2.2. Reversing Prisms

The ability of the vestibular ocular reflex to change its gain is enormous, as has been shown in experiments where people were wearing prisms (lenses) that inverted the image they saw of their environment. Wearing spectacles (prisms) that invert the image the wearer sees makes the environment appear backwards (right being left) on the retina. Movements that go from left to right will be perceived as going from right to left, hence in the opposite direction. To keep an image steady on the retina while wearing inverting prisms not only requires a change in the amount of the gain of the vestibular ocular reflex, but it also requires that the eyes move in the opposite direction of what they normally do -- (without the prisms). The gain must therefore be changed from its normal value of -1.0 to

+1.0. However, the vestibular ocular reflex can adapt to these changes within a few days and it was reported that the participants in these experiments could play tennis wearing inverting prisms [18].

This kind of adaptation may not be of much practical importance; people do not usually wear inverting prisms, but it is a telling example of how enormously malleable the brain is. It is also an example of our ability to adapt to situations that never occur in nature. The animals from which we inherited the vestibular ocular reflex never encounter a situation where images appear differently.

Normally the balance system helps keep posture. Loss of function of the balance system makes it difficult to stand and to walk if the loss has occurred rapidly. When the deficits of the balance system persist the symptoms decrease with time because of activation of neural plasticity that makes other systems take over. The systems that can take over what the balance system normally does, regarding keeping balance when standing and walking, are vision and body senses such as receptors in joints, tendons, and to some extent receptors in the skin. Activating receptors in joints, muscles, and tendons are not felt but it helps keep balance. The senses that involve receptors in muscles, joints, and tendons are known as "proprioception" and act as feedback for movements of limbs and the entire body. These body senses can take over many of the normal functions of the balance system such as posture and the control of gait. The position of the eyes can be maintained while turning the head through signal from the visual system. There is just ample redundancy in the systems that keep posture.

The ability to replace the function of the balance system by that of other systems is different for people of different ages. Young people may recover from sudden loss of function of the balance system within weeks; adults younger than 50 years of age may take many months, and after age 60 they do not totally recover. If the function of the balance organ or the balance nerve changes rapidly, the reactions are often violent symptoms. Inflammation of the balance nerve (vestibular neuritis) can totally prevent signals from the balance organ from reaching the brain. Insufficient recovery is most pronounced regarding the gait, and people with incomplete recovery walk with a wide gait. (Compare that to the critical age, discussed on page 78).

If the damage to the balance system occurs slowly it may not give any symptoms at all because other systems have time to take over the various functions, such as the control of the position of the eyes and help in keeping posture.

A slowly growing tumor on the balance nerve (vestibular schwannoma) can destroy the balance nerve slowly and that often does not cause any symptoms from the balance system.

3.2.3. Enriched Sound Environment

Exposure to moderately loud sounds (an enriched sound environment) is beneficial in various ways. The damage that occurs to the receptors in the ear from noise exposure and from aging has been documented by many studies but it has also been shown that a part of age-related hearing loss may also come from changes in the brain, parts of which could possibly be caused by activation of neural plasticity. This has become evident through studies in mice that have shown that exposure to moderately loud sounds can reduce (or rather stall the progression of) the "normal" occurring hearing loss with age. Dr. James Willott [54] and co-workers have shown that the hearing loss that normally increases with age did so more slowly in mice that lived in an "enriched sound environment" than in mice that lived in a quiet environment.

Other studies have shown that after noise trauma a similar enriched sound environment can reduce the hearing loss and prevent the effect of noise exposure on the organization of the cortex [38]. It is not proven that these effects of exposure to sound are caused by activation of neural plasticity, but it seems to be a likely explanation.

It is possible that the degree of damage to receptors in the ear may to some extent be affected by signals from the brain that reach these receptors through the descending hearing pathways [33] (see Chapter I). Again, research regarding such matters has been slow and it has been difficult to imagine that the brain could have any control over damage to sensory cells in the ear.

The effect of sound exposure on the sensory cells in the inner ear as discussed above is probably not affected by the content of the sound. This would mean that the benefit from exposure to meaningless (noise) sounds would be the same as from exposure to, for example, speech sounds and music.

There are other effects of hearing sounds where the content matters. It has been suggested that sounds can improve mental capabilities. Listening to music enhances recovery of cognitive (mental) functions in victims of some kinds of strokes [43]. It has also been shown that rats became better in finding their way in a labyrinth after they were exposed to music [41].

3.2.4. Toughening of the Ear

A common cause of hearing loss is from exposure to excessive noise and the resulting hearing loss has been ascribed to damage to the sensory cells in the cochlea. However, it has become evident that the hearing loss to some degree, in fact, can be related to changes in the central nervous system and possible involvement of neural plasticity. One of the first signs of an involvement of the nervous system on hearing loss came from a study by Dr. Joseph Miller, who in 1963 showed that hearing loss from noise exposure could be decreased by exposure to quieter sounds before being exposed to intense noise [30]. This surprising finding was perhaps the first sign that hearing loss from noise exposure is not just caused by damage to the sensory cells in the ear (hair cells) from mechanical stress from sound exposure. It also showed that the nervous system has some control over what happens to the hair cells in the cochlea from exposure to loud sounds.

That the risk of noise induced hearing loss could be affected by prior exposure to moderately loud sounds was looked upon with great skepticism for many years. Only much later were studies of this effect repeated and many investigators have now confirmed Dr. Miller's findings. The cause of this "toughening of the ear" was unknown at the time it was discovered, and is still not completely understood, but at least some part of the effect seems to be caused by plastic changes in the brain [33,55], probably in connection with the ability of the brain to influence how the sensory cells in the ear works through the descending pathways (see Chapter I) [33] (the outer hair cells that works as "motors that amplify the motion of the basilar membrane). This kind of "toughening" of the ear is just another example of how malleable the brain is even in adult life.

3.2.5. Changes in Muscle Reflexes

The benefits from activation of neural plasticity are not limited to sensory systems. The use of movement systems can also benefit. Control of movement is highly adaptable to changing demands and that is a result of neural plasticity being turned on.

We have many different kinds of muscle reflexes. Most of our reflexes are controlled by neural circuits in the spinal cord and some are located in the brainstem. Frequent use of reflexes can increase the ease with which they are turned on and making them react faster and stronger. It is also possible to suppress reflexes by training; all because the control of reflexes is plastic. Changing the ease with which reflexes are elicited can have a general effect on control of movements because control of muscles is to a great extent done by controlling reflexes by signals from the motor cortex [35].

That muscle reflexes can be made more active and easier to elicit by training is another sign of how use can affect the function, which can be explained by neural plasticity being turned on strengthening the synapses that activate the reflexes. The opposite can also be accomplished by training where activation of neural plasticity can make synapses less effective and thereby weakening reflexes. Muscles that are normally acting together at the same time can be made to act independently by training, which means that activation of neural plasticity has weakened some synapses.

There are many other examples of how training can increase motor skills. Learning to speak as a child involves neural plasticity that is activated through training. Later in life, learning to pronounce unfamiliar words requires involvement of neural plasticity for proper activation of the many different muscles that are involved in speech production. Training is necessary for being able to pronounce unfamiliar words, but after some attempts it becomes natural. That means neural circuits have been changed appropriately to produce a new series of commands to muscles. Training of muscle functions involved in speaking can make it easy to pronounce such unfamiliar words. The skill remains for a long time, often forever. Learning to ride a bicycle is common example of learning motor skills that can last a lifetime.

We may call this learning but it is in fact a matter of neural plasticity because activation of the skills does not involve conscious recall as does memorization of telephone numbers, etc. (see page 27 regarding the difference between learning and neural plasticity).

3.2.6. Increased Use of Motor Function Expand Sensory Cortical Areas

Increased use of a finger causes an expansion of the sensory cortical areas involved in control of the finger [12] (see page 39). This "steal" of cortical regions normally belonging to other fingers is a sign that connections that are normally dormant have become active through activation of neural plasticity.

4. THE IMPORTANCE OF NEURAL PLASTICITY
FOR MATURATION OF THE BRAIN

At birth the brain is not complete and extensive changes must occur in order to achieve what we regard as a normally functioning brain. Much needs to be done for the brain and the spinal cord to fully mature. The changes that normally occur early in life are extensive; consisting of re-arranging the circuits of nerve cells, creation of new synapses, elimination of synapses, elimination of nerve fibers, creation of new nerve fibers, and even elimination of entire cells (*programmed cell death (PCD)*, or apoptosis) (I have called that "midcourse correction", see page 42, 62, 67, 86, 92, 111, 157). Later in childhood exposure to sensory signals becomes important for further development of the nervous system. In adult life changes in the nervous system can occur as a result of exposure to sensory signals or from adaptation to changing demands.

4.1. Childhood Development

The blueprint for how the nervous system is organized is laid down by genetics but it needs a correction in order to function normally. Neural plasticity is normally turned on in early childhood to make the necessary changes for normal development. During the first years of life the brain changes in many ways; the number of nerve cells is reduced and there is competition in making connections between nerve cells. Many connections between nerve cells are eliminated during childhood development. I call this childhood re-organization of the brain a "midcourse correction". If this process does not proceed correctly abnormalities in many functions may occur and these are what we call developmental diseases (discussed in detail in Chapter IV).

4.2. "Midcourse Correction" of Anatomical Organization and Function

During the first years of life extensive reorganization of the brain occurs. The programmed plastic changes that provide "midcourse corrections" of genetically controlled (Darwinian) development consist of competition for synaptic space causing elimination of synapses, elimination of connections between nerve cells (pruning of axons and dendrites) and elimination of entire nerve cells (apoptosis or programmed cell death, PCD). New connections are also created in the spinal cord and the brain during early childhood.

Childhood development is originally programmed and controlled by genetic factors. Genes (hereditary factors) lay down a blueprint of the organization ("wiring") and function of the brain. The genes that program development before birth can be modified by epigenetics[18] (see page 246). Environmental factors affecting the fetus in the womb may interfere with development in positive as well as negative ways. After birth, environmental factors can also

---

[18] *Epigenetics: Regulation of the expression of gene activity without alteration of genetic structure.* (Stedman's Electronic Medical Dictionary Version 7.0).

interfere with childhood development. Activation of neural plasticity can correct or modify this blueprint that was laid down by genetics. The "midcourse correction" that normally takes place early in life is an example.

During the first few years of life as many as 50% of all nerve cells in the brain die and connections between nerve cells are interrupted either by elimination of nerve fibers that connect nerve cells with each other, by eliminating dendrites and synapses, or by making it impossible to activate connections which therefore become dormant. Dormant connections can be re-activated (turned on) by activation of neural plasticity. Making connections inactive or activating dormant connections may switch information from one group of nerve cells to another and thereby rearrange neural circuits.

This "mid-course correction" of the brain's organization is absolutely necessary for normal childhood development. Faults in this process are involved in causing developmental diseases such as, perhaps, autism [36]. (Discussed in Chapter IV, and a description of autism and various suggestions about its cause are found in Appendix C.) However, published studies regarding the damage that may occur early in life through faulty development have mostly concerned structure (morphology). Little is known about the functional changes that occur.

The changes that occur in the central nervous system early in life have similarities to the changes that occur when neural plasticity in turned on for other reasons. There is a difference, however, in that plastic changes that occur early in life are probably not turned on by external factors as other forms of neural plasticity are. Instead, the changes are most likely controlled by internal factors. External factors can most likely interfere with these normal processes.

It is poorly understood what exactly controls these structural and functional changes that occur during the period of normal development. It seems clear that these changes are *programmed*, but we know little about the actual programs, when and where they are created and how they are executed. We do not know what can affect these programs. If we knew more about them we might be able to find more efficient ways to affect and treat developmental diseases.

Chemicals that may have affected the brain at the time the symptoms of developmental diseases occur could naturally be the cause of the faulty development. It, however, seems more likely that interference with development occurred before birth – when the programs were created (se Figure 3.4). If this is the case, it may explain why there has been so little success in treating developmental diseases such as autism. There is evidence from studies in animals that exposure to some chemicals (PCB) before birth can cause severe faults in the development of the nervous system that occur after birth [19].

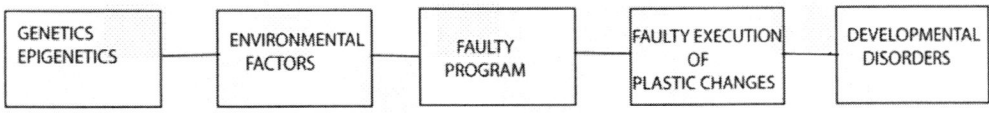

Figure 3.4. Hypothetical flowchart of the normal "midcourse correction" that occurs early in life. Programs laid down by genetics and epigenetics are affected by environmental factors before birth. After birth, these programs (rules) control the development of the nervous system. If the programs are faulty, the development does not proceed normally and the results are developmental disorders.

4.3. Cause of Developmental Diseases

Are the programs that control childhood development flawed or are the programs correct but executed incorrectly (because of the presence of factors that interfere with their implementation)? These two questions are of fundamental importance for understanding what causes many developmental diseases and for finding ways for treatment and prevention.

The "midcourse correction" that occurs during the few years after birth is extensive, but many parts of the brain are not fully developed until the age of 18 to 20 years. The maturation of the frontal parts of the brain, which deal with decision-making and other higher functions, are the last one to be completed - it does not seem to be fully developed until about 18 years of age. This may explain why an 18 year old suddenly begins to make decent decisions, and perhaps even gains the good judgment to ask his/her parents for advice--and more remarkably, even considers the advice and follows it. Little is known about the mechanisms that control this development, but it seems natural to assume that neural plasticity is involved and the progression of plastic changes are somehow controlled by internal control systems that may be affected by environmental factors including sensory stimulation and intellectual challenges.

Faults in the programs or in the execution of normal programs may cause abnormalities that are so extensive we call the outcome "diseases", but there are also abnormalities that are small and which just prevent optimal performance. This means that the definition of disease is important and it is important to distinguish between diseases and abnormalities that are no larger than the normal variations.

4.4. Plastic Changes Later in Childhood

Activation of neural plasticity is also necessary for further maturation of the brain. After the corrections that occur immediately after birth have been completed, the way the brain is wired can still change because it is plastic. Changes occur when children are exposed to an "enriched sensory environment", and sensory signals help to develop the nervous system to the best possible usage.

For example, the cells of the hearing nervous system are normally tuned to different frequencies and the cells are anatomically arranged according to the frequency of the sounds that reach the ear. However, this "tonotopic" organization does not occur in individuals who are deaf at birth.

The normal "tonotopic organization" of nerve cells evolves because of the ability of the cochlea to separate sounds according to their frequency. This causes sounds of different frequencies to activate nerve cells in the hearing pathways according to the frequency of the sounds. Through exposure to sounds, nerve cells become "tagged" and they become anatomically organized according to the frequencies to which they respond best. This is what we call tonotopic organization. This form of neural plasticity is turned on by signals from the ear that is elicited when sound from the entire audible frequency range of hearing activate the ear. This means that the tonotopic organization is directed by sound but requires many different kinds of sound.

In the absence of signals from the ear at birth there is only a rudimentary organization of the hearing nervous system [14,27]. Without activation of neural plasticity by sounds, the normal tonotopic organization cannot evolve. There are other abnormalities in the hearing nervous system in animals that are born deaf; synaptic activity in the hearing cortex is reduced [24]. This means that the development of normal synaptic activity requires stimulation of the sensory system. Absence of normal signals from the ear can be caused by faults in the function of the ear (not only total deafness but also reduced sensitivity) or by absence of normal exposure to a variation of natural sounds.

It has been shown that electrical stimulation of the cochlea in animals that were born deaf can establish a tonotopic organization [20,22]. These studies confirm that signals from the ear must be established within a narrow time window, the "critical period", in order to create a normal tonotopic organization (see page 144).

Being able to distinguish sounds with different frequencies is important for normal use of the hearing sense, such as for understanding speech. This ability depends on the function of the cochlea. As I discussed in Chapter I, the cochlea separates sounds according to their frequency. This frequency selectivity of the cochlea makes nerve cells in the hearing nervous system become arranged anatomically according to the frequency to which they respond best. Nerve cells that respond to tones of a certain frequency are located close to each other. This tonotopic organization is present in the classical pathways throughout the hearing nervous system. One can therefore map the frequency to which nerve cells respond best on nuclei and the cerebral cortex (Figure 3.5).

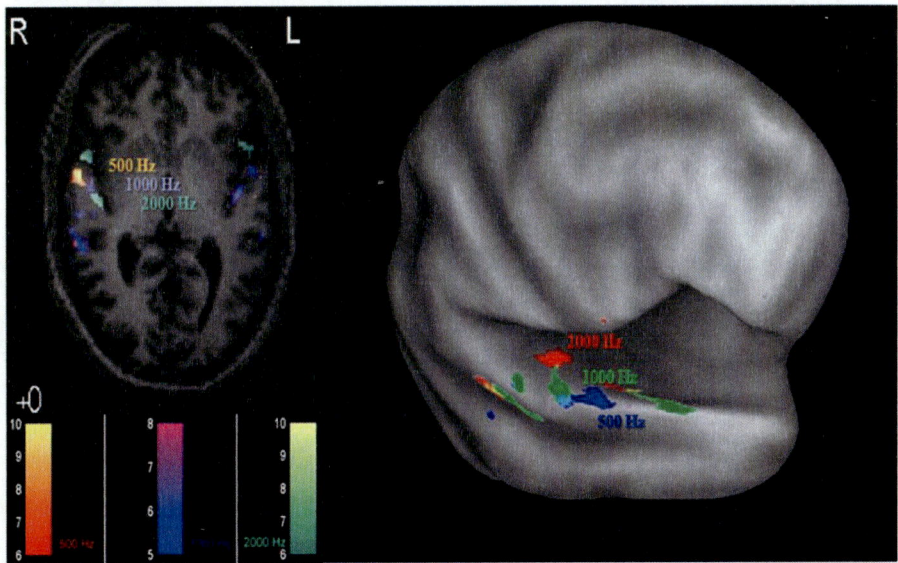

Figure 3.5. Tonotopic map of the hearing cortex, showing the location on the cortex of nerve cells that respond best to the frequencies shown. Images are based on functional MRI. Using headphones, 500Hz, 1,000Hz and 2,000Hz tones were presented inside the scanner. Changes in blood oxygen level (BOLD signal) localized at the tonotopic area in the auditory cortex for each frequency is depicted. Note the presence of multiple tonotopic maps in the auditory cortex. Courtesy Professors Sunaert and De Ridder, Antwerp, Belgium.

It is not only the representation of the frequency of sounds that is lacking in animals that are born deaf but also the organizations that are involved in directional hearing are abnormal if the hearing nervous system does not receive any signals from the ear [42].

4.5. Re-Organization of the Nerve Cells in the Brain in Children Born Deaf

I have pointed out in several places of this book that it is important to receive sensory signals to turn on beneficial neural plasticity which promotes the development of normal function of sensory systems. I have discussed how lack of sensory signals can cause abnormalities (because of faults in devolvement) in the nervous system that result in symptoms of diseases. If animals or humans are born deaf it leaves some parts of the brain deprived of their normal signals from the ear making these parts unused. Animal studies by Dr. Mriganka Sur of MIT, Cambridge MA and his co-workers have shown that absence of signals that can activate the auditory nervous system before or just after birth may cause other senses to invade the unused parts of the hearing nervous system [15] (see Figure 3.6).

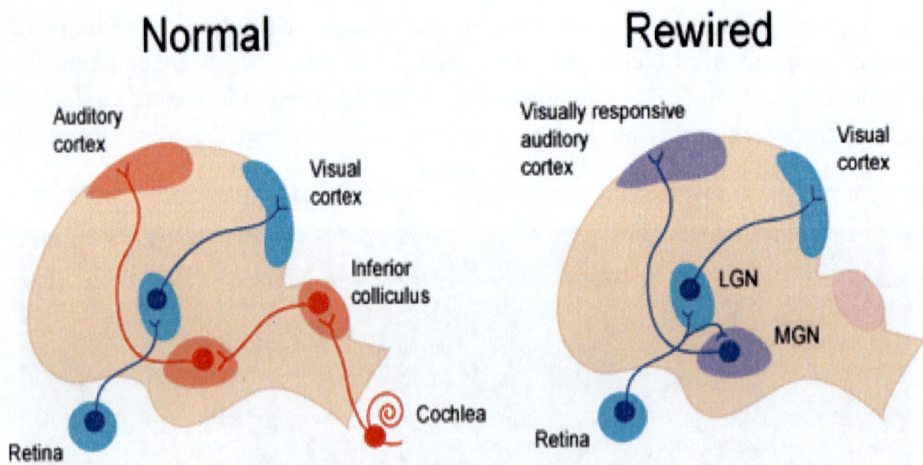

Figure 3.6. Illustration of how other senses such as vision can take over an unused hearing cortex [15]. LGN: Lateral geniculate nucleus, visual thalamic nucleus; MGM: Medial geniculate nucleus, hearing thalamic nucleus. (Reproduced from Horng, S.H., Sur, M. 2006. Visual activity and cortical rewiring: Activity-dependent plasticity of cortical networks. In: Møller, A.R., (Ed.), *Reprogramming the Brain, Progress in Brain Research* Vol. 157. Elsevier, Amsterdam pp. 3-11. (Reproduced with permission from Elsevier).

The absence of hearing signals in the nuclei of the hearing pathways can cause connections from the visual system to invade the part of the thalamus that normally is involved in hearing. The re-wiring causes changes in the nucleus of the thalamus that is normally involved in hearing, so it can process signals from the eye instead of processing signals from the ear as it does in individuals with intact hearing. The thalamus supplies the cerebral cortex with signals, and when the thalamus is re-arranged it reflects on the cerebral cortex. When parts of the thalamus that normally is involved with hearing become taken over by vision, the hearing cortex also becomes taken over by vision [15].

Normally, the different parts of the cerebral cortex are arranged into separate regions that receive signals from different sense organs. There is a part that receives signals from the ears, another part that receives signals from the eyes, and other parts receive signals from receptors in the skin and so on. In the same way, nuclei in the sensory pathways are dedicated to specific senses. For example, the different sensory nuclei of the thalamus receive input from different senses.

The signals from the eyes that cause this re-organization seem to come from the part of the visual nervous system that serves the peripheral vision. This is the part of the visual nervous system that is known as the non-classical visual system (see Chapter I and in Appendix B).

This is again an example that shows how powerful signals from the sense organs are in modifying the normal organization of the nervous system, and it confirms clearly that our genes only control and guide a part of the organization of the nervous system.

5. How Can Beneficial Plasticity be Activated?

I have already mentioned several factors that can activate neural plasticity. Many of these may activate neural plasticity that is beneficial to the individual person, but the same factors may also activate plasticity that is harmful, causing symptoms and signs of diseases. This will be discussed in Chapter IV.

I have pointed out earlier in this book the most powerful factor that can activate neural plasticity is lack of signals such as those that may occur in sensory systems where the sense organs have been damaged or disconnected. Injury that has destroyed parts of the brain or spinal cord may also turn on neural plasticity. Subsequent therapy in the form of training may activate neural plasticity further. Many unknown factors can probably also turn on neural plasticity. It is hence not known what activates neural plasticity that causes maturation of the nervous system through the "midcourse correction" that occurs immediately after birth and which was discussed above.

6. Limitations in the Benefits from Plastic Changes

There are limitations in the amount of beneficial effects that can be achieved through activation of neural plasticity. I have already discussed one important limitation, namely age. The possibility to change the function of the nervous system is greatest at a young age. After the "critical period" many functions become established and difficult to change.

Neural plasticity can open connections to brain regions not usually used and thereby replace functions that have been impaired by disease processes such as strokes and other causes of permanent damage to parts of the brain or spinal cord. The beneficial effect from redirecting functions that have suffered damage such as in strokes is limited by the availability of other structures that can perform the functions of the damaged structures.

Adaptation to change in demands is limited by the extent of the flexibility of neural circuits (mainly the number of dormant synapses) and the ability to create new synapses.

6.1. Redundancy

In order to replace functions that are lost because of strokes or injury to the brain, other parts of the brain must be available that can do the same functions. This means that *redundancy,* or a duplication of functions, is required.

Many functions can be performed with more than one part of the brain. We have two kidneys and we can do well with only one, we have two adrenal glands, men have two testicles, women two ovaries, but we have only one liver and one heart. We have also two ears and two eyes, but while we can hear with one ear and see with one eye there are functions that are lost when an eye or an ear is lost --namely our ability to hear from which direction a sound comes (directional hearing). Our ability of perception of depth in what we see at a short distance depends on stereoscopic vision, and this depends on the use of two eyes.

The brain has two similar, but not identical, halves. Not all functions are replicated in the two halves. The redundancy is limited in many parts of the brain, and while some tasks can be done equally well by either half, other functions can only be done by one of the two halves of the brain. Movements, such as of the limbs, is controlled from the motor cortex on one side of the brain. Therefore, loss of functions of the motor cortex (such as from strokes or traumatic injuries) cannot be replaced by other parts of the brain.

Control of speech cannot easily be shifted from the left side, which is normally used, to the right side when the left side of the brain is damaged. The two regions of the brain that control speech are Broca's area in the frontal part of the brain near the temporal lobe and Wernicke's area located in the parietal lobe (Figure 4.8). Broca's area controls the muscles of the speech organs. Wernicke's area is more involved in planning speech and it plays an important role in understanding speech. It has connections to and from the hearing cortex and it sends its signals to Broca's area. Damage to these two regions causes two different kinds of aphasia, namely expressive (Broca) and receptive aphasia (Wernicke). These two regions of the brain (see Chapter I, Figure 1.1) are normally found only on the left side of the brain. The function of these two regions is therefore difficult to replace if damaged by strokes, tumors or trauma.

There are considerable individual variations in the anatomical locations of these areas. Surgeons who operate on the left side of the brain therefore want to avoid damaging speech regions by testing exactly where these critical regions are located before and during an operation [39]. This is often done during the operation, in which the patient is awake, by electrically stimulating different areas of the brain that are to be removed. If the electrical stimulation blocks the ability to speak or to understand speech it can be assumed that the area that is stimulated is involved in speech production and it should not be removed.

Some functions are normally done by both halves of the brain and loss of one side has little noticeable effect. One example is from hearing, where the part of the cerebral cortex that is first reached by signals from the ear (primary hearing cortex) can be damaged with very little effect on the person's ability to hear and understand normal speech. If the hearing cortex that is located deep in temporal lobe is damaged by strokes or tumors a person can understand normal speech perfectly well and have little other symptoms. Only when some of the redundancy of the speech signals has been removed does deficit become apparent [37].

Sensory pathways are generally crossed so that sensory signals from sense organs on one side of the body activate the cerebral cortices on the other side. But there are connections between the hearing pathways on the left and the right side of the brain (at the midbrain level). Sounds that reach the left ear can therefore activate cells in the cortex on both sides and sounds that reach the right ear not only reach the hearing cortex on the left side but also activate cells in the cortex on the right side (see Chapter I). The cortices on both sides therefore receive signals from both ears. This explains why injuries to the cortex on one side cause very few symptoms. In fact, it requires sophisticated tests to reveal that one side's hearing cortex does not function [37], which can occur as a result of a tumor or a stroke. Activation of neural plasticity is therefore not necessary for maintaining near normal hearing after injuries to the hearing cortex on one side. Injuries to hearing structures in the brainstem have different effects.

6.2. Systems that are Not Needed for (Nearly) Normal Function

There are systems that are not necessary for normal function of the body and that are special forms of redundancy. Systems in the brain, the function of which can be totally absent without any noticeable signs of deficits, are examples of such redundancy.

One such example is the balance (vestibular) system. As I mentioned earlier, the absence of the function of the balance system produces few signs and symptoms if the deficit occurs gradually and at young age. If it occurs rapidly it produces violent symptoms of vertigo and other forms of dizziness. These changes in function activate neural plasticity that gradually transfers the balance system's normal functions in maintaining posture, etc. to other systems. The balance system also controls the position of the eyes during head movements, which serve to keep an image steady on the retina when the head is turned. Information from the visual system can replace this function of the balance system. This means that the balance system is generally redundant and all its functions can be taken over by other systems in the brain.

Even absence of neural transmitters such as the family known as prostaglandins gives no noticeable symptoms. This is experienced whenever taking an aspirin because the ingredient in aspirin (and for that matter in may other generally available medications) is acetylsalicylate, which stops production of prostaglandins.

6.3. Reserves

The nervous system, as does other parts of the body, has reserves. This means that some parts of nerves, the brain, and the spinal cord can be lost without any symptoms, but when the reserves are used up symptoms will occur. Reserves are slowly used up during normal aging but disease processes can accelerate the decrease in reserves. Reserves are forms of redundancy. When plasticity is turned on it may use some of these reserves to shift functions from damaged nerve fibers or nerve cells in the brain.

Nerves, the spinal cord, and the brain in young individuals have many forms of reserves. This means there are more nerve fibers and more nerve cells than necessary for normal function and loss of a small fraction of nerve fibers or nerve cells does not give any symptoms or signs. Because peripheral nerves in young healthy individual have more fibers than necessary for performing normal functions it will not cause any signs or symptoms if some fibers are damaged or eliminated. With age the number of nerve fibers that can function decreases, and at a certain point signs of deficits begin to occur. Therefore, if a disease produces a slow and gradual destruction of nerve fibers, at first there are no symptoms because the reserves keep functions normal. Symptoms only start after that the reserves are used up which occurs when a certain number of nerve fibers have been damaged.

The time the reserves are used up may be incorrectly interpreted as the time the disease first starts. When a person appears at a physician's office with symptoms, the physician will always ask when the symptoms were first noticed. The purpose is to find events in the patient's life that occurred at the time the symptoms first occurred and which could be regarded as the cause of the disease. In case of peripheral nerve damage the symptoms (normally) do not occur until a long time after the process of damage to the nerve has begun, and information about when the symptoms were first noticed will therefore not tell when the disease began. Not recognizing the influence of reserves may therefore cause erroneous diagnoses.

The precise rate with which nerve fibers normally deteriorate and die is not known, because few studies have concentrated on the physiology of normal aging process, if there at all is such a thing as normal aging. It is likely that there are great individual variations in the "normal" loss of nerve fibers. Diseases of various kinds most often accompany aging, and these may affect the reduction of nerve fibers and nerve cells in the brain. In particular, diseases such as diabetes affect peripheral nerves and causes death of nerve fibers. Diseases such as poliomyelitis may have destructed a portion of nerve fibers. If only the reserves were destroyed, symptoms would not occur immediately after recovery from the disease. When normal aging reduces the number of nerve fibers the reserves may be used up and symptoms may become manifest. The occurrence of symptoms may erroneously be interpreted as the signs of the occurrence of a neurological disease. The amount of reserves that a person has affects treatments of various kinds (see Chapter V).

7. REFERENCES

[1]   Adkins-Muir DL, Jones TA. Cortical electrical stimulation combined with rehabilitative training: Enhanced functional recovery and dendritic plasticity following focal cortical ischemia in rats. *Neurol Res.* 2003;25:780-8.

[2]   Baloh RW, Honrubia V. *Clinical neurophysiology of the vestibular system.* Philadelphia: F.A.Davis Company; 1990.

[3]   Brach JS, Van Swearingen JM, Lenert J, Johnson PC. Facial Neuromuscular Retraining for Oral Synkinesis. *Plastic and Reconstructive Surgery.* 1997;99(7):1922-31.

[4]   Brown JA, Lutsep HL, Cramer SC, Weinand M. Motor cortex stimulation for enhancement of recovery after stroke: Case report. *Neurol Res.* 2003;25:815-8.

[5]   Colletti V. Auditory Outcomes in Tumor vs. Nontumor Patients Fitted with Auditory Brainstem Implants. In: Møller AR, editor. *Cochlear and Brainstem Implants.* Basel: Karger; Adv. Oto Rinol Laryngol 2006;64:167-85.

[6]   Colletti V, Carner M, Miorelli V, Guida M, Colletti L, Fiorino F. Auditory brainstem implant (ABI): new frontiers in adults and children. *Otolaryngol Head Neck Surg* 2005;133:126-38..

[7]   Colletti V, Shannon RV. Open set of speech perception with auditory brainstem implant? *Laryngoscope.* 2005;115:1974-8.

[8]   Dancause N. Vicarious function of remote cortex following stroke: recent evidence from human and animal studies. *Neuroscientist.* 2006;12:489-99.

[9]   Djourno A, Eyries C. Prothese auditive par excitatiob electrique a distance du nerf sensoriel a l'aide d'un bobinage inclus a demeure. *Presse Med.* 1957;35:1417.

[10] Dorman M, Loizou P, Rainey R. Speech intelligibility as a function of the number of channels of stimulation for signal processors using sine-wave and noise-band outputs. *J Acoust Soc Am.* 1997;102(4):2403-11.

[11] Dorman MF. Speech Perception by Adults. In: Walzman SB, Cohen NL, editors. *Cochlear Implants.* New York: Thieme; 2000.

[12] Elbert T, Pantev C, Wienbruch C, Rockstroh B, Taub E. Increased cortical representation of the fingers of the left hand in string players. *Science.* 1995;270(5234):305-7.

[13] Hall EJ, Flament D, Fraser C, Lemon R. Non-invasive brain stimulation reveals reorganized cortical outputs in amputees. *Neurosci Lett.* 1990;116:379-86.

[14] Hartmann R, Shepherd RK, Heid S, Klinke R. Response of the primary auditory cortex to electrical stimulation of the auditory nerve in the congenitally deaf white cat. *Hear Res.* 1997;112:115-33.

[15] Horng SH, Sur M. Visual activity and cortical rewiring: Activity-dependent plasticity of cortical networks. In: Møller AR, editor. *Reprogramming the brain.* Amsterdam: Elsevier; *Progress in Brain Research* 2006;157:3-11.

[16] House WH. Cochlear implants. *Ann Otol RhinolLaryngol.* 1976;85, (Suppl. 27):3-91.

[17] Hubel DH. *Eye, Brain, and Vision.* New York: Scientific American Library; 1988.

[18] Keller EL, Precht W. Adaptive modification of central vestibular neurons in response to visual stimulation through reversing prisms. *J Neurophys.* 1979;42(3):896-911.

[19] Kenet T, Froemke RC, Schreiner CE, Pessah IN, Merzenich MM. Perinatal exposure to a noncoplanar polychlorinated biphenyl alters tonotopy, receptive fields, and plasticity in rat primary auditory cortex. *Proc Natl Acad Sci U S A*. 2007;104(18):7646-51.

[20] Klinke R, Hartmann R, Heid S, Tillein J, Kral A. Plastic changes in the auditory cortex of congenitally deaf cats following cochlear implantation. *Audiol Neurootol*. 2001;6:203-6.

[21] Knudsen EI. Sensitive periods in the development of the brain and behavior. *J Cogn NeurosciJ Cogn Neurosci*. 2004;16(8):1412-25.

[22] Kral A, Eggermont JJ. What's to lose and what's to learn: Development under auditory deprivation, cochlear implants and limits of cortical plasticity. *Brain Res Rev*. 2007;56:259-69.

[23] Kral A, Hartmann R, Tillein J, Heid S, Klinke R. Delayed maturation and sensitive periods in the auditory cortex. *Audiol Neurootol*. 2001;6:346-62.

[24] Kral A, Hartmann R, Tillrin J, Heid S, Klinke R. Congenital auditory deprivation reduces synaptic activity within the auditory cortex in layer specific manner. *Cerebral Cortex*. 2000;10:714-26.

[25] Kral A, Tillein J. Brain plasticity under cochlear implant stimulation. In: Møller AR, editor. *Cochlear and Brainstem Implants*. Basel: Karger; Adv. Oto Rinol Laryngol 2006;64:89-108.

[26] Kral A, Tillein J, Heid S, Klinke R, Hartmann R. Cochlear implants: cortical plasticity in congenital deprivation. In: Møller AR, editor. *Reprogramming the brain*. Amsterdam: Elsevier; *Progress in Brain Research* 2006;157:283-313.

[27] Leake PA, Snyder RL, Rebscher SJ, Moore CM, Vollmer M. Plasticity in central representation in the inferior colliculus induced by chronic single- vs. two-channel electrical stimulation by cochlear implant after neonatal deafness. *Hear Res*. 2000;147:221-41.

[28] Loizou PC. Speech Processing in Vocoder-Centric Cochlear Implants. In: Møller AR, editor. *Cochlear and Brainstem Implants*. Basel: Karger; Adv. Oto Rinol Laryngol 2006;64:109-143

[29] Michelson RP. Stimulation of the human cochlea. *Arch Otolaryngol*. 1971;93:317-23.

[30] Miller JM, Watson CS, Covell WP. Deafening effects of noise on the cat. *Acta Oto Laryng Suppl 176*. 1963:1-91.

[31] Møller AR. Cranial nerve dysfunction syndromes: Pathophysiology of microvascular compression. In: Barrow DL, editor. *Neurosurgical Topics Book 13, Surgery of Cranial Nerves of the Posterior Fossa, Chapter 2*. Park Ridge. IL: American Association of Neurological Surgeons; 1993. p. 105-29.

[32] Møller AR, editor. *Cochlear and Brainstem Implants,* Basel: Karger; Adv. Oto Rinol Laryngol 2006;64:1-228

[33] Møller AR. *Hearing: Anatomy, Physiology, and Disorders of the Auditory System, 2nd Ed.* Amsterdam: Academic Press; 2006.

[34] Møller AR. History of Cochlear Implants and Auditory Brainstem Implants. In: Møller AR, editor. *Cochlear and Brainstem Implants*. In: Møller AR, editor. *Cochlear and Brainstem Implants*. Basel: Karger; Adv. Oto Rinol Laryngol 2006;64:1-10.

[35] Møller AR. *Neural plasticity and disorders of the nervous system.* Cambridge: Cambridge University Press 2006.

[36] Møller AR. Neurophysiologic abnormalities in autism. In: Mesmere BS, editor. *New Autism Research Developments.* New York: Nova Science Publishers; 2007.

[37] Møller MB. (Korsan-Bengtsen, M.). Distorted Speech Audiometry. *Acta Otolaryng (Stockholm).* 1973;Suppl. 310.

[38] Norena AJ, Eggermont JJ. Enriched acoustic environment after noise trauma reduces hearing loss and prevents cortical map reorganization. *J Neurosci* 2005;25(3):699-705.

[39] Ojemann G, Ojemann J, Lettich E, Berger M. Cortical language localization in left, dominant hemisphere. *J Neurosurg.* 2008;108(2):411-21.

[40] Porter R, Lemon R. *Cortical function and voluntary movement.* Oxford: Clarendon Press; 1993.

[41] Raucher FH, Robinson KD, Jens JJ. Improved maze learning through early music exposure in rate. *Neurol Res* 1998;20:427-32.

[42] Reale RA, Brugge JF, Chan JCK. Maps of auditory cortex in cats reared after unilateral cochlear ablation in the neonatal period. *Dev Brain Res.* 1987;34:281-90.

[43] Särkämö T, Tervaniemi M, Laitinen S, Forsblom A, Soinila S, Mikkonen M, et al. Music listening enhances cognitive recovery and mood after middle cerebral artery stroke. *Brain.* 2008;131:866-76.

[44] Schroeder M. Vocoders: Analysis and synthesis of speech. *Proc IEEE.* 1966;54:720-34.

[45] Shannon RV, Zeng F-G, Kamath V, Wygonski J, Ekelid M. Speech recognition with primarily temporal cues. *Science.* 1995;270:303-4.

[46] Sharma A, Dorman MF. Central Auditory Development in Children with Cochlear Implants: Clinical Implications. In: Møller AR, editor. *Cochlear and Brainstem Implants.* Basel: Karger; Adv. Oto Rinol Laryngol 2006;64:66-88.

[47] Sharma A, Dorman MF, Spahr AJ. A sensitive period for the development of the central auditory system in children with cochlear implants: implications for age of implantation. *Ear Hear.* 2002;23(6):532-9.

[48] Sharma A, Dorman MF, Spahr AJ. Rapid development of cortical auditory evoked potentials after early cochlear implantation. *Neuroreport.* 2002;13(10):1365-8.

[49] Simmons FB. Electrical stimulation of the auditory nerve in man. *Arch Otolaryngol.* 1966;84:22-76.

[50] Taub E, Uswatte G, Elbert T. New treatments in neurorehabilitation founded on basic research. *Nature Rev Neurosci.* 2002;3(3):228-36.

[51] Wiesel TN, Hubel DH. Effects of visual deprivation on morphology and physiology of cells in the cats lateral geniculate body. *J Neurophysiol.* 1963;26:973-93.

[52] Wiesel TN, Hubel DH. Effects of monocular deprivation in kittens. *Naunyn Schmiedebergs Arch Pharmacol.* 1964;248:492-7.

[53] Wiesel TN, Hubel DH. Extent of recovery from the effects of visual deprivation in kittens. *J Neurophysiol.* 1965;28:1060-72.

[54] Willott JF, Turner JG, Sundin VS. Effects of exposure to an augmented acoustic environment on auditory function in mice: roles of hearing loss and age during treatment. *Hear Res.* 2000;142:79–88.

[55] Yoshida N, Liberman MC. Sound conditioning reduces noise-induced permanent threshold shift in mice. *Hear Res.* 2000;148:213-9.

Chapter IV

PLASTICITY DISEASES

ABSTRACT

Activation of neural plasticity can cause symptoms and signs of disease; we call such disorders plasticity diseases. The most prominent examples are phantom limb syndrome, some forms of pain, and tinnitus. However, activation of neural plasticity causes or contributes to many other symptoms such as spasticity and synkinesis, but is also believed to be involved in disorders such as fibromyalgia, myofascial pain as well as some forms of balance disorders. There are indications that activation of neural plasticity also plays a role in creating the symptoms of disorders such as dementia and Alzheimer's disease. Developmental disorders caused by failure in the pruning and reorganization of the nervous system that occurs in early childhood may be regarded as a plasticity disorder.

Plasticity diseases can be caused by plasticity that is normally beneficial being turned on incorrectly. Examples are the body's attempts to compensate for hearing by increasing the excitability of nerve cells in the hearing nervous system. This may lead to tinnitus, a kind of self-oscillation because of to much amplification. Spasticity in spinal cord injuries may be regarded as an attempt to compensate for a lost ability to activate muscles by increasing the excitability in the neural circuits in the spinal cord and the brain. In a similar way, it is difficult to distinguish which symptoms of developmental diseases are caused by genetic factors and which are caused by activation of neural plasticity. It could also be possible there is an incorrect activation, or lack thereof, of neural plasticity such as the "midcourse correction". The course of these diseases is also affected by environmental factors, such as sensory stimulation, that also activate neural plasticity.

The fact that it is important to have precise names for diseases is essential for treatment as well as for research purposes. For plasticity diseases the anatomical location of the symptoms is different from location of the abnormality that gives the symptoms. Many systems of the brain and spinal cord consist of cascades of groups of nerve cells. Abnormalities in one group of nerve cells will cause the cells to send abnormal neural activity to other nerve cells that then act abnormally although there is nothing wrong with them. Directing treatment to such structures will not cure plasticity diseases.

Various forms of pain caused by activation of neural plasticity or where it p
role is described, followed by discussions of phantom limb sensations and tinnitu
Chapter also discusses how different individuals perceive symptoms such pa

tinnitus differently and how it inflicts in their daily life. The role of neural plasticity in movement disease and specific diseases such as hemifacial spasm is discussed.

A section of this Chapter discusses developmental disorders where it is believed the symptoms are caused by a malfunction in the normal development after birth, causing disorders such as autism. Autism spectrum disorders are discussed in more detail in Appendix C. The last section discusses the cause of plasticity disorders and how to diagnose the disorders of plasticity (discussed in more detain in Chapter V).

1. INTRODUCTION

We have in the previous Chapters discussed examples of activation of plasticity that have a beneficial effect to an individual. However, activation of plastic changes can also cause symptoms and signs of illness, such as some forms of pain and tinnitus, and this is the topic of this Chapter. We call these forms of plasticity "bad" or "harmful" plasticity and the diseases they cause we call *"plasticity diseases"*.

Activation of neural plasticity works together with other factors causing many more diseases than previously assumed. Many diseases that are regarded to have an unknown cause (or causes) may in fact be plasticity diseases. There are also diseases where the assumed cause is incorrect and some of such diseases may also be plasticity diseases.

Plasticity diseases are caused by incorrect activation of neural plasticity, lack of activation, or too much activation. The symptoms are the result of abnormal activity in the brain and/or spinal cord such as hyperactivity (increased neural firing), hyperexcitability (increased ability to respond to a stimulus) and redirection of information. These alterations can cause change in processing sensory information and abnormal control of muscle activity.

There are many reasons why plastic changes are often overlooked as a cause of diseases. People, including physicians, want to find a cause of a disease they can either detect by examining the patient or, even more common, a cause which gives signs in the form of abnormal imaging tests (such as MRIs) or chemical changes (blood tests). Many patients with plasticity diseases show no objective signs at all of disease. Cancers, virus or bacterial infections and traumatic injuries are regarded as "real" reasons for diseases. Many physicians do not regard a change in function of the nervous system that occurs through activation of neural plasticity as a "real" reason for a patient's symptoms or complaints. After all, it does not show up on MRIs or produce changes in blood tests that can be detected. These so-called objective signs take priority over what a patient describes. This is a great disadvantage in diagnosing plasticity diseases, as we will see later in this Chapter. Activation of neural plasticity is also involved in some diseases of muscle control such as spasm[19] and spasticity[20] and some balance disorders. These diseases have signs that can help in diagnosis although

---

[19] Spasm: *A sudden involuntary contraction of one or more muscles; includes cramps, and contractures.* (Stedman's Electronic Medical Dictionary, Version 7.0).

[20] Spasticity: *One type of increase in muscle tone at rest; characterized by increased resistance to passive stretch, velocity dependent and asymmetric about joints (i.e., greater in the flexor muscles at the elbow and the extensor muscles at the knee). Exaggerated deep tendon reflexes and clonus are additional manifestations* (Stedman's Electronic Medical Dictionary, Version 7.0).

they rarely points towards neural plasticity as the cause of the symptoms. To date, neural plasticity has mostly been neglected as a cause of disorders.

In this Chapter I will discuss the role of activation of neural plasticity in causing disorders such as central neuropathic pain[21], tinnitus[22] and the phantom limb[23] symptoms.

I will show evidence that neural plasticity not only plays an important role in diseases such as chronic pain and tinnitus but that it also plays an important role in many other diseases. Neural plasticity plays an important role in the normal childhood development of the nervous system as was discussed in Chapter III. If not carried out in the normal way, developmental diseases may result.

Last, I will speculate about other diseases where activation of neural plasticity may play a role.

2. WHAT ARE PLASTICITY DISEASES?

There are two main kinds of plasticity diseases: One where the cause is faulty expression of neural plasticity, and another kind is caused by lack of, or incorrect expression of neural plasticity. The first kind causes hyperactive diseases such as central neuropathic pain, tinnitus and hyperactive movement diseases (spasm and spasticity). The second kind is suspected to be involved in the cause of developmental diseases such as some forms of autism.

Plasticity diseases typically have many forms and many different degrees of severity. Plasticity diseases are not deadly but they can make life miserable and deemed not being worth living. Most plasticity diseases such as central neuropathic pain and some forms of tinnitus are related to perception. However, a few involve abnormal muscle activity such as spasm, spasticity and synkinesis. Only the person who has plasticity diseases that involve perception such as pain or tinnitus is aware of the disease; there are no signs that can be detected by someone else, and no clinical test can detect and evaluate the existence or the severity.

Central neuropathic pain and tinnitus have many forms and the severity varies widely. Both of these diseases are common although the exact prevalence[24] is not known because different investigators have used different definitions of severity. We will discuss pain and tinnitus in more detail below.

Plasticity diseases are caused by something going wrong at a different location (the spinal cord or the brain) than where the symptoms are felt. Symptoms such as tinnitus are not psychological but caused by disease related changes in the ear or parts of the nervous system. These changes may involve the connections between nerve cells (changes in synaptic efficacy) or changes in the function of individual nerve cells (change in excitability) through activation of neural plasticity. Such changes in functions may cause tinnitus (hearing sounds

---

[21] Central neuropathic pain: pain generated in the brain without signals from pain receptors.

[22] Tinnitus: ringing in the ears.

[23] Phantom limb: sensations such as pain and tingling that are felt as coming from an amputated limb.

[24] In epidemiology, prevalence of a disease means the total number of a disease that exists at a given time in a certain population. The Incidence is the number of new occurrences of the disease during a certain period (often one year).

 sounds reach the ear). Changes in other parts of the nervous system cause the pain (central neuropathic pain).

For many years, patients and physicians alike believed tinnitus was caused by something wrong in the ear. It was therefore a major step forward when it became evident that most forms of tinnitus are caused by abnormal neural activity in the brain. In a similar way, pain that is felt as it comes from a certain location on the body may be caused by abnormal neural activity in the spinal cord and the brain, and not caused by something being wrong at the place where it hurts. There are still much misconception regarding the cause of such common forms of plasticity disorders as lower back pain and pain from spinal stenosis.

That the symptoms are not referred to the location where the fault is may result in incorrect diagnosis and treatment directed at the incorrect body part making the treatment ineffective. When a patient consults a physician about pain the first thing the physician asks is: where does it hurt? Now we understand that the answer to this question may lead the physician to make a wrong diagnosis and direct treatment to the wrong part of the body. This is also the reason why it is often not possible to find the cause of plasticity diseases. This is discussed in more detail in Chapter V.

The clearest demonstration of the role of neural plasticity in creating symptoms and signs is *phantom sensations* such as phantom pain. The term "phantom sensations" has been used most often to explain the odd feeling many individuals have after amputation of a leg or an arm [86] (see page 99). However, it is also a valid term for many forms of plasticity diseases such as pain and tinnitus. In phantom sensations, abnormal neural activity in the spinal cord and brain causes sensations that are similar to those caused by natural activation of receptors in the sense organs or in the body (skin, joints, tendons, muscles and internal organs).

A person with an amputated limb often can feel tingling or pain that is referred to the amputated limb. The fact that phantom sensations such as the pain and tingling are felt as if they were coming from the amputated limb is strong evidence that sensations are not necessarily generated in the structure where it is felt. The symptoms that are felt in an amputated leg cannot possible be generated in the leg but must generated somewhere else, and that is the spinal cord or the brain [86].

As we shall see later in this Chapter it is difficult to convince patients, physicians and surgeons alike that the problem is not always where the symptoms are felt [96]. Tinnitus definitely seems to come from the ear but the fault is often in the brain where some abnormal functions cause the sensation of sounds despite no sounds are reaching the ear. Tinnitus that is felt as coming from an ear after the hearing nerve has been severed is an equally strong sign that a sensation that is referred to a location on the body may be generated in the central nervous system and not in the ear [64,93,95,97], thus a phantom sensation.

Many forms of pain are plasticity diseases caused by changes in the function and reorganization of neural circuits. However, the pain seems to come from distinct parts of the body such as the leg or back. Lower back pain is an example of a disease where treatment often has been directed to the wrong structures. In this group of diseases it has in most cases been impossible to find any anatomical abnormality that could explain the pain [80]. Some claim the cause is compression of nerve roots that enter the spinal cord possibly caused by ruptured spinal disks. Such claims have been difficult to prove [79,80]. Studies have shown that many people with no symptoms of back pain have similar abnormal discs and nerve root compressions [11] (discussed in more detail later, page 120).

It seems likely that in most cases lower back pain is caused by activation of neural plasticity, and we may therefore regard most forms of lower back pain to be plasticity diseases. The abnormal vertebral discs and compression of nerve roots evident from MRIs may only be the cause of the pain in a few individuals and it occurs coincidentally in most other individuals who do not have lower back pain.

It is less well known that disorders that involve control of muscles (movement diseases) may also be caused by activation of neural plasticity causing different forms of spasm and spasticity. These diseases do indeed have visible signs but the faults consist of plastic changes in the function of the spinal cord or the brain and that is difficult to study. Hyperactive diseases of muscle control such as spasticity, tremor, synkinesis and ataxia may be caused by activation of neural plasticity. Spasmodic dysphonia is not a disease of the vocal cords although the symptoms are related to the vocal cords [96]. It is instead a disease of the brain. Hemifacial spasm [39] is not a disease of facial muscles or a fault in the facial nerve as was previously believed but a disease of the facial motonucleus[25] [91]. The involvement of neural plasticity in diseases of the spinal cord or the brain causing spasm or spasticity is not obvious from the symptoms or from results of tests. Neural plasticity has rarely been considered when the cause of such diseases has been sought and usually other causes are suggested for such diseases.

Activation of neural plasticity is also involved in synkinesis[26] that occurs after peripheral nerve injuries.

Damage to peripheral nerves can cause hyperactivity of the respective motonucleus [71]. It is perhaps surprising that severing a motor nerve can influence the function of its motonucleus [144].

Damage to the spinal cord and brain causes activation of neural plasticity. In most situations, such activation of neural plasticity has beneficial effects as we discussed in Chapter III, but activation of neural plasticity can go awry and cause symptoms and signs of disease [25].

As we discussed in Chapter II, plasticity diseases can be caused by abnormal neural activity in different regions of the spinal cord and brain. Plasticity diseases are also likely to cause more than one region of the brain or spinal cord to behave abnormally. The abnormal brain activity can have two causes, one being that there are faults in the neural circuits in a certain region of the spinal cord or the brain. Another reason for abnormal neural activity is that nerve cells in parts of the spinal cord and the brain may receive abnormal signals from a faulty region and therefore act abnormally although there is nothing wrong with the part of the nervous system in question; it just received bad signals and therefore its activity became abnormal.

Neural plasticity is also suspected to be involved in other disorders such as fibromyalgia but direct proof that may be the case is so far lacking. Fibromyalgia presents muscle pain but

---

[25] Motonucleus: Cluster of nerve cells the nerve fibers (axons) of which innervate muscles.

[26] Synkinesis: *Involuntary movement accompanying a voluntary one, as the movement of a closed eye following that of the uncovered one, or the movement occurring in a paralyzed muscle accompanying motion in another part.* (Stedman's Electronic Medical Dictionary, Version 7.0).

nothing is wrong with the muscles. It is an enigmatic disorder that has earlier been classified as a rheumatic disease. It is now assumed that the symptoms are in fact caused by faults in processing of sensory signals in some parts of the spinal cord and the brain [126], which also points towards central mechanisms such as plastic changes.

This means that fibromyalgia would best be classified as a plasticity disease and treated accordingly. This is supported by the fact that the symptoms respond poorly to traditional pain relievers but can be reversed by medications used to treat epileptic seizures (see Chapter V) such as gabapentin and pregabalin (Lyrica) [3] and old tricyclic antidepressants such as nortriptyline. These medications affect the nervous system (see Chapter V). The only medication that is approved by the FDA (Food and Drug Administration) for treating fibromyalgia is pregabalin (Lyrica).

The fact that these medications have beneficial effect on fibromyalgia [28] supports the suggestion that fibromyalgia is a plasticity disease. We will discuss these diseases later (page 124).

Neural plasticity may also be involved in myofascial pain syndrome. Both of these diseases present muscle pain without any abnormalities in the muscles to be found [96].

There are other diseases where activation of neural plasticity plays a role in creating symptoms and signs. One is related to the balance system. Many forms of balance diseases are caused by changes in the function of the brain and not caused by diseases of the balance organ in the inner ear.

Turning the head activates the sensors in the balance organ causing the eyes to move in the opposite direction to maintain a steady image on the retina. This normally is done without conscious awareness. Under certain circumstances turning the head is felt, and sometimes gives an unpleasant feeling (dizziness) and even vomiting. This is an example of induced neural plasticity that redirects the information from the balance organ to parts of the brain that gives the feeling of movement of the head.

The fact that at least some forms of Ménière's disease[27] [82] can be treated successfully by applying pulses of air pressure to the inner ear and thereby activating the balance system [32] is a sign that plastic changes are involved in the cause of the disease. This means some forms of balance disorders are plasticity diseases.

The role of neural plasticity in creating symptoms and signs is perhaps best illustrated in the phantom limb syndrome. Phantom sensations such as pain and tingling that are felt from amputated limbs are forms of pain that are caused by abnormal function of the nervous system, therefore plasticity diseases. However, neural plasticity is also involved in other pain conditions in ways that are often poorly understood. The most studied plasticity disease is central neuropathic pain[28].

Some forms of tinnitus (hearing buzzing or other meaningless sounds without any sound reaching the ear) are also plasticity diseases. Some individuals experience sounds that are meaningful such as voices and music. This is normally known as hallucinations.

---

[27] Ménière's disease is defined as there symptoms: Fluctuating hearing loss, tinnitus and vertigo ("the world is spinning").

[28] Central neuropathic pain is pain caused by abnormal neural activity in the brain without any signals from pain receptors have reached the brain.

Hallucinations occur together with psychiatric diseases such as schizophrenia [94,97] but it may also occur in rare occurrences of temporal lobe disorders.

Disorders such as those affecting memory may also be regarded as plasticity diseases. This is because memory is based on long-term potentiation (LTP), which is a change of synaptic efficacy, therefore, similar to the changes that occur when neural plasticity is turned on. The symptoms of Alzheimer's disease and other forms of dementias improve by treatments similar to those effective for treating plasticity diseases such as physical exercise and an active intellectual and social life (see Chapter V).

This suggests that neural plasticity is also involved in causing the symptoms of Alzheimer's disease and some forms of dementia. Physical exercise is also effective for treatment of some forms of depression, a disorder in which there is a failure in normal sensory processing. This means that it may be valuable to view disorders such as dementia, Alzheimer's disease and depression as plasticity diseases.

Activation of neural plasticity is probably also involved in causing the symptoms and signs of other diseases which so far are not known to be plasticity diseases. It is possible that neural plasticity plays a role in diseases such as schizophrenia and addiction.

It was mentioned earlier in this book that neural plasticity is normally turned on immediately after birth causing re-arranging of the neural circuitry in the brain and the spinal cord, including elimination of synapses and nerve fibers and even entire nerve cells (Chapter III). This "pruning" that normally occurs during the first years of life is absolutely necessary. Failure in activating this kind of neural plasticity (or activating it incorrectly) is involved in the cause of developmental diseases of various kinds, including autism [99]. This means some developmental disorders are plasticity diseases.

We are just beginning to understand some of the aspects of plasticity diseases and it will take some time before the concepts win recognition by researchers and those who treat patients with such diseases. It requires accepting that some patients have no visible signs from physical examinations, or signs that can be detected using current imaging techniques or other clinical tests. We may need to develop new methods for studying diseases in order to be able to diagnose plasticity disorders properly. Diagnosis of plasticity diseases will be discussed in Chapter V that concerns treatment of these disorders.

2.1. How do We Usually Study Diseases?

In diagnosis and scientific studies of diseases we often focus on what we can see. Diagnosis is often based on imaging studies (such as MRIs), but it is often ignored that such tests can only detect abnormalities in structure. Activation of neural plasticity mainly causes changes in function of synapses, which cannot be seen in the imaging methods that are available now. Some forms of neural plasticity include change in structure such as formation of nerve fibers and elimination of cells (see Chapter II), but such changes do not show up in imaging studies either.

MRIs are given more value than they deserve. To some extent it is because MRIs produce pretty pictures and because it seems as everybody can interpret and understand MRIs because of their resemblance with the anatomy of the brain. That the changes caused by expression of neural plasticity do not show up on MRIs does not make the symptoms less real.

There are also really no blood tests that can diagnose plasticity diseases. In addition to that, these shortcomings, of our investigative tools, we tend only to see what we are looking for.

There are many examples where obvious irregularities in MRIs were missed because the radiologists simply did not look for such abnormalities.

Plasticity diseases are complex and have different forms. Common for all plasticity diseases is that they occur with great variation in their symptoms and the different components of the symptoms vary from one individual to another. Different examiners of patients with such symptoms often come to different diagnoses. Research in these diseases is hampered by the ambiguity to distinguish between the different diseases and their different forms.

2.2. How do Patients and their Physicians Perceive Symptoms of Plasticity Disease?

Each individual has the potential to perceive symptoms of plasticity diseases very differently. Some individuals with central pain or tinnitus, for example, find their symptoms controlling their entire daily lives; while others will say "I have pain (or tinnitus) but pain (or tinnitus) does not have me".

Different health care professionals and scientists view plasticity diseases (as well as many other diseases) in different ways. The physician may view plasticity diseases as a medical problem that requires a diagnosis and a treatment. Some aim at possibly curing the disease a patient has. Others aim at an often more realistic goal of managing the disease in a way that makes it possible for the patient to live a life that is as close to normal as possible. Some health care specialists may see these diseases as a psychological problem and try to educate the patient in how to live with their symptoms. Yet another will come to the conclusion that the disease is caused by the patient's lifestyle and recommend a change (exercising, eating well but not too much, lose weight if overweight, etc).

A patient's expectations are important for successful management of a disease. If a patient expects to be cured, he/she may be unhappy with any treatment that does not cure the disease-- even if the treatment has reduced the symptoms and signs to a level where the patient will have a decent life. Side effects of treatments are very important to consider. Often a treatment turns out to be worse than the disease. We will discuss these matters in more detail in Chapter V.

The scientist will look for abnormalities in the way the nervous system functions and ask questions such as are there structural abnormalities or only functional ones? Which parts of the brain is involved? In which way is the current function different from normal function?

Plasticity diseases are neurological diseases. The ways many neurological diseases are approached are similar to the story about the six blind men and an elephant by John Godfrey Saxe (1816-87) based on a fable told in India:

2.2.1. The Blind Men and an Elephant

Once upon a time, there lived six blind men in a village. One day the villagers told them, "Hey, there is an elephant in the village today."

They had no idea what an elephant is. They decided, "Even though we would not be able to see it, let us go and feel it anyway." All of them went where the elephant was. Everyone of them touched the elephant.

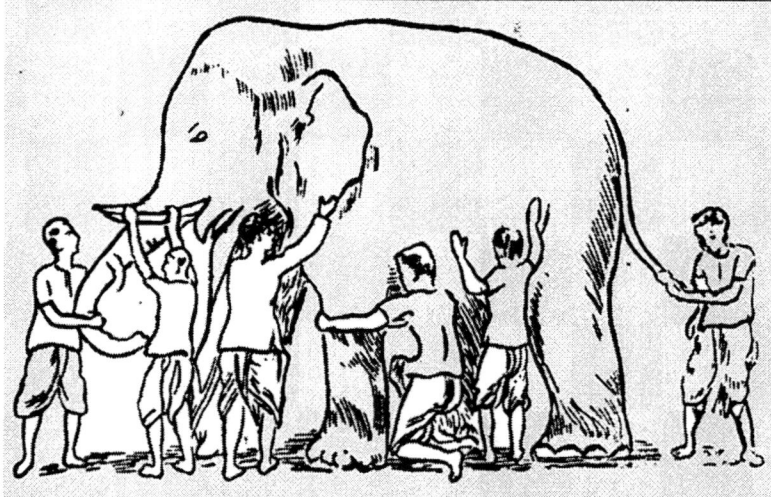

"Hey, the elephant is a pillar," said the first man who touched his leg.

"Oh, no! it is like a rope," said the second man who touched the tail.

"Oh, no! it is like a thick branch of a tree," said the third man who touched the trunk of the elephant.

"It is like a big hand fan" said the fourth man who touched the ear of the elephant.

"It is like a huge wall," said the fifth man who touched the belly of the elephant.

"It is like a solid pipe," Said the sixth man who touched the tusk of the elephant.

They began to argue about the elephant and everyone of them insisted that he was right. It looked like they were getting agitated. A wise man was passing by and he saw this. He stopped and asked them, "What is the matter?" They said, "We cannot agree to what the elephant is like." Each one of them told what he thought the elephant was like. The wise man calmly explained to them, "All of you are right. The reason every one of you is telling it differently because each one of you touched the different part of the elephant. So, actually the elephant has all those features what you all said."

"Oh!" everyone said. There was no more fight. They felt happy that they were all right.

The moral of the story is that there may be some truth to what someone says. Sometimes we see that truth, sometimes not because they may have different perspective which we may not agree too. So, rather than arguing like the blind men, we should say, "Maybe you have your reasons." This way we don't get in arguments. In Jainism, it is explained that truth can be stated in seven different ways. You can see how broad our religion is. It teaches us to be tolerant towards others for their viewpoints. This allows us to live in harmony with people of different thinking. This is known as the Syadvada, Anekantvad, the theory of Manifold Predictions.

Source: Jainism Global Resource Center http://www.jainworld.com/

2.3. Names of Diseases are Important

It is important that the names we use for diseases are related to the disease uniqueness. Some of the common plasticity diseases have many different forms, and in fact may be regarded as different diseases. This is especially the case for central pain and for tinnitus. The symptoms of plasticity diseases such as pain and tinnitus vary from mild annoyances to severe sufferings destroying the life of the person in question and may lead to suicide. The different forms of tinnitus are simply called 'tinnitus' and the different forms of pain always are referred to as 'pain'.

Such broad use of a single term makes it unclear what it specifically means. When an individual says he or she has pain it can represent very different things. It is not meaningful to use the same name for pain that is a minor nuisance and for pain that is unbearable. It does not seem meaningful to use the name for tinnitus that consists of occasional weak sounds to having a roaring sound 24 hours a day, 7 days a week.

We cannot think about matters that do not have names. Using the same names for fundamentally different forms of a disease is a disadvantage both in studying and treating such diseases as pain and tinnitus. Pain that lasts a short time (acute pain) is different from chronic pain, which goes on and on. Somatic (body) and visceral pain (from inner organs), caused by activation of nociceptors[29], and which ceases when the activation ceases is fundamentally different from central neuropathic pain, which is chronic pain caused by plastic changes in the spinal cord or brain. Central neuropathic pain is not caused by stimulation of pain receptors and it does not cease by itself and available treatments may be insufficient to cause relief.

Using the same name for different diseases can be directly misleading. For example, calling Asperger's disease autism is misleading. The symptoms that Asperger's disease have in common with other forms of autism is mainly impairment of social skills (see Appendix C). Other forms of autism involve serious deficits and signs of abnormalities that prevent a normal life. In fact, some cannot even take care of themselves in daily routines. Individuals with Asperger's disease are often very intelligent and many achieve great intellectual accomplishments. It has, in fact, been said that Albert Einstein had signs of Asperger's disease.

It is also common that a disease does not become studied to any great extent before it gets its own name. This underlines the importance of getting precise and well defined names for the different forms of neural plasticity that the professional community can agree upon.

Not having precise and unmistakable names for different diseases can have bad consequences, for example, those that may occur when treatments are tested. For instance if a new treatment for tinnitus is tested by the standard double blind technique[30] on a group of people with several different kinds of tinnitus, the treatment may only be beneficial to individuals with one of these several kinds.

Double blind tests have several problems, some of which are constantly overlooked. The test presumes that patients in whom a medication is tested have the same disease. However,

---

[29] Nociceptors: A receptor that mediates pain.

[30] Double blind tests consist of comparing the effect of a medication with an inactive substance in treatment of a certain well defined disease.

this is not always the case, especially when plasticity diseases are concerned. Let us say that a third of the individuals who are participating in a test of new medication for tinnitus have one kind of tinnitus and another third have a different form and the last third have yet another form of tinnitus. If the treatment is 100% effective for treating only one of these three kinds of tinnitus but ineffective for the other two thirds of the study group, then the results will be that the treatment is only effective in one third of individuals with tinnitus. Such treatment will often be regarded to be useless although it was very effective in treating one form of tinnitus.

In double blind testing, the participants do not know if they are given the medication that is assumed to be active or an inactive tablet. If people are treated with a medication they believe will help them many will experience an improvement. This is what is known as the placebo[31] effect. For diseases such as tinnitus and chronic pain, the placebo effect is large. The reason is that the person with such a disease feels they are being taken care of and that has a beneficial effect on how they perceive his/her disease. If a medication has the same effect as an inactive tablet it is regarded useless, which may be a mistake because the placebo effect is a short timed effect. We will discuss the effect of the placebo later in this Chapter (page 197).

2.4. What Causes the Symptoms and Signs of Plasticity Diseases?

The symptoms and signs of plasticity diseases are caused by abnormal neural activity in the parts of the brain that cause conscious awareness. This has traditionally been assumed to be certain regions of the cerebral cortex but there are indications that it may also be other structures such as certain parts of the limbic system (the amygdala, cingulate gyrus etc.).

2.4.1. Two Causes of Abnormal Neural Activity

The abnormal neural activity that causes symptoms of plasticity diseases may be caused by something being wrong with the nerve cells that generate this abnormal activity. However, nerve cells can also have abnormal activity without anything being wrong with them; the abnormal activity can be caused because the nerve cells receive abnormal activity from other nerve cells. For example, pain is often caused by plastic changes in the function of nerve cells in certain parts of the spinal cord, and these nerve cells send abnormal neural activity to other nerve cells such as those of the next stations of the ascending pain pathways. The nerve cells of the dorsal and medial nuclei of the thalamus and other regions of the brain may thereby have abnormal neural activity although there is nothing wrong with these nerve cells (see Figure 4.1) and they are functioning normally; the reason for their abnormal activity is they receive abnormal signals.

The nerve cells in the faulty nucleus send abnormal neural activity to the next nucleus. This nucleus may function normally but when receiving abnormal signals it will also deliver abnormal signals to the next nucleus giving the impression that something is wrong with the nucleus.

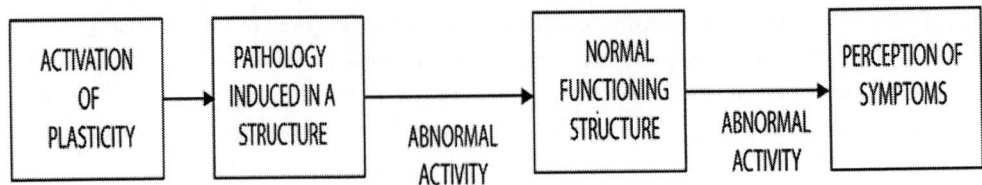

Figure 4.1. Hypothetical flowchart that shows how the neural activity in several nuclei can be affected when neural plasticity is turned on changing the function of one nucleus in a chain of nuclei.

If the chain of nuclei in this hypothetical example was the ascending pathway of the hearing nervous system it may be assumed that tinnitus could be caused by malfunction of a group of nerve cells that send information to many other groups of nerve cells that have no faults but their neural activity will be abnormal only because of the corrupted activity these nerve cells receive and that may be what give the sensation of sound (tinnitus).

The fact that nerve cells in normal regions of the brain can have abnormal activity can cause confusion about where the faulty structure is located. If treatment is directed to parts of the brain that behave abnormally only because the nerve cells receive faulty information the treatment will not be successful. Symptoms may therefore be referred to other parts of the body than those that are changed by the sickness. For successful treatment it is therefore important to identify the region of the brain that is faulty and to direct the treatment to this region of the brain or spinal cord in order to cure plasticity diseases. We will discuss that in more detail in Chapter V and compare it with situations in a common disease, diabetes type 2.

The word "cause" can mean what starts a disease, or it can mean from where in the body the symptoms originate. Plasticity diseases can have many causes. Reorganization of different parts of the nervous system causes the symptoms of many diseases. What starts such diseases is more difficult to determine and hampered by the fact that the sickness may begin before the symptoms starts to be noticeable.

2.4.2. Plasticity Turned on Incorrectly

Some plasticity diseases are caused by neural plasticity that has been turned on incorrectly (or when it should not have been activated) in response to internal or environmental (sensory) signals. Examples are some forms of tinnitus that can be caused by attempts to compensate for hearing loss by increasing the gain somewhere in the nervous system. Spasticity may be regarded as a response to a decrease in motor function such as that which occurs after spinal cord injuries. Spasticity may be regarded as an overdone attempt to compensate for lost or reduced control of muscles. The plastic changes that cause some forms of chronic pain (central neuropathic pain) may be started by inflammation or injuries to peripheral nerves, but the symptoms (pain) are caused by abnormal activity in the nervous system brought about by plastic changes. It is often difficult to untangle what has caused certain symptoms; was it reorganization of neural circuits that caused the symptoms or was it the diseases that caused the reorganization?

---

[31] In testing medications placebo is defined as an innocuous or inert substance having no pharmacological effect, given as a control in tests of the effect of a new medication. The word actually means "I will please".

Damage to the brain, such as occurs in strokes and from accidents, causes symptoms directly because of the damage. It is often difficult to distinguish these symptoms from those caused by activation of neural plasticity that is done by the damage.

2.4.3. Developmental Diseases: Fault in Midcourse Correction

It is usually assumed that neural plasticity is induced by some abnormal event such as lack of sensory signals, but neural plasticity can also be programmed genetically and turned on as a part of normal childhood development. During childhood, plastic changes normally proceed according to a pattern characterized by programmed reorganization of the brain, including elimination of contacts (synapses) between nerve fibers and nerve cells and their dendrites and creation of new contacts as well as programmed cell death (PCD).

It is believed that some developmental diseases are caused by failure in this "midcourse correction" (see Chapter I) that normally takes place during the first years of life. Autism is an example of a developmental disease where the symptoms may be caused by incorrect execution of plastic changes in early childhood (see page 246).

2.5. Many Structures are Involved in Plasticity Diseases

It is not only in plasticity diseases that abnormalities occur in a cascade of structures causing many regions of the body to behave abnormally. An example of a common disease, which involves a cascade of events in several different structures, is diabetes type 2 (see Chapter V). Only one of the structures that behaves abnormally may be faulty and all other structures behave in a faulty way because they receive signals from faulty structures.

2.5.1. Similarities between Plasticity Diseases and Epilepsy

Plasticity diseases such as tinnitus, pain and muscle spasm may have similarities with epileptic seizures. "Run away" neural activity that occurs in epileptic seizures can explain many of the symptoms of plasticity diseases. Some medications that are used to treat epilepsy are beneficial in treatment of pain and to some degree tinnitus. Pregabalin (Lyrica), is approved for diabetes neuropathy and is also beneficial for other forms of central pain. Local anesthetics such as Lidocain are effective in treatment of tinnitus. Lidocain is also effective against some forms of pain. The problem with Lidocain is the difficulty in administrating the medication; it has to be given intravenously, although there are now skin patches available where the medication slowly passes through the skin into the blood stream. Lidocain was used for many years to break epileptic seizures [10]. Now, benzodiazepines and other medications are used instead. Benzodiazepines such as Valium (diazepam) and Xanex (alprasolam) can also reduce tinnitus in some individuals.

3. PAIN

Pain is common; it is the most common reason a person seeks medical help. Some forms of pain have been reported to occur in 86% of individuals above the age of 65 (Iowa study

1994), severe pain has been reported to occur in 33% of people at the age of 77 years [15]. Different studies show different results, mainly because different investigators have used different definitions of pain.

Pain can be caused by injury, inflammation (viral, bacterial or body reactions), and pressure on nerves, muscles or bones. Often no known cause can be found such as in most forms of headache.

This book is about neural plasticity which plays an important role in many forms of pain, but there are also many forms of pain that are caused by stimulation of pain receptors. This book takes a broad approach to pain. Pain that is a plasticity disease will be discussed in this section; pain caused by stimulation of pain receptors is discussed in Appendix A, which reviews the anatomy and physiology of acute pain. This is important to know to understand the forms of pain that are plasticity diseases (central neuropathic pain).

3.1. Cause of Pain

The word "cause" can have two meanings with regard to pain: It can mean what has started the pain, which can be injuries of various kinds such as accidents, ischemia (lack of oxygen), inflammation of nerves, osteoarthritis, cancer, etc. "Cause" can also mean the biochemical aspects of pain, how stimulation of pain receptors occurs, etc., or it can mean how abnormal neural activity in certain parts of the brain can cause sensation of pain.

Clinically, for treatment of pain it is most important to know how and what has started the neural activity that gives the perception of pain. While it is obvious pain can be caused by injuries to the body from accidents there are many kinds of pain that have no obvious cause. This must mean that we just do not know what the cause is. Physicians call such pain idiopathic[32] pain. Often no clear signs of the causes of the abnormal neural activity that causes the sensation of pain can be found. Neural plasticity in the spinal cord and brain are often contributing to the generation of abnormal neural activity that causes sensation of pain in diseases where there is no known cause (idiopathic pain). There are also diseases where we believe we know the cause but what we believe is the cause, is actually not.

A typical example of a common pain condition often incorrectly diagnosed and, as a result, treated in ways that are not beneficial to the patient is lower back pain. Lower back pain is often believed to be caused by abnormalities that can be seen on MRI (nerve compression etc.), but as we have discussed above often is misunderstood by believing it is the cause of the pain. Instead, pain in many instances is caused by plastic changes in the spinal cord or the brain. The fact that structural changes seen on MRIs are often not the cause of the pain is supported by poor outcome of surgical operations that correct these structural changes [79]. Despite this is well documented in many studies many people are still having surgical operations that do them no good and in fact may make things worse [98]. There may be two reasons for that: 1) our strong belief in what we see (on the MRI) ("I could see it with my own eyes"); 2) surgeons who make their income on such operations will often persuade

---

[32] Idiopathic means that the cause of the disease is not known or that the physician is unable to determine the cause of the disease. Actually, the word idiopathic means something like "a disease of its own kind", but the word is used in medicine to describe diseases with unknown cause.

the patients to have operations [98]. Another reason that surgical treatment is chosen for treatment of lower back pain is that it makes sense to correct what seem to be clear abnormalities. Changes in the function of the nervous system are much more difficult to understand as a cause of pain and the abnormalities that cause the pain cannot be seen on imaging tests.

We can therefore distinguish between two main kinds of pain: One that is caused by stimulation of pain receptors and one that is caused by change in the function of the nervous system through activation of neural plasticity.

Understanding the anatomy and physiology of acute pain is important for understanding other forms of pain including pain where neural plasticity plays an important role. Appendix A provides a brief description of the anatomy and physiology of acute pain.

Central neuropathic pain is caused by activation of neural plasticity. Neural plasticity is involved in other pain conditions without being the sole cause of the symptoms.

3.1.1. Pain is Poorly Understood

Pain is not regarded to be a sense such as hearing, vision and taste, but there is no doubt that pain reaches awareness in similar ways as our senses but also in many different ways. Because it is not recognized as a sense, education about pain is sporadic, especially in medical schools where is should really be required (about half of the number of people who seek help in emergency rooms does it for pain).

What causes pain, its impact on a person and its treatment are topics that are taught sparsely in medical schools. Basic science textbooks used in medical schools do not cover pain to any great extent and books on clinical topics do not include much about pain either. There is only limited coverage in clinical textbooks on neurology and pain takes up only a few pages. A major textbook, the well known "Wall and Melzack Textbook of Pain", with about 1200 pages is devoted to pain alone [84]. This book is scientifically oriented but with some clinical relevance. Weiner's "Pain Management" a big book with 1648 pages [13] and is much more clinically oriented than the Melzack and Wall book, providing practical information about how to treat different forms of pain.

The lack of suitable textbooks in the clinical field may be one of the reasons physicians often ignore pain. Another reason that the medical profession pays scant attention to patients who have pain may be that pain has no objective signs and there is no known diagnostic test such as imaging (MRI, X-ray), chemical (blood tests) or electrophysiological tests that can diagnose pain. Only the person who has the pain can assess nature and severity. That pain in itself is not regarded to be life threatening may be another reason the medical profession neglects pain. Only when pain is a sign of a life threatening disease does it get attention and then the attention is directed to what disease the pain signals. Pain no doubt reduces the quality of life and that can, in fact, be life threatening in itself because it can lead to suicide (studies have shown that suicide is at least twice as frequent in individuals with chronic pain compared with individual who do not have pain [142]).

Lack of objective signs also causes people to pay less attention to pain conditions of their relatives. A person with chronic pain does not get much sympathy from family members and friends. The old saying that "the only tolerable pain is someone else's pain" (René Leriche, French surgeon, 1879–1955), is still valid.

3.1.2. Pain is Subjective

Pain can be a nuisance, it can be troublesome and it can be disabling. It can last a short time (being acute) or it can be lasting a long time (being chronic).

Pain is always subjective and it is not exactly related to the amount of stimulation of pain receptors or to the amount of damage to parts of the body. The perception of pain depends on many psychological factors, and the tolerance level for pain has large individual variations and it depends on even more different factors such as cultural background. Attention to the pain, time of the day and other circumstances can affect (modulate) the way pain is perceived. The threshold of experimentally induced pain is rather stable but the perceived intensity of the pain and, in particular, the tolerance of pain depends on such factors. Even ineffective treatment ("sugar pills") can affect (decrease) pain to a great extent (placebo effect, see Chapter V page 197) because the patients believe they are receiving an effective treatment.

A committee of the International Association for the Study of Pain, chaired by the psychiatrist Harold Mersky, provided the following definition of pain: "Pain is an unpleasant sensory and emotional experience associated with actual or potential tissue damage or described in terms of such damage". They added: "Pain is always subjective".

The sensation of pain is often accompanied by emotional components and pain can cause affective signs such as anxiety, depression, and general changes in mood. Pain can also make it difficult to sleep and can cause several bodily reactions such as change in muscle reflexes, increased heart rate, raised blood pressure and it can even cause sweating – all signs of activation of the sympathetic nervous system (a part of the autonomic nervous system). Pain can cause increased muscle tonus (continuous, passive contraction of muscle), even spasm.

Pain is almost always regarded as unpleasant although a few people feel pleasure from pain. Some individuals with autism feel pleasure from self inflicted pain. A few individuals may inflict pain on themselves (masochism), a psychiatric condition where people get a gratification from self-inflicted pain. Pain in connection with sport activities may give pleasure ("no pain no gain").

Pain can occur at certain times such as menstrual pain; some have headaches that come regularly. Pain can be self-inflicted such as headache from excessive indulgence of alcohol. It can be a used as a punishment, it can be used for enjoyment (masochistic), it can enhance sexual enjoyment, and it can be used to obtain control over a person (torture).

Pain is not an isolated phenomenon, but a group of symptoms and signs may include increased muscle tension and prevention or disturbance of sleep. It may interfere with or prevent intellectual work. Severe pain may cause affective (emotional) symptoms such as depression and it may lead to suicide.

There is no pure pain. Pain is always part of a complete package that can cause fear and suffering, and which cannot be separated from other feelings such as that of fear or misery. The sensation of the pain is not always related to the severity of the injury that caused the pain. Some people report that they have excruciating pain from the same injury other people would report giving much less pain.

Pain is not a disease in itself but it is a symptom that can be a sign of something being wrong such as a disease or some form of bodily injury. Chronic pain often occurs without any known cause (idiopathic pain) or the symptoms (or signs) may be misleading regarding the location of the fault that causes the pain.

3.2. There are Many Kinds of Pain

Pain can be divided into two large groups: one kind is caused by signals from various kinds of pain receptors in the body (somatic pain) and the other kind is caused by signals from receptors in internal organs (visceral pain) (Figure 4.2). Pain that is not caused by activation of pain receptors is central neuropathic pain and that will be discussed later in this Chapter.

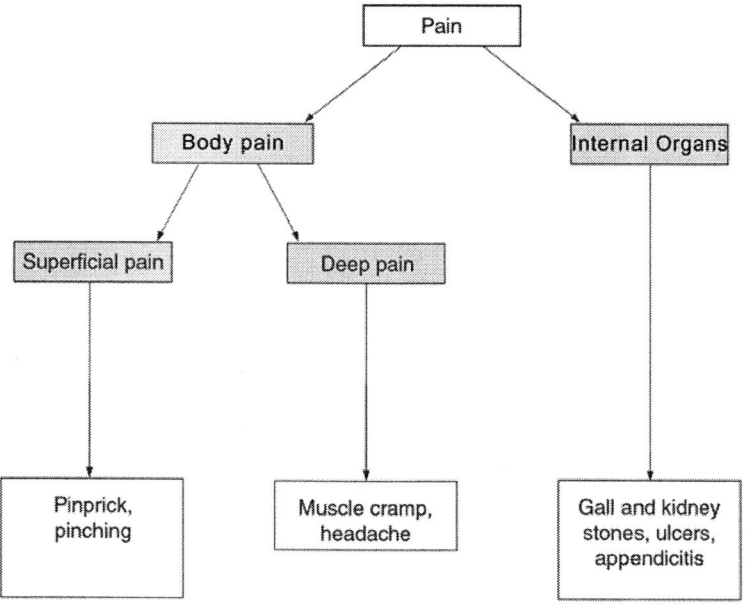

Figure 4.2. Illustration of the many different forms of pain.

Pain from the internal organs in the body (visceral pain) is different from other forms of acute pain and is often felt as if it was coming from a place on the surface of the body (referred pain). This means the place of the disease is not the same as that where the pain is felt. The nerve cells that receive signals from internal organs also receive signals from receptors in the skin and this is one explanation of referred pain where pain in internal organs is felt as originating from a place on the surface of the body.

Pain is not always related directly to bodily injuries. This is because pain signals are transformed and modulated as they climb towards central structures in the brain to reach our consciousness in the form of a sensation. Because of such modulation of pain signals, some injuries do not cause any pain sensation. People who have had serious injuries in accident or gunshot wounds may be totally pain free for a period after the event. Pain may occur even after complete healing of wounds where there should have been no pain any longer. Pain may even occur in a limb that has been amputated. These forms of pain are phantom sensations (see page 131).

Pain can be divided into two other large groups according to how long it lasts. Chronic pain is defined arbitrarily as pain that last more than 3 months. The cause of pain is not involved in the distinction between acute and chronic pain.

Pain caused by faults in the spinal cord and the brain is known as central neuropathic pain, and pain from injuries to peripheral nerves is known as neuralgia. However, neurologists usually restrict the use of the term "neuropathic pain" to the kinds of pain that are related to diseases of peripheral nerves and cranial nerves.

3.2.1. Acute Pain

Acute pain may be caused by activating certain receptors in the skin, muscles and joints. A slightly different form of pain is the one that is caused by activating pain receptors in the stomach, intestines, heart and other internal organs in the belly (known as visceral pain). Another variant of pain is caused by inflammation. Body pain can be divided into deep pain and superficial pain. Many forms of injuries, such as from trauma, can cause pain because of invasion of white blood cells and widening of blood vessels which also causes redness of the skin.

Acute pain has two main parts, the primary perception that gives awareness of the pain, almost like perception of sensory signals, and a secondary, emotional part that causes unpleasant feelings and often fear. Senses such as hearing, vision, taste and smell mainly cause awareness but may also cause emotional reactions in addition to perception of the particular sensory qualities of sound, images, taste and odors. This is because the neural pathways of all senses connect to the emotional brain. Pain pathways do that to a greater extent than sensory signals, as we will discuss a little later.

3.2.2. Chronic Pain

Pain that lasts more than 3 months is called chronic pain, although there may not be any certain features distinguishing such pain compared with that which last a shorter time. Chronic pain often involves suffering to a greater extent than acute pain.

There are two main forms of chronic pain, one that is caused by chronic stimulation of pain receptors such as in chronic inflammation (for ex arthritis) and one that is caused by abnormal neural activity in the spinal cord and brain that occurs without any known signals from receptors in the body. This kind of pain is known as central neuropathic pain and it is a plasticity disease because the changes in the function are caused by activation of neural plasticity.

Central neuropathic pain is another common form of chronic pain. It is caused by plastic changes in the spinal cord and the brain and therefore is a plasticity disease. Central neuropathic pain involves other qualities than just perception of pain, which is the main feature of acute pain. Neural plasticity is also involved in some other forms of chronic pain.

3.3. Different Causes of Pain

Pain that affects different parts of the body has special characteristics and therefore different names. Pain that originates in the nervous system, peripheral nerves, the spinal cord and the brain, is known as *neuropathic pain*. While the term may be used for all kinds of pain that are related to any part of the nervous system, neurologists use the term "neuropathic pain" only for pain that is caused by disorders of peripheral nerves and cranial nerves. Peripheral nerves have pain receptors and are therefore sensitive to pressure and mechanical manipulations. The spinal cord and the brain are not sensitive to injury; only the lining (dura mater) and some large blood vessels have pain receptors. Head injuries and strokes, however, often involve pain.

Viral or bacterial infections can give pain, for example the different strains of the Herpes virus can cause excruciating pain (neuralgia). Metabolic disorders such as diabetes can cause diseases of peripheral nerves (diabetes neuropathy).

The reaction to pain from injury is complex and can be divided into three main phases, namely the immediate one, the delayed one and the long term (chronic) phase. The immediate reactions include sensations of pressure, heat and cold and during this phase several chemicals appear in the region of injury. The pain felt later may be caused by chemicals (peptides) that widen the blood vessels. Other chemicals (enzymes) will break down debris in smaller molecules that may activate pain fibers. The long-term effects of injury may come from swelling (edema) caused by leakage of fluid into the wound and its surrounding areas. At this stage neural plasticity may be turned on and the changes in the spinal cord that follows contribute to the pain.

There are many causes of chronic pain. Chronic inflammation is probably the most common. Rheumatoid arthritis is a chronic inflammation of joints that causes constant pain. Normally inflammation is a condition where the body's defense system (immune system) attacks bacteria, virus or foreign substances. The defense system may also sometimes attack the body's own tissue, known as an autoimmune reaction. The inflammation that causes the symptoms of arthritis can affect different kinds of tissue, such as joints or tendons of the movement apparatus. Other autoimmune diseases are systemic lupus erythematosus causing inflammation that can affect inner organs. The heart, kidneys and the large intestine are common organs that are affected. This means activation of the body's defense system can go wrong in a similar way as activation of plasticity as we discuss in this Chapter.

A special form of pain caused by injuries to peripheral nerves is deafferentation pain, which is caused by activation of neural plasticity, therefore a plasticity disease.

3.4. Neuralgias

Neuralgias are defined as sharp shooting pain from the region that is innervated by a certain nerve. There are many forms of neuralgias and many causes, such as diabetes, viral infections, and trauma. Close contact between a nerve root and a blood vessel can promote neuralgias such as has been shown to occur in trigeminal neuralgia [49,62]. Nevertheless there are indications that the pain in neuralgias may be caused by changes in sensory structures in the brain and studies have shown signs that neural plasticity is involved in at least some forms of neuralgias (see [91]).

3.4.1. Trigeminal Neuralgia

A typical neuralgia is trigeminal neuralgia [46], also known as tic doulouroux or typical face pain. It is a rare disorder the average incidence is 47 new cases per year per 1 million people, occurring more often in women (59 per one million) than in men (34 per million) [68]. The incidence of the disease increases with age. The disease has been studied extensively and more is known about this disease than any other kind of neuralgia [46].

Trigeminal neuralgia starts with attacks of sharp shooting pain in one or more of the three areas of the face that are innervated by the three branches of the trigeminal nerve. These areas are usually labeled V1 for the upper face, V2 for the middle face and V3 for the lower face including inside the mouth (V stands for the number five referring to the trigeminal nerve being the fifth cranial nerve).

Between attacks there is no pain or other signs of disease. Pain attacks may come without any warning but more common, pain attacks are triggered by touch or applying cold to a certain spot (trigger point). The trigger point is often located in the mouth and people with trigeminal neuralgia often get pain attacks from eating something cold. Over years the attacks become more frequent and the extension and the intensity of the pain increases.

The medications that are effective in treating trigeminal neuralgia (see Chapter V) all act on the central nervous system and not on nerves. It may therefore be assumed that their effect in treating trigeminal neuralgia comes from their action on the trigeminal nucleus and not on the trigeminal nerve. The success in treating the disease with a medication that acts on the nervous system supports the suggestion that the pain in trigeminal neuralgia is caused by malfunction of the trigeminal nucleus rather than the trigeminal nerve.

The malfunction consists of hyperactivity or can be likened with epileptic seizure in the trigeminal nucleus. There are indications that activation of neural plasticity is involved in causing the malfunction. The fact that treatments with medications such as carbamazepine (Tegretol) [45] (see Chapter V) that are also known to control seizure activity are effective supports the suggestion that the disease is caused by abnormalities in the brain and not a fault of the trigeminal nerve despite it can be cured by moving a blood vessel that is in contact with the root of the nerve off the nerve. This operation is known as the microvascular decompression (MVD) operation [8,49,62] (see Chapter V). The disease is assumed to be a plasticity disease similar to hemifacial spasm (see page 126) that also can be cured by moving a blood vessel off the respective nerve's root. Studies of hemifacial spasm have shown that the facial motonucleus is functioning abnormally and causing the symptoms.

The treatments that are aimed at the trigeminal nerve or its root (microvascular decompression or injury to the nerve) [8,49,62]) may cure the disease because it reduces the signals that reach the trigeminal nucleus [91]. Trigeminal neuralgia is therefore another disease where neural plasticity plays an important role.

3.4.2. Viral Cause of Neuralgias

Viral infections in peripheral nerves are often causing neuralgias with unbearable pain. For example, the virus that causes chicken pox (Varicella Zoster virus, VZV) can cause excruciating pain later in life many years after an initial episode of chicken pox. The chicken pox virus causes pain that usually occurs in patches of skin (dermatomes) and the disease is called shingles. The occurrence increases with age and at age 85, about 50 percent of people have or have had shingles. The pain normally occurs in one or a few patches of skin that are innerved by a nerve root. (Such skin patches are known as dermatomes.)

It is not known how inflammation of a peripheral nerve can cause such violent symptoms. It seems clear from many studies that malfunction of the respective nuclei (groups of nerve cells) is involved in causing the pain and therefore neural plasticity is involved in creating the symptoms of these diseases, which may be called plasticity diseases. This may happen because the virus damages the respective nerve and this damage creates abnormal neural activity in the nerve. When the abnormal activity reaches the nucleus (group of nerve cells) that is the target of the nerve it changes the function of the nucleus by activating of neural plasticity.

3.4.3. Ramsay Hunt Syndrome

The Ramsay Hunt Syndrome is caused by the same member of the herpes family (herpes zoster), which actually destroys nerves and therefore causes permanent damage. The disease is slightly different from the other herpes diseases. It can cause deafness, most often in one ear only, or paralysis of face muscles on one side. Blisters on the skin in the ear canal and the outer ear often occur when the disease begins.

3.4.4. Cold Sores

Cold sores are painful blisters that often occur on the lips. Another member of the herpes family, herpes simplex, causes the symptoms. The same strain of virus causes genital herpes, a common sexually transmitted disease. The symptoms from herpes simplex infections come and go and may decrease with time but the virus is present for a lifetime. All these conditions are painful either constantly or with intervals.

3.4.5. Injuries to Peripheral Nerves

Acute injuries to peripheral nerves often occur in bodily injury of various kinds, including injury from surgical operations. It has recently been shown that nerves have pain receptors and it is possible that these receptors are involved in causing pain from injuries to nerves.

Diabetes neuropathy (disease of nerves) is becoming a common disorder of peripheral nerves because of the increase in the occurrence of diabetes type 2 in many countries of the industrialized world, most prominent in the US. Diabetes neuropathy (disease of nerves) is caused by damage to nerves because of changes in blood vessels induced by diabetes. Medications that are not analgesics (pain relievers) such as antiepileptic medications such as gabapentin (Neurontin), and the more modern version, pregabalin (Lyrica), sometimes together with a tricyclic antidepressant (nortriptyline) are now being used more and more to treat such diseases (see Chapter V). They act on the spinal cord and brain suggesting that abnormalities that cause the pain are in the spinal cord or brain and that neural plasticity is involved in creating the sensation of pain in these disorders. Diabetes neuropathy may therefore be regarded to be a plasticity disease.

Ingestion of poisonous substances can cause slowly developing injury to nerves. Vitamin deficits can also cause severe injuries to nerves. Vitamin B1 (thiamine) deficiency is the cause of Beriberi the occurrence of which increased rapidly in countries where rice is the main source of food after introduction of polished rice as replacement of the natural rice. Now it is seen in alcoholics with inadequate diets and in people whose digestive system is impaired such as after gastric bypass surgery. All these kinds of nerve injuries can cause pain.

Loss of nerve fibers (or loss of functioning nerve fibers) may cause what is known as deprivation syndromes, which include pain and other sensations such as tingling (paresthesia). The pain of this kind is caused by neural plasticity often turned on by reduction of the signals reaching the respective nuclei.

3.4.6. Pain from Neuroma

After injury to peripheral nerves [112] a neuroma[33] may form. When a nerve is injured and nerve fibers or an entire nerve is interrupted, sprouts forms. These sprouts would normally grow out and seek a target to which they can connect. A neuroma consists of sprouts of nerve fibers that have found nowhere to go. When there is no conduit that can guide the way these sprouts grow they just form a "ball" and that is what is known as a neuroma. When a nerve is cut such as occurs in amputations of limbs, neuroma may develop on the stump especially on the large nerves that often occur when a leg is amputated. Neuroma are sensitive to touch. The slightest touch can cause severe pain from the stump. The pain sensitivity in the stump may prevent the use of prosthesis.

There are ways to reduce the risk of creation of neuroma when nerves are cut in connection with amputation of limbs. By splitting the nerve at the cut end and connecting the two ends together (making an anastomosis) the risk of creation of a neuroma becomes less [7]. However, few orthopedic surgeons know about this method.

3.4.7. Spinal Cord Injuries

Injury to the spinal cord itself is often associated with pain, which may be caused by increased excitability of nerve cells in the spinal cord. It has been suggested that a surge of the neural transmitter glutamate causes central *sensitization* (see page 128) of nerve cells in the dorsal horn nuclei causing pain. It has also been suggested that pain receptors may contribute to pain following injury to the spinal cord or brain just reminding us that central neuropathic pain is a very complicated disease.

It has also been suggested that a reverberating central-peripheral nervous system loop may be established following spinal cord injury [21]. Damage to the spinal cord and the brain does not heal in the same way as damage to body parts. Damaged parts of the spinal cord or the brain cannot regenerate but their functions may be taken over by other parts of the spinal cord or brain through activation of neural plasticity (see Chapter III).

---

[33] Neuroma: a general term for abnormal growth or swelling in the nervous system.

3.5. Lower Back Pain

Lower back pain is one of the most common reasons to see a physician, its cause is poorly understood and the most common treatments have questionable benefit to most of the patients. Many of these patients suffer severe side effects too [79,80]. Lower back pain is one of the many examples where the first choice of treatment is often determined by what can be seen on imaging studies such as MRI. Using this method alone can lead to confused diagnosis and ineffective treatment.

The finding that many people with lower back pain have signs of damage to disks as seen on an MRI has been taken to support the assumption that the damage to vertebral disks and the compression of nerve roots is what causes the pain. Surgical treatment of these abnormalities rarely provides any benefit to the patients [79,80,150].

Is that an example of looking in the wrong place for the problems? MRIs are magnificent methods for detecting structural abnormalities but they cannot provide an answer to the question about what important factor is causing the pain.

Structural changes such as compression of nerves, although they look convincing, may not be what causes the patient's problems (pain); that they are present may just be a coincidence or a phenomenon that just occurs along with whatever is the cause of the pain. In fact, many people who do not have back pain have similar signs of damaged disks [57,11] and nerve compression. Drawing the conclusion that nerve root compression is the cause is often an example of confusing coincidence and causality – a mistake often made in medicine as well as in other sectors of life.

This means that nerve compression and vertebral discs that look abnormal on MRI may in fact not cause pain, or may not be the only factor necessary for causing the pain. That compressed nerve roots only rarely cause lower back pain is supported by the fact that operations to correct damage to spinal disks have poor outcome in most cases. The seduction from what can be seen (on MRI) often overrides information from scientific studies and the poor outcome of surgical treatment. Only a few patients have any long-term benefit from these kinds of operations [79]. The lack of success from common back operations often spurs new operations and it is not uncommon that patients have 3-5 operations only to find that their situation is just becoming worse.

It has been estimated that the reason for lower back pain is known only in 10-15 percent of all cases [79]. The cause is perhaps something we have never thought of. It is also possible that lower back pain in some individuals is referred pain that is caused by faults in other parts of the body (see page 115).

The common operation for lower back pain is reminds of the story about the intoxicated person who is looking for something under a streetlight. A policeman comes by and asks the man what he is looking for. He answers that he is looking for his keys. The policeman asks if he lost the keys here and the drunk man answers: No, but there is more light here.

Several facts support the suggestion that neural plasticity of central pain circuits are involved in creating the symptoms and signs of lower back pain. Many patients with lower back pain get relief from treatment with medications such as pregabalin (Lyrica) and nortriptyline, which are not pain relievers but affect the central nervous system (see Chapter V). These medications do not change the compression of nerve roots but instead act on the nervous system where they calm down excessive activity. Pregabalin (Lyrica) is also used to treat epileptic seizures and more recently treatment of diabetes neuropathy and fibromyalgia (see page 124).

The benefit from such medical treatment supports the suggestion that lower back pain is caused by faults in the nervous system (spinal cord and brain) and activation of neural plasticity. The experience that TENS (transderm electric nerve stimulation has a long-term beneficial effect on many forms of lower back pain is perhaps a more direct sign of involvement of neural plasticity. An immediate effect of TENS could be explained by its inhibitory effect on pain nerve cells in the dorsal horn. However, there is evidence that the pain relieving effect of TENS is achieved through its effect on the brain, therefore a sign of involvement of neural plasticity in the cause of lower back pain. The fact that behavioral interventions are beneficial in lower back pain [42] is a further sign that activation of neural plasticity is involved in creating this kind of pain.

Despite all the scientific evidence that points to plastic changes in the nervous system, many people have surgical treatment anyway to no avail. Surgical treatment often causes the pain to become worse. One reason may be misinterpreted MRIs, another may be that such operations are a substantial source of income for many orthopedic surgeons and neurosurgeons [98]. A very experienced neurosurgeon in treatment of lower back pain, Dr. Donlin Long, a neurosurgeon active at the Johns Hopkins University Hospital in Baltimore, has stated that conservative treatment can resolve most forms of lower back pain and only when failed should surgical treatment be considered [79]. Despite this strong evidence many people with classical lower back pain are being operated upon to no benefit – in fact often the opposite [135].

3.6. Other Forms of Back Pain

It is fair to state that we know little about the cause of other forms of back pain. Vertebral arthritis and spinal stenosis are common conditions in older people but there is also here little evidence that these structural changes are the cause of pain. Many people have these conditions but no pain.

As for lower back pain, there is no evidence that relieving the compression of a spinal nerve root can definitely cure these diseases (relieve the pain) or even provide any benefit to the patients.

3.7. Repetitive Stress Injury

One common kind of repetitive stress injury is known as the carpal tunnel syndrome. Repetitive stress injury occurs often in an industrialized society. It can occur in people who use keyboards or a computer mouse daily. It has no obvious signs of damage. Carpal tunnel syndrome is the most common peripheral entrapment neuropathy in the western world. It has been claimed that the symptoms, pain and tingling, are caused by compression of a nerve at the wrist and many people have been operated upon for the syndrome. It can be treated in many other ways than by surgical operations to release pressure on the median nerve, such as by rest and/or splinting the involved wrist, ice application, galvanic stimulation, or iontophoresis to reduce inflammation, or by exercising. Modifications to the hand and wrist positions while using a keyboard or mouse are also effective in relieving symptoms from carpal tunnel symptom.

Although it has been stated by the National Institute of Neurological Disorders and Stroke (NINDS) that the symptoms are caused by a compressed or squeezed nerve, the disease is more complex. There are signs that people with carpal tunnel syndrome have changes in central processing of pain signals [145], therefore signs of involvement of neural plasticity in generating the symptoms of the carpal tunnel syndrome. This could explain why so many different treatments are effective. Similar signs of abnormalities in temporal summation of pain signals that occur in individuals with central pain have been shown to occur in an individual with carpal tunnel syndrome [106].

3.8. Pain Diseases related to the Sympathetic Nervous System

Activation of the sympathetic nervous system is essential for normal life. A person would faint when getting out of bed if the sympathetic nervous system did not adjust the vascular system appropriately. Activation of the sympathetic nervous system in flight or fight reactions to threats is an important function of the sympathetic nervous system. However, too much activation of the sympathetic nervous system can cause symptoms of disease such as hypertension (abnormally elevated blood pressure), excessive sweating, tremor, etc.

Activation of the sympathetic nervous system can also affect the way pain is perceived. It can increase the severity of existing pain and it can cause pain. The sympathetic nervous system can also decrease and even abolish the sensation of pain in severe injuries and diseases such as heart infarcts. This is a part of the "flight and fight" situation causing the suppression of pain that often occur after trauma. This situation is created by changing the function of the pain circuits in the spinal cord (state II, see page129).

3.8.1. Sympathetic Maintained Pain
A common name for pain diseases that are caused by larger than normal activation of the sympathetic nervous system is sympathetic maintained pain (SMP). Two kinds of SMP have been identified, earlier known as reflex sympathetic dystrophy (RSD) and causalgia. Now the names commonly used for SMP diseases are complex regional pain syndrome CRPS type I for RSD and CRPS type II for causalgia. CRPS Type I is triggered by injuries of some kind, while CRPS Type II has similar symptoms but is not caused by any known injury.

Sympathetic maintained pain (SMP) is a group of diseases where the sympathetic nervous system influences the function of pain receptors and the processing that occurs in the central pain nervous system. Increased activity of the sympathetic nervous system normally increases the sensitivity of pain receptors by secretion of nor-epinephrine from the ends of the sympathetic nerve fibers that terminate near pain receptors. If the sensitivity of pain receptors is increased to an extent that the pain receptors begin to send pain signals to the brain without any other activation of the pain receptors then a person will feel pain without any normal cause. Pain increases the sympathetic activation, which then will increase the activation of the pain receptors creating a vicious cycle. The result is that the pain is maintained indefinitely if the vicious cycle is not broken.

SMP conditions are typically accompanied by changes of the skin, but not always. Other signs of increased sympathetic activity are increased sweating and increased heart rate. These symptoms and signs only occur at certain locations of the body as reflected in the name used now for these diseases (Complex *regional* pain syndrome). These diseases are difficult to diagnose and there are large variations in the symptoms often delaying effective treatment. Unfortunately, SMP diseases tend to become difficult (or perhaps impossible) to treat after some time, suggesting neural plasticity in one form or another may be involved in maintaining the disease [69,38].

What causes the sympathetic nervous system to cause such chronic pain conditions is not completely understood. There are signs that adrenergic "super sensitivity" is involved. One may wonder why these adverse effects are maintained through evolution. One explanation may be that these disorders often occur late in life and therefore do not influence reproduction (see Chapter VI).

3.9. Muscle Pain

Muscle pain may be acute or chronic. Muscles that are contracted repeatedly voluntarily or involuntarily may cause pain. Muscles may be contracted because motor nerve cells (*motoneurons*) in the spinal cord send signals to the muscles or muscles can contract without signals from the motoneurons because of diseases that affect the muscles in question.

People who have diseases that cause spasm often have pain because of muscle contractions. For example, individuals with spasmodic torticollis (se page 154, 171) often have severe pain in their neck muscles. Spasticity that can occur after spinal cord injuries is often associated with severe pain. Pain in itself may induce muscle contractions (increased muscle tone), which then can induce a vicious cycle. Tension headache is a typical example of pain from contraction of muscles [47]. Muscle contractions in connection with the classical low-back pain often cause some of the pain.

Muscles can also contract for other reasons and give rise to pain. Leg muscles in elderly people sometimes contract without any known signals from motor nerves. Muscle pain occurs in some diseases such as viral infections. The symptoms of the common influenza often are accompanied by muscle pain.

3.9.1. Fibromyalgia and Myofascial Pain

This group of complex disorders is associated with muscle pain but there is nothing wrong with the muscles. The pain that is referred to muscles in individuals with fibromyalgia and myofascial pain are forms of muscle pain that are fundamentally different from other forms of muscle pain. These disorders have been regarded to be psychiatric diseases similar to the chronic fatigue syndrome. Depression and other affective diseases are common together with these two groups of diseases. It is now believed that fibromyalgia and myofascial pain are caused by abnormal processing of sensory information. Myofascial pain is believed to be caused by dysfunction of the connection between the motor nerve fibers and the muscle fibers (muscle endplates) [126]. The incidence of fibromyalgia increases with age. It affects females more than males (9 to 1) [126] (Figure 4.3).

It is now accepted that the symptoms are caused by abnormal processing of sensory information [126]. Hypotheses about the cause of such abnormal processing range from abnormalities in the dopamine and serotonin systems to stress or psychosomatic factors.

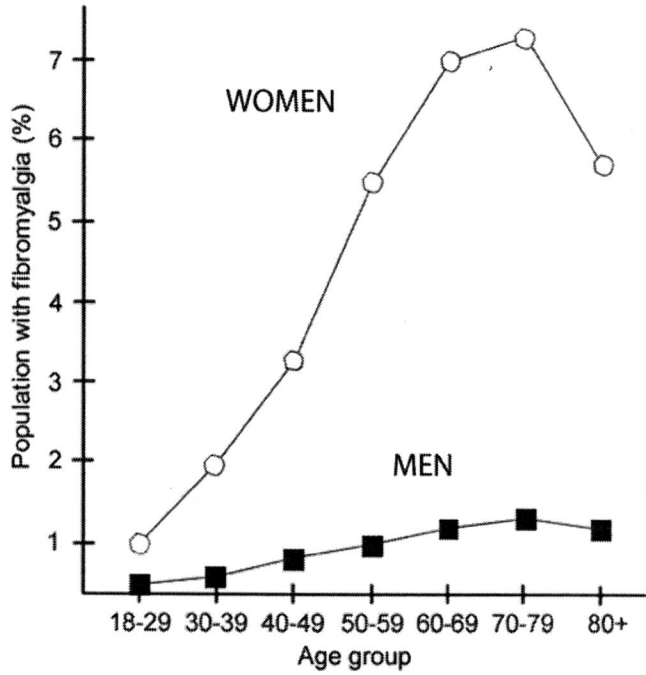

Figure 4.3. The incidence of fibromyalgia syndrome with age. Data from Wolfe et al 1995 [151].

Typical symptoms of fibromyalgia are widespread muscle pain, tenderness and sleep disturbance. There are also signs such as generalized pain, tender points in deep structures with no trigger points, general fatigue and sleep disturbances, irritable bowel symptoms, occipital headache (pain in the back of the head) and other diffuse sensations such as a swelling sensation. Morning stiffness is pronounced in most individuals with fibromyalgia and it lasts much longer than it does in inflammatory rheumatoid arthritis. Many patients with fibromyalgia have a persistent feeling of tiredness [126]. These symptoms are usually accompanied by many other often diffuse symptoms.

It is not known what starts these symptoms but genetics is likely to play an important role. Since many patients with fibromyalgia benefit from treatment with pregabalin (Lyrica) (currently the only FDA approved treatment for fibromyalgia), nortriptyline and other medications that affect the brain (see Chapter V) support the suggestion that neural plasticity is involved in creating the symptoms of fibromyalgia, indicating that fibromyalgia is a plasticity disease.

Myofascial pain is different from fibromyalgia in several ways. As for fibromyalgia, research on myofascial pain has also been focused on muscles perhaps because of the name of the disease and because the patients are told about pain in muscles. The cause of the disorder is unknown but there are signs that at least some of the symptoms are caused by plastic changes in the spinal cord and the brain.

> People who have myofascial pain experience pain from a single muscle, some spasm, stiffness, and limited range of motion. Attacks of pain can be elicited from certain points on the body (trigger points). Some patients also have moderate sleep disturbances and regional paresthesia and headache.

It is not known with certainty what causes these symptoms of myofascial spasm. It has been suggested that the symptoms are caused by dysfunction of the connection between the nerve fibers and the muscle fibers (muscle endplates). Numbing (by local anesthesia) of trigger points can resolve the problems [126].

3.10. Cranial Nerve Root Compression Disorders

Trigeminal neuralgia and hemifacial spasm are two disorders, which are associated with contacts between blood vessels and the roots of cranial nerves. It was earlier believed that these disorders were caused by compression of the respective nerve roots by an artery [61]. There is now evidence that moving any blood vessel (artery or vein), even small ones off the respective nerve root, can cure these diseases. However, there is also evidence that close contact between a cranial nerve root and a blood vessel is only a part of the cause of the symptoms and that a yet unknown other factor is necessary for generating the symptoms [91]. In fact, close contact between the root of a cranial nerve and a blood vessel is common [138] while disorders that were assumed to be caused by such close contact are very rare; hemifacial spasm occurs at a rate of 7.8 per one million per year [4] and trigeminal neuralgia has an incidence of about 47 per one million [68] (for a review of the pathophysiology of cranial nerve compression disorders, see [92]).

Here the effective treatment was introduced before the cause of the symptoms was understood (or rather at a time when the presumed cause later tuned out to be incorrect). A more correct understanding of the pathophysiology, nevertheless, did not change the way the disease was treated. Trigeminal neuralgia is discussed under neuralgias (page 179) and hemifacial spasm is discussed later (page 190).

4. CENTRAL NEUROPATHIC PAIN

Central neuropathic pain is pain that is not caused by signals from pain receptors. It is instead caused by nerve signals that are generated in the spinal cord and the brain through activation of neural plasticity. The abnormal neural activity in the spinal cord [153] and the brain [17] that causes the pain is created by activation of neural plasticity [96]. When such abnormal neural activity reaches consciousness it causes sensation of pain in a similar way as neural activity that is elicited by stimulation of pain receptors.

Central neuropathic pain, also known as *central pain*[34] is a neurological disease. Despite the fact that the pain seems to come from distinct parts of the body such as the leg or back, the pain is caused by faults in the brain from changes in function and by reorganization of the neural circuits in the brain.

Central neuropathic pain has only become recognized recently, but it is common and can be severe. The diagnosis of central neuropathic pain is often missed and the disease is difficult to treat and is often not treated in the best possible way (see Chapter V). Phantom pain is one particular kind of central neuropathic pain. Phantom pain occurs typically in amputations of a limb. These kinds of pain are plasticity diseases. Neural plasticity may also be involved in other forms of pain without directly causing the pain. In discussions about pain, it is important to remember it is a subjective sensation that is difficult to measure and quantify, and that its perceived intensity and character often varies from time to time.

Central neuropathic pain may begin because of acute pain from stimulation of pain receptors, for example, from bodily injuries of various kinds. Central pain occurs together with many major diseases such as injuries to the spinal cord and the brain, multiple sclerosis, strokes, epilepsy and Parkinson's disease.

Pain that continues after the signals from pain receptors have ceased is central neuropathic pain. This kind of pain may be chronic (last more than 3 months). Often central neuropathic pain is regarded to have no known cause (being idiopathic), either because the physician has not been able to find the cause or because the reason for the activity in the nervous system that cause the pain cannot be found by the methods we have available. Often the determined cause of the pain is incorrect (faulty diagnosis).

4.1. Incidence of Central Pain

Central neuropathic pain is more common than shown by available statistics because it is often overlooked as the cause of persistent pain (Table 4.1).

Table 4.1. Estimated prevalence of major disorders with central pain (Data from Bonica (1991) and Österberg et al 2005) [12,115]

Disease	Total patients (numbers)	Patients with CP (numbers)	(%)
Spinal cord injuries	225,000	68,000	30
Multiple sclerosis	150,000	42,000	28
Stroke	2,000,000	168,000	8.4
Epilepsy	1,600,000	44,800	2.8
Parkinson's disease	500,000	50,000	10

---

[34] Central neuropathic pain: The term "central neuropathic pain", or central pain, is used for pain related to the brain mostly but also to some extent to pain from the spinal cord. The term "central neuropathic pain" is mostly used to describe pain caused by neural activity in the brain where activation of neural plasticity is the (main) cause of the pain.

4.2. Abnormal Sensations in Central Neuropathic Pain

Individuals with central neuropathic pain may often find that light touch to the skin is painful. This is known as *allodynia*[35] and it seems to be caused by redirection of information from the receptors in the skin that normally mediate innocuous sensation to pain circuits in the brain [70,116,117]. The sensitization that often is present in central neuropathic pain may contribute to this phenomenon.

The tolerance to mild pain is often decreased. Small cuts or pin pricks that normally would cause only mild to moderate pain sensations may cause prolonged sensation of pain in individuals with central pain. These abnormal reactions to stimulations of pain receptors are known as hyperpathia. More rarely, some individuals with central pain may also experience an increased sensitivity to pain (lowered threshold), known as hyperalgesia.

Since pain caused by changes in the function of the nervous system is felt as if it came from a specific place on the body is common, it often causes physicians or surgeons to use the wrong form of treatment of central pain, and the result is that the pain is not relieved. This is what can cause central neuropathic pain to be a problem both for the patient and for the physician or surgeon.

4.3. A Patient with Pain

Here is a hypothetical history of a patient that illustrates many of the symptoms and signs of central neuropathic pain.

A nurse, who worked in a psychiatric clinic, was beaten by a patient who hit her arm with a bottle. Her resulting wound was treated by a surgeon. As expected, she had pain in her arm even after the surgery while the wound healed.

To her surprise, the pain continued even after the wound had healed. She therefore went back to her surgeon, who opened the wound to see if anything was wrong but could not find anything abnormal. The nurse went home and was asked to wait for the healing process again, and with the expectation that the pain would disappear. It did not, and being a nurse she looked for other doctors, unfortunately to little avail.

What caused her arm pain to continue after the injury healed? The pain or the injury had triggered changes in the way her brain functioned. From the beginning, her pain was caused by stimulation of receptors in her arm that signaled to the brain that something had happened to her arm and the activity in these nerve cells gave the feeling of pain.

The pain she felt in her arm after the wound healed was caused by activity in the same nerve cells that had signaled the pain in response to the injury. But now these nerve cells did not need the signals from the arm to become turned on. She had acquired central neuropathic pain; a plasticity disease.

---

[35] Allodynia: a condition where pain from normally non-painful stimuli causes pain.

Since the same nerve cells in the brain as were activated when the injury occurred now were activated because of plastic changes in the spinal cord or the brain, it was felt as if the pain came from the arm. The pain was no longer caused by signals from the arm and it did not help to open the wound. The pain was real but it was caused by activity in the nervous system and not by her arm. Because pain was felt coming from the wound the surgeon opened the wound but found nothing wrong. The reason was that the surgeon looked in the wrong part of the body for the cause. The fault was no longer in the wound but was now in the brain.

The pain from the wound had disappeared and had been replaced by central neuropathic pain caused by plastic changes. The reason the surgeon believed that there was something wrong in the wound was that the patient complained about pain from the wound. This is typical for central neuropathic pain that it is felt as it came from the location of the injury that started the pain.

The story about the nurse is an example of pain that is not unique nor is it uncommon that attempts to treat such pain is in vain because the treatment is often aimed at the wrong part of the body. The treatment should have been aimed at the nervous system instead of the arm and treated with medications (see Chapter V).

4.4. Causes of Central Neuropathic Pain

While central neuropathic pain may be started by injury to an arm, leg or any other part of the body the pain is caused by sensitization of nerve cells and re-organization in the dorsal horn. Injury to a peripheral nerve causing decrease in the signals from receptors can cause such changes in the function of some nerve cells in the dorsal horn of the spinal cord.

4.4.1. Abnormalities in the Dorsal Horn

Activation of neural plasticity can change the way neural circuits in the spinal cord that are involved in pain work as described by Doubell, 1999, who assumed that these pain circuits can operate in four different ways (modes, also known as states) [34]. Which one of these four states circuits operates determines the symptoms. The pain cells in the dorsal horn of the spinal cord receive pain signals from pain receptors through Aδ and C fibers.

State I is the normal state where only stimulation of pain receptors can give a sensation of pain. If the receptors are not activated the person does not feel any pain.

In state II, the sensibility to signals from Aδ and C fibers is lower than normal. The pain sensitivity is also lower than normal and that is the "flight and fight" situation where pain is suppressed. This happens often immediately after major injuries such as gunshot wounds but only for a short time.

In state III, persistent pain occurs. In addition to hyperpathia, allodynia and hyperalgesia pain occurs when signals from different kinds of nerve fibers (Aβ, Aδ and C) arrive at the dorsal horn. This condition is caused by plastic changes that are reversible.

In stage IV, the malfunction is the same as it is in stage III but it is not reversible as it is in stage II and III. The reason is that structural alterations have occurred, with cells dying and nerve fibers and dendrites degenerating. New nerve fibers may appear and synapses may be altered.

The changes in function of the nerve cells in the dorsal horn can be started by injury to a peripheral nerve, by inflammation or other traumatic injuries that cause expression of neural plasticity. The abnormal state three can be maintained without the events that caused the change from stage one (the normal one) to stage three remain present. This means that activation of neural plasticity has switched the state of the neural circuits in the dorsal horn from a stable normal condition to an equally stable state of disorder.

The neural circuits in the dorsal horn therefore have two stable states and we call the system a bistable system. That the neural circuits have bistable functions is important for treatment. It is obviously not sufficient to remove whatever has caused the circuits in the dorsal horn to become faulty, but some other intervention is necessary to bring these neural circuits back to their normal function. That the abnormalities in state four are permanent because of structural changes is of course also a severe obstacle in treatment of pain conditions.

Pain and abnormalities in function such as allodynia, hyperalgesia and hyperpathia have been linked to processes in the dorsal horn [153]. For example, allodynia may be caused by Aβ fibers (that respond to light touch) invading areas of the dorsal horn that are normally restricted to Aδ and C fibers (lamina I and II) where they make contacts with cells that are involved in pain, therefore a form of re-routing. Sensitization may also be involved in the cause of allodynia.

Understanding the molecular and cellular mechanisms for these processes have increased lately, and we now begin to understand the basis for many of the pain phenomena related to neural plasticity. For example, the role of some kinds of glia cells has recently become known. Three main kinds of glia cells, astrocytes, oligodendrocytes and microglia are present in the brain. There are about 10 times more glia cells than nerve cells. For a long time, glia cells were regarded only to take care of "house keeping tasks" in the brain and the spinal cord, but more recently it has become evident that they may play important roles in the function of nerve cells. Chemicals that are released by microglia cells have been implicated in processes that are elicited by damage to peripheral nerves such as pain, hyperalgesia and allodynia [153].

The abnormal neural activity in the neural circuits in the dorsal horn (and those of the trigeminal nucleus) climbs in the pain pathways and reaches nuclei in the brain. These central structures are not malfunctioning, but they just relay and process the abnormal neural activity from other (peripheral) structures that are faulty. This is important to keep in mind for treatment because treatment aimed at the structures in the brain that behave abnormally just because they receive abnormal signals from the spinal cord will not cause permanent relief of the pain nor will it relieve the other symptoms of central neuropathic pain. Treatment aimed at such structures may block the abnormal signals that cause pain and therefore relieve the pain temporarily. The pain will return when the treatment wears off. Only by aiming the treatment at the faulty neural structure in the spinal cord is it possible to achieve lasting relief. (This will be discussed in more detail in Chapter V).

The abnormal activity may reach many parts of the brain such as the amygdala where it may cause emotional reactions (depression etc.). Awareness of the pain occurs when the abnormal activity reaches certain regions in the brain.

5. PHANTOM LIMB SENSATIONS

The sensations of pain and tingling that are not caused by physical activation of pain receptors are known as phantom sensations. The term describes conditions that are often associated with pain and other feelings that people who have had limbs amputated perceive as coming from the limb that they no longer have [86]. This form of pain is clearly produced by activity in the nervous system that occurs without signals from the body part to which the sensation is referred, therefore a plasticity disease.

The term phantom limb is assumed to have been coined by Silas Weir Mitchell (1829-1914) [112]. It has been reported that between 50 and 80 percent of individuals who have had a limb amputated have phantom sensations, mostly these sensations are painful [133].

Phantom limb sensations give the impression that a missing limb is still attached to the body and is still moving [86,120].

Phantom limb sensations are mostly feelings of pain and tingling, but sensations such as warmth, cold, itching, squeezing and burning are also common. The phantom limb symptoms are generally unpleasant. Occasionally, the pain can be made worse by stress, anxiety and weather changes. Some people with amputated limbs feel that the missing limb is still attached to the body and is moving together with other body parts [112]. The missing limb often feels shorter and may feel as if it is in a distorted and painful position. Phantom limb sensations are more common after unexpected losses of a body part than from planned amputations.

Phantom sensations are best known from amputated legs but may also occur after the removal of body parts such as after amputation of the breast, extraction of a tooth (phantom tooth pain) or removal of an eye (phantom eye syndrome). People who are born without limbs and people who are paralyzed may also experience phantom pain and other forms of discomfort may be referred to the missing limb [112,119,127].

Disconnecting muscles through cutting peripheral nerves also give symptoms that are unpleasant. Phantom limb signs can occur after blocking a nerve such as is done for dental work. These signs can include a feeling that the lip is much larger than it really is. Spinal anesthesia can also cause distorted impressions of the size and the location of body parts.

Amputations turn on neural plasticity causing changes in the function of certain parts of the spinal cord and the brain, and it may re-organize neural circuits. Maps of the body surface on structures in the brain such as on the cerebral cortex (the familiar homunculus) are altered after amputations to an extent that is related to the strength of the phantom pain (see Chapter II). The phantom limb phenomenon is therefore a fascinating demonstration of how the human adult brain can re-organize and how new functional connections can be created through activation of neural plasticity.

Dr Dirk De Ridder, a neurosurgeon in Antwerp, Belgium has reported on a lady who perceived her right eye had been displaced to a location below her right maxillary arc [31] (Figure 4.4).

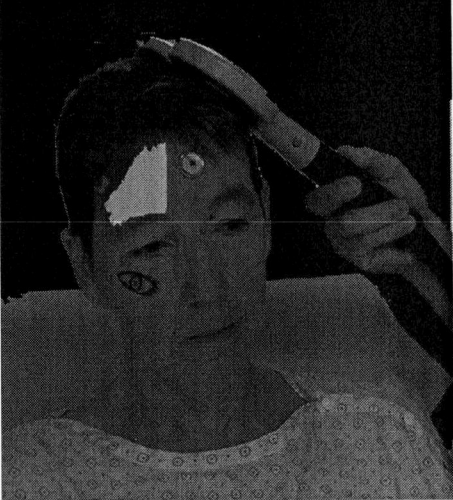

Figure 4.4. Drawing of the phantom eye, and showing the placement of the magnetic activating coil. The phantom eye is located in the area of the second branch of the trigeminal nerve, below and to the side of the real eye, slightly tilted. (Reprinted from De Ridder, D., De Mulder, G., Menovsky, T., Sunaert, S., Kovacs, S. 2007. Electrical stimulation of hearing and somatosensory (bodysensory) cortices for treatment of tinnitus and pain. In: Langguth, B., Hajak, G., Kleinjung, T., Cacace, A.T., Møller, A.R., (Eds.), *Tinnitus, Pathophysiology and Treatment, Progress in Brain Research* Vol. 166. Elsevier, Amsterdam. pp. 377-388. [31], with permission from Elsevier).

She had normal vision when examined by an ophthalmologist but she often bumped into objects because of a misconception of the position of surrounding objects. The lady also had central neuropathic pain with the pain sensation located to a region above her eye. Magnetically induced stimulation of her left cerebral cortex using a magnetic coil placed as seen in Figure 5.1 (Chapter V) reduced her pain by 80% and her phantom eye perception disappeared totally.

The results of examination of her eye by an ophthalmologist, was normal and that was probably correct; there was nothing wrong with her eye, and it was just another example of looking in the wrong place for a problem. The problem was not in the eyes, but in the brain.

5.1. Cause of Phantom Limb Symptoms

Earlier it was believed that phantom limb symptoms were caused by irritation of the nerve fibers in the stump of the nerves that were severed, but more recent evidence has supported the suggestion that the phantom limb symptoms are caused by the sudden absence of sensory signals from the amputated body part turning on neural plasticity and causing an unfortunate reorganizing of the sensory system of the spinal cord and the brain.

The deprivation of signals is assumed to have induced neural plasticity in the part of the brain that normally deals with sensations from the limb that has been amputated. For example, the amount of pain is related to the degree of reorganization of the cerebral cortex [42].

The development of phantom limb pain depends on the pain the patient has experienced before the operation in addition to genetic and other factors. The amount of nerve activity that is caused during the operation to amputate the limb is also a contributing factor for phantom limb pain. Applying local anesthetics before the amputation to the nerves that are to be cut can reduce the risk of phantom limb symptoms.

Reorganization can also occur in a motonucleus after it has been disconnected from muscles by severing the motor nerve, as has been shown in experiments in animals. In this way Kreutzberg has shown that the organization of the facial motor nuclei changes after injuries to the facial nerve [71].

Formation of neuroma at the stump of nerves that are cut during an operation may also cause pain (see page 120) in addition to the phantom pain.

6. PEOPLE'S DESCRIPTION OF THEIR PAIN

The description of a sensation as being no more than a mental representations of a stimulus in accordance with the Cartesians view on sensory perception is not valid for pain. When the International Association for the Study of pain asked a group of people, with the psychiatrist Harold Merskey as chairman they said: "Pain is an unpleasant sensory and emotional experience associated with actual or potential tissue damage or described in terms of such damage" They added that "Pain is always subjective... This definition avoids tying pain to the stimulus" [149]. Notice that this organization did not take into account that pain can be caused in other ways than by trauma to the body ("tissue damage") omitting causes that are dealt with in this book namely activation of neural plasticity that is known to cause neuropathic pain including central pain and other plasticity diseases.

6.1. Perception of Pain is Individual

People who seek medical help describe their pain in different ways. In a study by Dr. Ronald Melzack [85], patients who came to his clinic for their pain were asked to describe their pain in their own words. Table 4.2 lists some of the words these patients used to describe how they perceived their pain and how it affected them emotionally. The participants in Dr. Melzack's study also tried to judge the meaning of the pain signals such as whether they are signs of something that is a risk to the body, dangerous, frightening, or just making them miserable. The information from was the basis for the McGill University pain questionnaire.

**Table 4.2. Examples of how patients described their pain in the emergency room
as recorded by Dr. Melzack [85] as reported by Dr. Wall [149]**

TEMPORAL	SPATIAL	PRESSURE	SENSORY	AFFECTIVE	EVALUATIVE
POUNDING	SHOOTING	LANCINATING	SPLITTING	KILLING	EXCRUCIATING
BEATING	FLASHING	LACERATING	HEAVY	VICIOUS	UNBEARABLE
THROBBING	JUMPING	STABBING	ACHING	CRUEL	HORRIBLE
QUIVERING		DRILLING	HURTING	TERRIFYING	MISERABLE ,
FLICKERING			SORE	FEARFUL	DISCOMFORTING

Pain is perceived differently under different circumstances, time of the day, and whether it is suspected that the pain may be a sign of a serious disease. Even a person's ethnicity plays a role in how they perceive pain [20,152]. That people use different words to describe their pain is just one sign that pain is more complex than the five normal senses.

Some diseases are associated with abnormal perception of pain. For example, many autistic individuals have reduced sensitivity and may even enjoy pain. The most dramatic abnormalities occur in people who are born without pain sensation (congenital analgesia).

6.2. Reactions to Pain

Pain can cause symptoms that are not directly related to the sensation itself. Pain activates the autonomic nervous system, mainly the sympathetic nervous system, causing elevated blood pressure and increased heart rate, perspiration, etc. High blood pressure (hypertension) increases the risk of heart attacks (myocardial infarction) and strokes. It is a serious "side-effect" to pain that is often ignored, but which means that treatment not only relieves suffering but it also reduces the risk of serious diseases and death.

6.2.1. Emotional Reactions to Pain

Pain is complex, it is never a single experience and it often causes distress and it may involve fear and anxiety. Pain is not just a sensation such as hearing a sound or smelling an odor but pain has emotional (affective) components. The effects of pain on an individual person can be numerous, from depression to distraction from other aspects of life. Pain affects the entire body and the entire person [27].   .

How pain affects an individual person naturally depends on the circumstances and the severity of the pain, but it also depends on how the person handles the pain emotionally.

Pain can evoke fear because of what is associated with it such as signs of severe illness, failure of treatment for a serious disease and even risk of death. Most people are afraid of pain; in fact many people are afraid of dying because they believe it will be painful.

These affective (emotional) reactions may not always be caused by worry and fear of the possible consequences of the pain, but such reactions may also be explained by the routing of pain signals to the emotional brain (limbic system, mainly the amygdala). Signals of pain that can reach the amygdala without having to travel through the cerebral cortex may not be under voluntary (conscious) control (see Appendix A) to the same degree as pain signals that have to pass through the cerebral cortex.

People who feel that they can escape their pain in one way or another or have hope of relief cope much better than those who feel that there is no hope of relief. Pain that is escapable and pain that is inescapable are not only perceived differently, but these two kinds of pain are processed in two different parts of the brain (known as the periaquaductal gray, PAG) (see Appendix A).

Pain is often accompanied by depression, and in fact, depression can exaggerate pain and perhaps emotional distress. Anxiety and anger can even cause new pain or activate old pain. Depression in connection with pain may be related to the degree of activation of the emotional brain (especially the amygdala) by the pain signals or it may be related to how the individual perceives and interprets the pain.

6.2.2. Suffering and Coping

Pain almost always causes some forms of suffering, and different people have different abilities of coping with suffering. Coping is not a passive skill but a learned one, where people learn to live with their pain. How a person copes with the suffering from pain depends on many factors, such as whether the pain is escapable or inescapable. A person who can live according to the concept: "I have pain but pain does not have me" is a lucky person. Learning about pain is an effective part of treatment (see Chapter V).

Pain signals reach the parts of the brain that normally deal with decision-making (prefrontal cortex) and other higher brain functions. Here, the pain signals may cause interruptions to life's activities. The signals from these regions of the brain may also elicit such feelings as depression, frustration, anxiety and anger by the ample connections to the emotional brain (limbic system).

6.3. Altered Perception of other Sensations

Acute pain can elicit various kinds of reflexes. The aim of pain reflexes is to avoid injury by moving away from, for example, touching something that is hot ("the withdrawal reflex"). The withdrawal reflex is elicited by pain signals; it contracts muscles that flex arms or legs. The reflex is controlled by nerve cells in the dorsal horn of the spinal cord activating the nerve cells in the ventral horn controlling muscles. These very simple bodily reactions have often been taken as a central and fundamental property of pain but, as we have seen from the discussion above, the withdrawal reflex is one small part of the reactions to pain.

Pain often causes contractions of muscles in general and muscle contractions can cause pain. This means that a vicious cycle may be established. Lower back pain that is typically associated with muscle contractions is an example. Whether these muscle contractions are regarded to be pain reflexes is a matter of semantics.

Many forms of chronic pain are accompanied with other sensations such as pain from light touch to the skin (allodynia), exaggerated and prolonged reaction to mild pain (hyperpathia), and less common, increased sensitivity to painful stimuli (hyperalgesia). These abnormalities were discussed earlier in this Chapter.

A phenomenon that often occurs together with chronic pain is known as the "wind-up" phenomenon. The wind-up phenomenon means that there is a stronger reaction to a painful stimulus that follows another painful stimulus; the reaction to a series of painful stimuli is stronger than that to a single stimulus. The wind-up phenomenon is caused by abnormalities in how pain signals are added over time (temporal summation). The phenomenon appears to be associated with chronic pain and it therefore seems as signals from pain receptors are processed differently in individuals with neuropathic pain compared with people who do not have such pain.

Sensation of pain may have similarities to other sensations such as hunger, thirst, sleepiness, fatigue and the sensation of just plain feeling ill. We discussed earlier (page 124) how pain from internal organs (visceral pain) such as that from infarction of the heart could be experienced as just feeling ill, almost like flu.

6.4. Assessment of the Severity of Pain

It has been difficult to get reliable measures of the severity of pain. One attempt to classify pain consists of just dividing pain into three different degrees of severity: mild, moderate and severe chronic pain. According to this definition, mild pain does not noticeably interfere with everyday life, moderate pain causes some annoyance and is definitely perceived as being unpleasant. Severe pain affects most aspects of a person's life, with difficulties to sleep and work.

For studies of pain in the laboratory and for monitoring treatment it is common to ask the person who has pain to rate the strength on a scale from 1 to 10, known as a visual analog scale (VAS). Other methods use hand pressure measured by a dynamometer to scale pain.

6.5. Tolerance to Pain

Heat applied to the skin is often used in laboratory studies aimed at determining a person's pain tolerance. The heat used in such studies may be generated by an infrared laser. The lowest heat that gives a sensation of pain is called its threshold and that is a measure of the sensitivity to pain. When the heat is increased there will be a point where the person can no longer tolerate the pain, and that is a measure of the tolerance. Unlike the threshold for pain the tolerance for pain is different in different individuals and it depends on the circumstances during which the pain occurs.

People of different ethnicities seem to perceive pain differently [152]. Italians and Jews seem to have lower tolerance for experimentally induced pain than people of northern Europe and Northern America. Finnish people are known to have a very high tolerance for pain. However the pain sensitivity does not seem to differ. Laboratory studies have shown there is no difference in pain sensitivity between people of different ethnic groups [20].

6.6. Development of the Experience of Pain

Some studies have suggested that pain awareness requires previous experience, therefore actions of neural plasticity [141]. This suggests that activation of neural plasticity is important for developing normal awareness of pain. We discussed earlier that sensory stimulation is necessary for normal development of the sensory nervous system. Recent studies have indicated that normal ability to feel pain also require exposure to pain for normal childhood development [131]. There are also signs that children's attitude to pain is influenced by their parents' attitude to pain, another form of learning that is involved in developing a normal sense of pain.

These findings may be interpreted as signs that the normal ability to perceive pain is acquired after birth or at least it is necessary to shape the ability after birth in order to develop normal awareness of pain. The question is then to what extent is our perception of pain based on genetics and to what extent is the ability to perceive pain acquired after birth. Clarification of these questions would be important for understanding to what extent unborn or newly born children have pain awareness.

7. TINNITUS

Tinnitus is hearing meaningless sounds that may resemble tones or more often sounds similar to those of crickets, a high whistling or it can be a roaring noise. Tinnitus may be felt as a sound but there are many differences between the perception of tinnitus and sounds that reach the ear.

There are two broad kinds of tinnitus. One is caused by an actual sound that is generated in the body (sometimes known as objective tinnitus). This kind of tinnitus may be caused by the noise from blood passing a constriction in a vessel where the flow of blood become turbulent, or it can be caused by muscle contractions giving clicking sounds. The other kind of tinnitus is generated by nerve activity in the hearing nerve or the brain without any sound has reached the ear. This kind of tinnitus is by far the most common and it is sometimes known as subjective tinnitus; it is different from sound hallucinations, which is the hearing of voices, music and other meaningful sounds. We will in this book only discuss subjective tinnitus.

Tinnitus has no objective signs and there is no known diagnostic test such as imaging (MRI, X-ray), chemical (blood tests) or electrophysiology that can be used to study and evaluate a person's tinnitus. Recently, however, some studies have indicated that some forms of tinnitus are associated with subtle abnormalities in the EEG pattern[36] and in some forms of evoked potentials[37] in individuals with tinnitus [37].

The lack of clear signs suitable for diagnosis is one of the reasons the medical profession pays scant attention to patients with tinnitus. Another reason treatment of tinnitus is neglected

---

[36] EEG: Electroencephalography, recording of electrical activity in the brain, performed by placing electrodes on the scalp.

[37] Evoked potentials: Electrical activity in the brain that is caused by activation of senses such as hearing, vision and body senses and which can be recorded by placing electrodes on the scalp.

is perhaps because tinnitus in itself is not life threatening; only when it leads to suicide can tinnitus cause death.

Tinnitus, its physiology, its impact on a person and its treatment, is taught sparsely, if at all, in medical schools. Few books cover the basic science of tinnitus [72,136,146] and few if any of these are used in medical schools. Books on clinical topics do not include much about tinnitus either. There is no major textbook devoted to the clinical aspects on tinnitus. However, some textbooks on the basics of hearing have a section on tinnitus [95]. Lack of suitable textbooks on tinnitus and its management is another reason why physicians often ignore this disorder. This causes severe chronic tinnitus to have many similarities with chronic pain [101].

Tinnitus is often caused by activation of neural plasticity and is therefore a plasticity disease. Tinnitus can be a symptom of a few different diseases but more often it is a symptom in itself with no known cause. In this book I will concentrate on this form of tinnitus.

7.1. There are Many Forms of Subjective Tinnitus

Tinnitus can be felt as if it is coming from one ear or from both ears and it can be felt as coming from the center of the head. Tinnitus can occur only at certain times, or it can be constant (chronic tinnitus). It can be barely noticeable or it can be a roaring noise that is bothersome and prevent intellectual work and sleep. Such distinctions can be important for selecting treatment (see Chapter V).

The way people perceive their tinnitus has been used to distinguish between different severities of tinnitus. Classification in three groups, mild, moderate and severe, has been suggested [123]. Mild forms rarely cause any problems; moderate tinnitus can interfere with intellectual work and sleep and often causes suffering. Severe tinnitus can have a major effect on a person's entire life, making it difficult to sleep, and making intellectual work impossible and cause severe suffering. Tinnitus that involves suffering has been called "bothersome tinnitus" or "problem tinnitus" by some investigators [52].

7.1.1. Tinnitus Is often Accompanied by Altered Perception of Sounds

Tinnitus, especially severe tinnitus, is often accompanied by changes in the ways sounds that reach the ear are perceived. Individuals with some forms of tinnitus often hear normal sounds to be distorted. Everybody finds that some loud sounds are not only unpleasant but also intolerable. However, individuals with tinnitus often have a lower tolerance level for sounds than people who do not have this disorder. Many people with tinnitus perceive even normal sounds to be so unpleasant that they are intolerable. This is known as hyperacusis, which is defined as a lowered tolerance for sounds, meaning that often even moderately loud sounds create discomfort [5,102]. Repeating an unpleasant sound may be felt as excessively unpleasant to a person with severe tinnitus, therefore similar to the wind-up phenomenon in central neuropathic pain (see page 135). Some individuals with tinnitus find that sounds may invoke fear (phonophobia).

The cause of such change in the way sounds are perceived is not completely understood. It is, however, believed that reorganization of the brain through activation of neural plasticity may have caused a change in the way sounds are processed in the brain or perhaps it has caused information to be sent to the wrong part of the brain (re-wiring). Such plastic changes in the brain can explain why some sounds are perceived differently from what is normal.

7.2. Prevalence of Tinnitus

Tinnitus is common. Most people over the age of 60 have some form of tinnitus at one time or another. Different studies have arrived at very different numbers of persons who have noticeable or bothersome tinnitus; the differences mostly caused by different definitions of tinnitus. The prevalence of tinnitus in individuals over the age of 50 reported by different studies varies from 7.6-20.1% [58].

It is often assumed that children do not have tinnitus. However, a recent study in children (5-12 years) regarded to have normal hearing found a prevalence of tinnitus of 37.7%, with 17% reporting annoyance from the tinnitus [26]. Different studies have reported widely different values, again probably because different investigators define tinnitus differently. Children do not seem to be bothered by their tinnitus to the same extent as adults and children do not seem to complain about tinnitus as adults do. In general, published studies show that tinnitus in children is often associated with exposure to loud sounds and hearing loss. Again, it should be kept in mind that different studies use different definitions of both tinnitus and of suffering from tinnitus. This is likely to account for a part of the differences in the results from different studies.

When discussing children and tinnitus it must be pointed out that children are not just small adults. Studies have shown signs of involvement of the non-classical hearing pathways in children [107] and that may be one reason why they observe their tinnitus to be different from that of adults.

7.3. Tinnitus as a Sign of Ailment

Tinnitus is rarely a sign of a serious ailment. Many people get worried that it is a sign that something is seriously wrong. Tinnitus is one of the symptoms of William's disease (infantile hypocalcaemia), which has many other symptoms and signs. Tinnitus is also one of the three signs of Ménière's disease (the other two are fluctuating hearing loss and vertigo, a feeling that the surroundings are spinning).

Some may have heard that tumors, on the hearing and balance nerve, vestibular schwannoma, are associated with tinnitus and therefore are afraid that they may have a brain tumor. That almost all individuals with vestibular schwannoma have tinnitus does not mean everybody who has tinnitus has a vestibular schwannoma – on the contrary, the risk of having vestibular schwannoma for people with tinnitus is very small. Only about 9 people out of 1 million get such tumors every year. These tumors are not cancerous and should therefore perhaps not be called brain tumors. They grow very slowly, on an average 0.2 cm per year, and even sometimes disappear without any treatment [23,137]. They are only a danger because they grow in a place with little room.

It is easy to exclude a vestibular schwannoma (by MRI or audiologic tests), but it is far more difficult to find out what causes tinnitus in the great majority of individuals who have it.

7.4. Causes of Tinnitus

Tinnitus can be caused by injuries to the hearing nerve most often caused by head trauma, or surgically induced damage or from viral inflammation. Closed head injuries including concussions, are often followed by tinnitus, which may last a lifetime. (Head injuries are also often followed by oversensitivity to light).

Exposure to loud sounds (noise) may cause tinnitus. For example, a strong sound such as that of emergency vehicles' sirens can start severe tinnitus in some people while exposure to similar sounds does not cause tinnitus in other individuals. Tinnitus most often decreases after the end of exposure to loud sounds, over minutes, hours or perhaps days. A few people acquire strong tinnitus after a single exposure to a loud sound and the tinnitus may last a lifetime.

Perhaps the most common cause of tinnitus is lack of signals to the hearing nervous system, either caused by hearing loss because of disorders of the ear of by lack of sound exposure. Many older people experience tinnitus when in a quiet environment.

It was earlier believed that tinnitus was a result of damage to the ear but it is now believed that most forms of tinnitus instead are caused by changes in the nervous system through activation of neural plasticity. Many reports on studies in animals have shown evidence that exposure to loud sounds can cause changes in the function of the hearing nervous system [139,140] and in other systems of the brain [53]. It is therefore not only silence that can cause tinnitus, but paradoxically also exposure to strong sounds can cause tinnitus.

Damage to the hearing nerve can cause tinnitus. Tumors on the hearing and vestibular nerve (acoustic tumors, or vestibular Schwannoma) are almost always accompanied by tinnitus. Traumatic injuries to the hearing such as may occur in head trauma and as a result of surgical operations often cause tinnitus.

Medications such as salicylates (Aspirin) [110,65] can cause tinnitus when administrated in large dosages [77]. Some antibiotics can cause hearing loss [43] and also administration of quinine[38] [77,154] often causes tinnitus. These medications also cause hearing loss which has been studied extensively in animal experiments by Dr. Jochen Schacht and his co-workers [154].

It is now understood that a harmful form of neural plasticity being turned on causes many, probably most forms of tinnitus. Most forms of chronic tinnitus are therefore plasticity diseases [100], which means that many forms of tinnitus are caused by nerve cells that have changed the way they function but nothing is damaged as occurs after strokes or head injury. We want to find out what changes in the nervous system would favor the "run-away" neural

---

[38] Quinine: The first effective treatment for malaria, it is used to treat leg cramp and arthritis.

activity that would be interpreted as a sound, when no sound reaches the ear. These are important questions that need to be answered to understand tinnitus.

7.4.1. Where Is Tinnitus Generated?

It is obvious that tinnitus is caused by neural activity that is not normal or which occurs when it should not occur. The first thing one would ask is probably where in the body is this neural activity generated. Or rather, what structures cause the abnormal neural activity. Tinnitus is felt as something coming from the ears; it was therefore natural to search the ear for the cause. Much research on the cause of tinnitus and its treatment has focused on the ear.

The ear can cause tinnitus in two ways: 1) It can generate abnormal impulse traffic in the hearing nerve that is interpreted by the brain as a sound although no sound is reaching the ear, or 2) it can cause reduced activity in the hearing nerve, which can induce neural plasticity because lack of signals to the brain can activate neural plasticity. This could occur because of diseases of the cochlea or the structures the conduct the sound to the cochlea (ear canal and middle ear) (see Appendix B).

Lack of signals to the brain in general is a strong promoter of neural plasticity. This means that hearing loss from disorders of the ear can cause tinnitus and treating the hearing loss by treating middle ear diseases or by hearing aids or cochlear implants can help alleviate tinnitus in some individuals (see Chapter V).

While the abnormal neural activity that causes tinnitus in some individuals is generated in the ear, tinnitus in most people is generated somewhere in the brain without the ear being involved. In that way tinnitus has many similarities with some forms of pain [101] as discussed earlier in this Chapter. Perhaps the most convincing evidence of the involvement of the hearing nervous system comes from the knowledge that people whose hearing nerve has been cut can still have tinnitus because of lack of signals to the brain from the ear [59]. This means many forms of tinnitus are phantom sounds in a similar way as many forms of pain are phantom sensations from an amputated limb (see page 103). In order to understand what causes tinnitus it is important to know about the function of the ear and the hearing nervous system (see Appendix A).

We know little about where in the brain the conscious perception of sounds is created. I have pointed out earlier in this Chapter that symptoms such as pain involve abnormal neural activity in a chain of structures and that it is the abnormal neural activity in one of these structures that gives the sensation of pain. The same is the case for some forms of tinnitus. It may be abnormal neural activity from some certain nerve cells that are faulty that causes the sensation of tinnitus. On the other hand, some of the structures that are abnormally activated in individuals with tinnitus may not contribute to the sensation of tinnitus. The activation may be a secondary phenomenon (an epiphenomenon). Also, the re-organization of tonotopic maps may be secondary (an "epiphenomenon") to tinnitus.

It has often been assumed that conscious awareness was generated somewhere in the cerebral cortex, but perhaps other parts of the brain, such as nuclei of the amygdala play a role in perception of some sensory signals under some circumstances. For example, the major target of the pathways of the sense of smell (the olfactory system) is the central nucleus of the amygdala and the sense of smell has very little cortical representation [16].

Parts of the emotional brain (limbic system) are involved in abnormal ways in some forms of tinnitus [78], perhaps a nucleus of the amygdala may be involved in sensory perception and awareness of tinnitus.

7.5. What Changes in the Hearing Nervous System can Cause Tinnitus?

It seems reasonable to assume that tinnitus is caused by neural activity somewhere in the hearing nervous system and that such nerve activity is interpreted as a sign that sounds are present. When trying to find out what causes tinnitus it would be natural to ask how the ear normally tells the brain when a sound within the range of hearing has arrived at the ear. Tinnitus can be regarded as being caused by the brain having misunderstood the message that normally tells it when a sound has been received by the ear. It would therefore be valuable to find out which unique properties of nerve signals provide information about the presence of a sound.

One can therefore ask the question: What features of the impulse pattern of nerve cells tells the brain that a sound is present? The same question can be asked for the normal activity that is elicited by sounds that have reached the ear by some process in the nervous system that generates the particular pattern of nerve impulses without any signals coming from the ear. Is it the rate (frequency) of nerve impulses, or is it the pattern of nerve impulses (bursts or a continuous stream) that is important, or is it the relationship between the impulse pattern generated by different cells in a large population of nerve cells that matter. These different possibilities will be discussed below. First let's consider how the brain interpret nerve signals from the ear that are evoked by sound that have reached the ear.

7.5.1. How Does the Brain Interpret Signals from the Ear?

It would be natural to suggest a sound is only perceived when the rate (frequency) of the nerve fibers' impulses exceeds a certain value. The nerve fibers in the hearing nerve normally have considerable activity without any sound reaching the ear (silence) and without causing tinnitus (we call such activity *spontaneous* activity). This means it may not be the presence of nerve activity that tells the brain a sound is present but some other property of the nerve signals that carry the message about a sound's presence at the ear.

Nonetheless, experiments in animals have shown that the discharge rate of nerve fibers in the hearing nerve is only related to a sound's intensity over a small range [95]. It therefore seems as it is not the frequency (rate) of nerve impulses in hearing nerve fibers that tells the brain how strong a sound is or for that matter, when a sound has reached the ear.

With that in mind it seems unlikely that tinnitus would be caused by increased neural activity in the hearing nerve. It may be some other properties of neural activity that tells the brain when a sound has reached the ear and how loud the sound was.

A better candidate for providing information about the presence of a sound seems to be the pattern of nerve impulses. It has been suggested that the way the pattern in one nerve fiber is related to that of another that communicates the message that a sound has arrived at the ear [35,89].

The neural activity that cause tinnitus may be similar to the activity elicited by sounds, with the difference that it occurs without any sounds reaching the ear, or the neural activity that causes tinnitus may be different from that caused by normal sounds that reaches the ear. The neural activity that cause tinnitus may occur in nerve cells that normally become active when sounds reach the ear or occur in nerve cells that are not normally activated by sounds.

7.5.2. Abnormal Neural Activity May Cause Tinnitus

The hypothesis that some forms of tinnitus is caused by nerve cells in the brain that either functions in an abnormal way or have become active by themselves is supported by an observation of a person whose tinnitus disappeared after a stroke [81]. The person was an ear-nose and throat physician who should be able to adequately assess his tinnitus, which he had had for many years ("lifelong"). A stroke obviously destroys brain cells and it seems logical to conclude that the cells that were destroyed by the stroke had caused the tinnitus.

The suggestion that the relationship between neural activity in different nerve fibers in the hearing nerve carries important information about sounds has been further developed by researchers in hearing such as Dr. Jos Eggermont for the purpose of providing understanding of what causes tinnitus and for finding out what has gone wrong in the nervous system of individuals with tinnitus [36,37]. He has proposed that the way the nerve impulses of the different members of a population of nerve cells are related to each other is important for signaling the presence of a sound. This means that the relationship between the neural activity in the members of a population of many nerve cells is more important for telling the brain that a sound has reached the ear and how loud it is than the frequency of the nerve impulses in individual nerve cells [35,37,89].

Understanding how the ear tells the brain that a sound has arrive is naturally important for understanding of tinnitus, because tinnitus is caused by false indications that a sound has arrived at the ear.

Tinnitus would occur if similar nerve activity as caused by a sound was generated without sound reaching the ear. If we assume that the relations between neural activity in many nerve cells is important we would look for ways that could (falsely) occur. One way is through direct communication between nerve cells. Such direct communication could occur through what is known as ephaptic transmission[39] between nerve cells. Ephaptic transmission between bare (denuded) nerve fibers in injured nerves have been suggested a long time ago as an explanation of different kinds of diseases (hemifacial spasm [48], (see page 153), and pain [121]). More recently similar hypotheses have been presented to explain some forms of epileptic seizures where many nerve cells fire in synchrony, which may be caused by an abnormal direct communication between nerve cells (ephaptic transmission) [83].

Noise induced hearing loss has been shown to promote plastic changes in the form of kindling[40] and it has been shown that within a short time after exposure to strong noise (that cause hearing loss) synchrony of firing of nerve cells increases. Studies have shown that this increase continued to progress during noise exposure [113]. If synchrony, or correlation,

---

[39] Ephaptic transmission: Neural transmission between bare nerve fibers or between the bodies of nerve cells without any chemicals (transmitter substances) involved.

[40] Kindling: The term "kindling" was used by Goddard in 1964 to describe seizure activity in rats after daily activation of the amygdala with electrical impulses [54].

between neural activities in groups of nerve cells is the factor that provides information about sounds then it may explain how noise exposure can cause tinnitus.

Eggermont and his co-workers also showed that the changes normally brought about by noise exposure could be reduced if the animals had been exposed to sounds of lower intensity ("enriched acoustic environment") before the noise exposure [114]. This shows some of the complexity regarding tinnitus and its relationship to noise exposure but it also opens up possibilities for treatment and prevention of tinnitus.

7.5.3. Changes in Frequency Maps

Each nerve cell throughout the hearing nervous system is tuned to a certain frequency of sound (see Appendix B) which means that each cell and nerve fiber respond best to a certain frequency. Nerve cells are organized anatomically according to which frequency they respond best and cells that are tuned to similar frequencies are located close together. This organization of nerve cells according to the frequency to which they respond best (*tonotopic maps*) is affected by activation of neural plasticity. Distortion of the frequency maps on the hearing cortices (tonotopic maps) are some of other signs of plastic changes in the brain that occur in some forms of tinnitus. The tonotopic maps of the cerebral cortex are distorted as a result of tinnitus as shown in studies using *magnetoencephalograpic* (MEG)[41] recordings [109].

It is not known if the distortion of the tonotopic maps causes tinnitus or if the distortion is caused by the tinnitus and therefore being a secondary phenomenon to the cause of the tinnitus. Exposure to loud noise causes changes in the tonotopic maps of the cerebral cortex [113]. Several other studies have shown reorganization after exposure to loud sounds [124] and that has been suggested to be involved in tinnitus [122].

The changes in the tonotopic maps are similar to the changes observed in the maps that show the projection of the body surface onto the surface of the cerebral cortex that receive signals from receptors in the skin and other parts of the body (somatosensory cortex) that occur after amputation of body parts such as a finger [66,87,148]. Regions of the cortex that are neighbors to areas that do not receive any signals from skin receptors because of the amputation will expand and take over the cortical areas that do not receive any signals. These reorganizations are caused by activation of neural plasticity.

7.6. What Causes Tinnitus?

· It seems obvious that tinnitus is caused by abnormal neural activity or neural activity that occurs when it should not occur. The question is where and how is this neural activity generated and what has caused it to be generated. The ear has been in focus for many year for causing the neural activity that causes tinnitus but more recently the search for a cause of tinnitus has been directed to the nervous system.

---

[41] Magnetoencephalograpic (MEG): recordings of the magnetic fields that are generated by the electrical currents from neural activity in the brain.

7.6.1. Diseases of the Ear

One would imagine that if the ear's sensitivity would be abnormally increased it would cause tinnitus. Such an increase could be caused by stress, which would increase the activity of the sympathetic nervous system and cause autonomic (sympathetic) nerve fibers to secrete a substance known as norepinephrine. Such sympathetic nerve fibers are located near the receptor cells (known as hair cells) in the cochlea [33], and when these nerve fibers become activated they secrete norepinephrine and that increases the sensitivity of the receptors. This is similar to what happens in other parts of the body such as in pain receptors (page 123). Other disorders of the ear may cause abnormal neural activity in the hearing nerve being interpreted by the brain as a sound (tinnitus).

Tinnitus often occurs together with hearing loss caused by something being wrong with the sensory cells in the cochlea. Hearing loss means reduction of sensory signals to the brain, and this reduction can activate neural plasticity. The reduced signals from the ear to the brain caused by disorders of the cochlea (cochlear hearing loss) may turn on neural plasticity and thereby cause tinnitus.

Hearing loss caused by problems in getting sound to the cochlea (conductive hearing loss) can also promote plastic changes because it reduces the intensity of the sound that reaches the cochlea, and thereby reduce the signals that the ear sends to the brain.

These two common ear problems decrease the signals that reach the brain. This can turn on neural plasticity because deprivation of sensory signals is a strong promoter of plastic changes. Activation of neural plasticity can increase the sensitivity of the ear and certain parts of the hearing nervous systems to compensate for the loss in sensitivity in hearing loss. Too much of an increase in sensitivity can cause tinnitus ("self oscillation" in neural circuits). Activation of neural plasticity can also re-organize (re-wire) neural circuits that process the neural activity that is elicited by sounds.

That most people who have tinnitus also have hearing loss does not mean hearing loss causes tinnitus. There are many people with hearing loss who do not have tinnitus. There are a few people who have tinnitus and no hearing loss or at least very little hearing loss. This is just another example of the complexity of tinnitus.

Hearing loss, especially for high frequencies, increases with age. This may contribute to tinnitus because it reduces the signals from the ear to the hearing nervous system. In fact, most elderly individuals who do not have tinnitus in a normal environment will experience tinnitus after a short while when placed in a silent environment such as a sound insulated room used for hearing tests.

That the natural *reserves* of the nervous system are gradually depleted with age may be the factor, or one of the factors that promote plastic changes in the brain. This may also be the reason that central pain occurs more frequently in older people than in young people. Central pain has many similarities with tinnitus (see also Chapter III [101]).

7.6.2. Imbalance between Inhibition and Excitation

It seems logical to suggest that some kind of imbalance in the hearing nervous system could cause abnormal neural activity that was interpreted to be a sound by the brain. Upset of the balance between inhibition and excitation would seem as a good candidate for causing odd neural activity.

Almost all nerve cells receive two different kinds of signals--one that can activate the nerve cell (excitation) and one that reduce the activation (inhibition) (see Chapter I). Nerve cells in the hearing nervous system are naturally activated by sound, but almost all such nerve cells also receive inhibitory signals that decrease the activation. Reduced inhibition causes nerve cells to be activated more easily and less excitatory signals are needed – the results are increased sensitivity to sounds. If the inhibition is further decreased, the nerve cells may become active even without sound reaching the ear. The result is that the person will hear a sound even when no sounds reach the ear, which means tinnitus. Tinnitus could therefore be caused be an imbalance between inhibition and excitation that made nerve cells react as if they received signals from the ear.

To make things even more complicated, most nerve cells receive both excitatory and inhibitory signals from large descending pathways that run in parallel with the ascending pathway, but in the opposite direction (see Appendix B). We know very little about the function of this top-down influence but in general the impulse traffic in the descending pathways allow higher centers to influence the way nerve cells lower down in the ascending pathways process sounds. For example, the most peripheral (lowest) part of the descending pathways, the olivocochlear efferent system, has influence on the function of the hair cells in the cochlea [95]. This has been suspected to play a role in creating tinnitus but, so far no solid evidence for this suggestion has been presented.

Nerve cells in the hearing nervous system also receive influence from many parts of the brain that are not directly involved with hearing. This opens many different possibilities for altering the way the hearing nervous system works, some of which may cause or promote the development of tinnitus. It has been suggested that signals from other parts of the brain may cause tinnitus or make tinnitus be affected by factors such as emotions and stress. These theories are plausible but it has been difficult to gain direct experimental proofs of their validity.

7.6.3. Involvement of the Non-classical Hearing Pathways

Reorganization of some kind of the nervous system may also be involved in causing tinnitus. This suggestion is supported by studies that have shown that stimulation of a nerve that innervate the skin (the median nerve at the wrist) can change the way tinnitus is perceived in 40% of individuals [105]. In this study the nerve was stimulated by applying electrical impulses through electrodes placed on the skin.

Other studies have reported that some individuals can modulate the intensity of their tinnitus and how it sounds by activation of other senses. Many individuals with tinnitus can modulate their tinnitus by activation of receptors in the skin and other parts of the body (the somatic system) [19]. Since the median nerve innervates receptors in the hand, stimulation of the median nerve with electrical impulses is similar to activating receptors in the skin of the hand.

Some people can change their tinnitus by touching their skin or by making muscle contractions of various kinds. A few individuals with tinnitus have mentioned that they heard sounds when they touched the skin on their arm. A patient once mentioned he heard a swishing sound when he dried his back with a towel. These observations are also signs of interaction between senses.

It has been reported that as much as 80% of individuals with tinnitus can change their tinnitus by contracting head and neck muscles [74,75]. Some individuals can change the way their tinnitus sounds by changing their gaze as has been shown by Dr. Anthony Cacace and his co-workers [18]. Looking in different directions therefore changes the tinnitus in some individuals. This kind of tinnitus is often called somatic tinnitus because of its relation with body functions. In another study 33% of individuals with tinnitus could change their perception of tinnitus by moving their jaws [125]. These findings are supported by clinical experience that temporomandibular joint disorders (TMJ) often are associated with tinnitus, and treating the TMJ problems also decreases the tinnitus [88].

There is evidence that these abnormalities that occur in connection with some forms of tinnitus are caused by an abnormal involvement of the non-classical ascending pathways (see Appendix B). Perception of tinnitus can be affected by activating receptors in the skin and this is a sign of interaction between two senses (hearing and body senses). It is known as "cross-modal" interaction. Involvement of the non-classical pathways may explain such cross-modal interaction because it, unlike the classical pathways, receives sensory signals of more than one modality (see Appendix B).

This interaction between hearing and body senses has been further explored recently and several explanations have been suggested. One is that there are newly discovered connections between nerve cells in the spinal cord and the cochlear nucleus$$$. There are also connections between the trigeminal nucleus and the ventral cochlear nucleus and that may explain these interactions; for a review, see Shore, 2007 [134].

Studies using electrical stimulation of a nerve at the wrist have found that children's perception of sounds could be changed by electrical stimulation of the medical nerve at the wrist [107] and this has been taken as an indication that the non-classical pathways are active. The effect decreased gradually with age and most had disappeared when the children reached their late teens. Involvement of non-classical hearing pathways therefore seems to be "phased out" as a part of normal childhood development and it is not normally active in adults, except in some who have tinnitus [105].

These studies indicate that the connections between the ear (or peripheral parts of the hearing nervous system) and the non-classical pathways are open in young children [107] and that these connections close during childhood development. There are also indications that some individuals with autism have similar cross-modal interaction [99,104] and that has been ascribed to an abnormal use of the non-classical pathways caused by faults in childhood development. It is known that some autistic individuals have a more emotional reaction to sensory signals than non-autistic individuals.

That some individuals with tinnitus have signs of cross-modal interaction [105] between hearing and body senses means that these (dormant) connections can be re-opened through activation of neural plasticity. The abnormal involvement of the non-classical hearing pathways in connection with tinnitus is likely brought about by activation of neural plasticity and therefore a further indication that some forms of tinnitus are plasticity diseases.

Hearing sounds from touching the skin is likewise an indication that the non-classical hearing pathways are involved in some forms of tinnitus because the classical hearing pathways only receive signals from the ear (see Appendix B).

Involvement of the non-classical pathways implies that a different part of the thalamus (the dorsal or medial part) is activated while only the ventral part is activated by the classical pathways. This may explain some observed changes in the EEG pattern such as increased delta waves [37]. The fact that the non-classical pathways bypass the primary hearing cortex and project directly to the secondary cortex (and association cortices) may also play a role in tinnitus.

8. DISEASES OF HEARING AND BALANCE

The balance (vestibular) system is closely associated with hearing because the sensory organ for balance is a part of the inner ear. Hearing and balance share the eighth cranial nerve. Also many disorders of the balance system are plasticity diseases. Some diseases such as Ménière's disease involve symptoms from both hearing and balance systems and there are indications that neural plasticity is involved in creation of these symptoms.

8.1. Balance Diseases (Dizziness)

There are many different kinds of diseases of the balance system [6] and they have different names, mostly related to the symptoms of balance diseases. The symptoms of balance disorders are vertigo[42], unsteadiness[43] and dizziness[44] and signs such as nystagmus[45].

A common kind of balance disorder is benign positional vertigo (BPV) or benign paroxysmal positional vertigo (BPPV), which is characterized by vertigo, lightheadedness and nausea [6]. The symptoms are worse when the position of the head is changed. Disabling positional vertigo (DPV) is characterized by constant vertigo, unsteadiness and nausea [108]. These symptoms get worse with movements of the head. Many individuals with disabling positional vertigo spend most of their time in bed because that is the position in which they have fewest symptoms.

Neural plasticity is most likely involved in causing at least some of the symptoms of these diseases. The fact that DPV can be cured by moving a blood vessel off the balance nerve in a similar way as in hemifacial spasm and trigeminal neuralgia (typical face pain) can be cured (see Chapter V), indicates that neural plasticity is involved in creating its symptoms.

> The balance system with its sense organ in the inner ear helps keep balance when standing or walking. When the head is turned the balance system moves the eyes in the opposite direction so that an image is kept still on the retina (see page 82). Normally the balance system does its job without causing any awareness of what it is doing. This is why it is normally regarded to be a *proprioceptive* system (propius is Latin meaning "ones

---

[42] Vertigo: A feeling that the world is spinning, often associated with nausea and vomiting when intense.

[43] Unsteadiness: difficult to maintain balance when standing.

[44] Dizziness is an imprecise term that covers many symptoms from the balance system.

[45] Nystagmus: involuntary movements of the eyes, is a sign used to diagnoses such diseases showing that the function of the vestibular ocular reflex is not normal (see page 82).

own") and it is not regarded to be a sensory system (*exteroception*) (exteroception means "what we perceive from the outside world").

Under certain circumstances, however, turning the head can give clear symptoms. This can occur because of diseases such as viral infections, intoxication from for example alcohol or diseases such as disabling positional vertigo. Side effects of treatments such as those for cancer (cytostatica) are associated with nausea.

When movements of the head reaches awareness it must mean that information from the balance organs in the inner ear has been re-directed to centers of the brain different from where the information normally goes. The symptoms can begin suddenly and disappear equally quickly, which means the symptoms are caused by changes in function. This suggests that the re-routing of information that brings about the symptoms most likely is caused by opening dormant synapses that lead to brain regions involved in conscious perception. Activation of neural plasticity can cause such redirection of information by unmasking of dormant synapses.

8.2. *Ménière's* Disease

People with Ménière's disease have symptoms from both the hearing and the balance parts of the inner ear. Three symptoms define Ménière's disease: fluctuating (low frequency) hearing loss, tinnitus and attacks of vertigo. The symptoms are believed to be caused by an imbalance in the pressure (or actually the volume) [130] in the two different fluid filled compartments of the inner ear where the receptors for hearing and balance are located (see Figure 4.5).

The fluid system is made up of two different compartments, the perilymphatic space and the endolymphatic space. The fluids in these two compartments have different (ionic) composition and these two fluids are separated by thin membranes. There must therefore be perfect balance between the volumes in these two compartments. It is believed that imbalance between the volumes in these two compartments causes the symptoms of Ménière's disease [6]. It is not known how this balance is kept and it is not known what may cause the imbalance that occurs in Ménière's disease.

It is interesting that Drs. Barbara and Ove Densert, MDs, a research couple from Sweden, have shown that applying air puffs to the inner ear [32] can relieve the symptoms of Ménière's disease. Such air puffs activate the balance system, but they do not affect the imbalance in the fluid systems directly. Rather, these air puffs activates the receptors in the balance organ. By activating receptors in the balance part of the inner ear, the air puffs may act in a similar way as TENS used in treatment of central neuropathic pain (see page 122). That such activation of the balance system can lessen the symptoms of Ménière's disease suggests the symptoms of this disease are caused by activation of neural plasticity in a similar way as many forms of tinnitus and central neuropathic pain. This means that Ménière's disease may be regarded to be a plasticity disease.

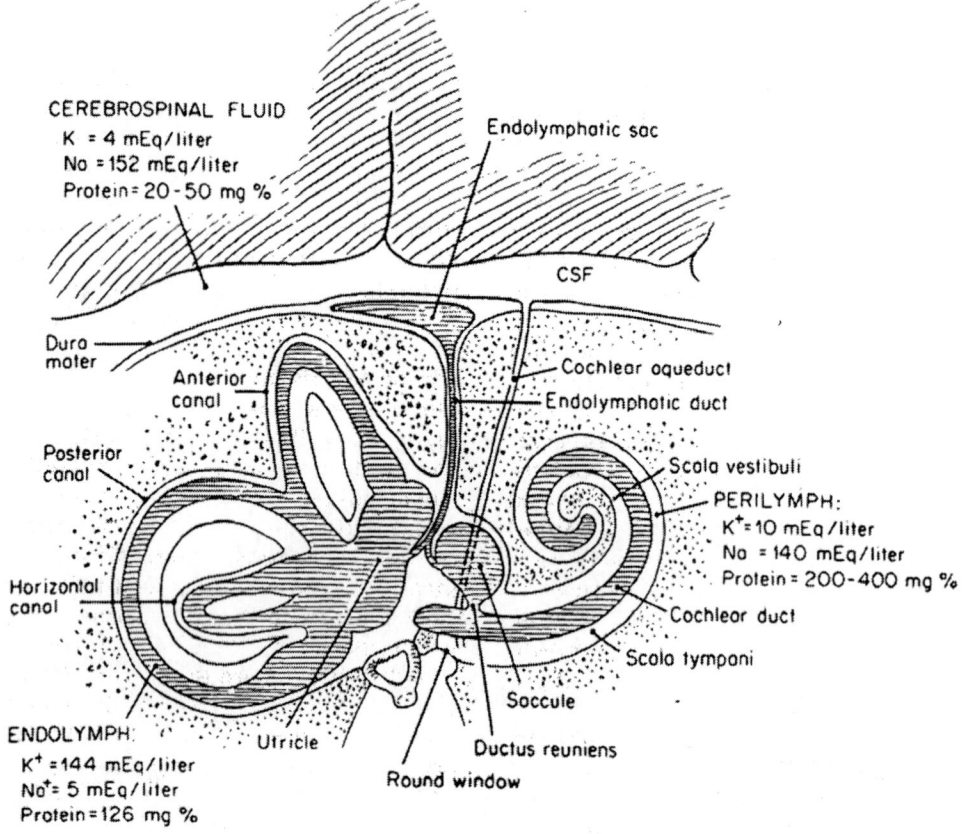

Figure 4.5. Schematic drawing of the fluid system in the inner ear. The different compartments communicate with each other through narrow canals, some of which are bare patent. (From: Baloh, R.W., Honrubia, V. 1990. *Clinical neurophysiology of the vestibular system* F.A.Davis Company, Philadelphia. (Reproduced with permission from the F.A. Davis Company) [6].

9. THE ROLE OF NEURAL PLASTICITY IN MOVEMENT DISEASES

Movement diseases can include several kinds of symptoms and signs. Complete loss of muscle function (paralysis) or partial lack of function (paresis) is common forms of movement diseases. Other signs of movement diseases are the opposite, namely unintentional muscle activity (spasm and spasticity). Spinal cord injuries may naturally cause pareses and paralysis, but such injuries are often followed by increased muscle activity such as spasticity and some reflexes may become exaggerated. Activation of neural plasticity is involved in causing these symptoms.

Periodic muscle contractions (tremor) also occur in connection with many kinds of movement diseases such as Parkinson's disease. Inability to contract muscles correctly, for example involuntarily contractions of other muscles than those anticipated (synkinesis[46]), are common after nerve injuries. Deficits in coordination of movements (ataxia[47]) also occur. Movement diseases are different from pain and diseases of sensory systems such as tinnitus in that there are visible and measurable signs of the disease.

Traditionally, neural plasticity was regarded to be involved in causing the symptoms and signs of only a few movement disorders, but it has recently become evident that the changes in function that cause the symptoms of many movement diseases occur because of activation of neural plasticity. Neural plasticity is most likely involved in many more yet to be identified. Plastic changes in the nervous system may cause increased tonus of muscles and increased reflexes such as in spasticity. There are also signs that synkinesis can be caused by activation of neural plasticity. Reflexes play an important role in normal function of the motor system. The ease with which reflexes are activated may be increased through activation of neural plasticity. Such changes in the spinal cord and the brain may be a way to compensate for lost or decreased motor function such as occurs in spinal cord injuries.

9.1. Muscle Spasm and Spasticity

People who have had injuries to their spinal cord often develop muscle spasm and spasticity some time after the injury has occurred. Spasticity is often regarded as a more bothersome complication to spinal cord injuries than the loss of functions (pareses and paralysis). Neural plasticity being turned on by signals from the injured spinal cord is involved in causing these symptoms.

9.1.1. Hemifacial Spasm

Individuals with hemifacial spasm have attacks of involuntary muscle contractions in one side of their face [39] and often synkinesis of facial muscles. Hemifacial spasm is a rare disease; it occurs in 7.4 per one million men per year and 8.1 for women [4]. The spasm usually starts around the eye and over time more and more of the facial mimic muscles become involved. After 10-15 years most facial muscles on one side of the face may be involved, including the platysma (muscles on the front side of the neck). However, muscles of the forehead are rarely involved.

Hemifacial spasm is in many ways similar to trigeminal neuralgia (page 118): moving a blood vessel of the respective nerve root can effectively treat both, but there are also differences. One is that trigeminal can be treated effectively by medications [45] but so far little effect has been shown from known medications on hemifacial spasm [1].

Two hypotheses regarding the cause of hemifacial spasm and trigeminal neuralgia (typical face pain) have prevailed. One claims that the symptoms are caused by close contact

---

[46] Synkinesis: *Involuntary movement accompanying a voluntary one, as the movement of a closed eye following that of the uncovered one, or the movement occurring in a paralyzed muscle accompanying motion in another part.* (Stedman's Electronic Medical Dictionary, Version 7.0).

[47] Ataxia: *An inability to coordinate muscle activity during voluntary movement; most often results from disorders of the cerebellum or the posterior columns of the spinal cord; may involve the limbs, head, or trunk.* (Stedman's Electronic Medical Dictionary, Version 7.0).

between nerve fibers through ephaptic[48] transmission causing "cross-talk" between nerve fibers of the respective nerves that have lost their myelin covering [48,111].

It was earlier believed that the close contact between the facial nerve root and a blood vessel (an artery) destroyed the myelin of the nerve fibers and that the bare nerve fibers that had lost their myelin coverage would communicate directly with each other (known as "ephaptic" transmission) [48,51,111]. Hemifacial spasm may engage most of the mimic muscles of the face and in order to explain how ephaptic transmission between facial nerve fibers can involve most face muscles (mimic muscles) including the platysma (the muscle on the front side of the neck) all nerve fibers of the facial nerve would need to have their myelin removed (being denuded) and brought in contact with each other. No evidence whatsoever has been presented that this would occur and common sense makes it seems utterly unlikely to occur even if there was serious injury to the facial nerve. Nevertheless, nobody had ever shown that the blood vessel that was in close contact with nerve root did any damage to the nerve's myelin.

The other theory claims that the symptoms are caused by hyperactivity (and re-organization) of the respective nucleus (the facial nucleus) [41]. These hypotheses have been tested in clinical examinations of patients [111,147], in studies on hemifacial spasm during microvascular decompression operations [91,103] and in animal models [128,132].

> Studies of hemifacial spasm using electrophysiological recording techniques during microvascular decompression operations to treat the disease indicated that the facial motonucleus was involved in causing the symptoms (spasm and synkinesis) [91,103]. This supported the theory proposed by Ferguson [41] many years ago. We saw similarities with the "kindling" phenomenon, described by Goddard [54]. Other studies performed in the operating room on patients undergoing microvascular decompression operations for hemifacial spasm [90] have indicated that it was unlikely that these symptoms could be caused by direct communication between nerve fibers of the facial nerve.

Since moving a blood vessel off the facial nerve is very effective in curing the disease (the cure rate was 85 % [9]) much attention has been directed to this vascular contact with the facial nerve root as a cause of the symptoms and signs of the disease. On the other hand, studies such as those by the Australian anatomist Dr. Sunderland have shown that blood vessels in close contact with the roots of cranial nerves (see Figure 4.6), including the facial nerve, is common as studied in autopsies [138]. In fact, close contact between a blood vessel and the facial nerve root occurs in over half of the individuals who do not have any symptoms from the facial nerve [138], see also Møller, 1993 [91]). This means the close contact with a blood vessel with the facial nerve root cannot be *sufficient* to cause of the symptoms of hemifacial spasm – if it had been most of us would have had hemifacial spasm. The fact that moving a blood vessel off the facial nerve where it leaves the brainstem can cure the disease means this irritation of the facial nerve root is *necessary* for the symptoms to

---

[48] Ephaptic transmission: Transmission directly between axons that have lost their myelin and are located close together.

occur. Something else is also needed, but we do not know what that second factor is [91]. It is obvious that each factor alone does not give any noticeable signs.

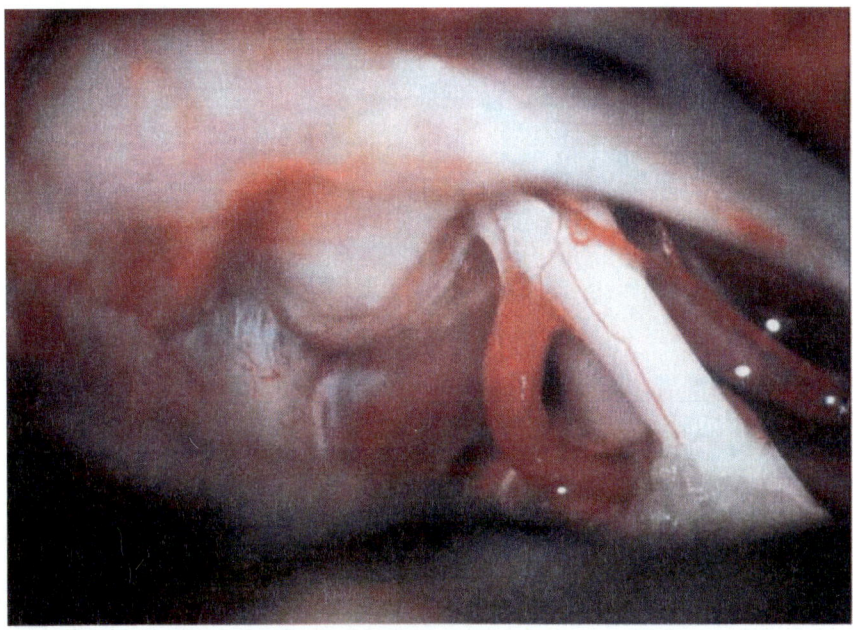

Figure 4.6. Example of vascular contacts with a cranial nerve (the balance and hearing nerve).

9.1.2. Synkinesis

Synkinesis often occurs after injuries to peripheral nerves and it has often been assumed to be caused by nerve fibers not finding their correct targets (muscles) when they grow out after injuries and making connections to the wrong muscles. Studies of injuries to the facial nerve have indicated that synkinesis is affected by training [14]. Therefore, it may be assumed that it is caused by changes in function, most likely of the motonucleus that controls the muscle contractions.

> Studies of patients who have recovered function of their facial muscles after injuries to branches of the facial nerve and who have synkinesis have shown that the synkinesis can be treated successfully by training [14,67]. Training does not change which muscle the outgrowing nerve fibers have reached, but training or exercise can alter how the nervous system works. These studies therefore show evidence that synkinesis is caused by changes in neural circuits in the brain and in particular the facial motonucleus which controls the mimic muscles of the face.

The studies of patients with injuries to the facial nerve supports the suggestion that synkinesis is caused by incorrect connections between nerve cells that control different groups of face muscles, most likely caused by the opening of dormant connections (synapses) between nerve cells in the motonucleus that allow commands aimed at one group of muscles to also go to other muscles than those intended. The studies of patients with hemifacial spasm discussed above makes it unlikely that *ephaptic* transmission in the facial nerve could cause the synkinesis that often is a part of the symptoms of hemifacial spasm. That synkinesis of facial muscles can be caused by abnormalities in the facial motonucleus is also supported by the observation that the spasm attacks of facial muscles in patients with hemifacial spasm are affected by stress [39,51,91].

The reorganization of the motonucleus is probably caused by neural plasticity being turned on by the irritation of the facial nerve by the close contact with a blood vessel. Synkinesis is therefore another example of how adverse effects can be caused by neural activation of neural plasticity.

The finding that moving very small arteries (arterioles) and even small veins off the facial nerve root could cure hemifacial spasm [63] made it further unlikely that ephaptic transmission between facial nerve fibers could cause the spasm and synkinesis in hemifacial spasm.

9.1.3. Other Hyperactive Disorders

Neural plasticity is most likely also involved in other diseases that have hyperactive symptoms such as spasmodic dysphonia and some forms of spasmodic torticollis [129].

9.2. Brain and Spinal Cord Injury

Movement deficits after traumatic injuries or strokes and other forms of damage to the brain and spinal cord include paresis (weakness of movement) and paralysis (inability to move). Injury to the brain or spinal cord can turn on neural plasticity causing re-organization of many regions of the spinal cord and the brain, which is mostly beneficial in that it can help restore and replace lost functions as discussed in Chapter III. However, these efforts sometimes go wrong and the induced plastic changes can be harmful by causing disease-like symptoms and signs. For example, lesions to the primary motor cortex (M1) may cause re-organizations of neural circuits in areas close to the lesion as well as in structures that are far from the lesions such as in the pre-motor areas and even in regions on the opposite side of the brain [29]. Some of the reorganizations that occur in structures that are far away from the primary cortex, where the lesions were made, such as in the premotor areas have a negative effect on recovery from damage of primary motor cortices [29]. This is just another example of how plastic changes in response to lesions can have complex consequences, some of which are harmful. These widespread changes in function affect the results of training a limb with weakness from a stroke. For example, when one arm has weakness and the other has normal function it is beneficial to restrict the movement of the normally functioning arm during training of the one that has weakness [143] (see Chapter V).

9.3. Disorders of Basal Ganglia

Many movement disorders have been linked to faults in a group of nuclei known as the basal ganglia[49]. The symptoms and signs of these diseases are complex and poorly understood. The basal ganglia process commands from the motor cortex before they are sent to the muscles through the pathways down through the spinal cord to the alpha motoneurons that control muscles of the body. Faults in the nuclei of the basal ganglia[30] can give many different symptoms and have been regarded to be the cause of many diseases of which Parkinson's disease is the best known and most common of these diseases. It affects 2% of the population over 60 years of age. The signs of Parkinson's disease vary from individual to individual with rigidity[50], slow movements and tremor as the most characteristic signs. It has been a general assumption that the symptoms are caused by degeneration of the nerve cells in one of the nuclei of the basal ganglia, the substantia nigra compacta, which produces dopamine, an important transmitter substance in the brain. It has therefore been assumed that the cause of the symptoms was a deficit in this transmitter substance. People with Parkinson's disease are treated with a substance, L-dopamine that supplies dopamine to the brain with good results, at least in early stages of the disease (see Chapter V).

Neural plasticity is involved in creating the side effects of the treatment with L-dopamine, when used for a long time in high-dose, by inducing dyskinesia (tradive dyskinesia[51]) [22].

10. THE ROLE OF NEURAL PLASTICITY IN AFFECTIVE DISEASES

Pain (and tinnitus) has both a sensory and an affective[52] component [116,44,73]. There is also evidence that plastic changes may be involved in causing the symptoms of some affective diseases such as depression. It is generally assumed that affective diseases are caused by abnormalities in a neural transmitter substance, serotonin, but attempts to correct such presumed defects have not had the beneficial effect that was expected [24].

Medications that are commonly used in treatment of depression, such as the selective serotonin re-uptake inhibitors (SSRIs, known under names such as Prozac, Paxil, Zoloft and many more) are supposed to correct a deficit in serotonin. However, these medications have been disappointing in that they have only had satisfactory beneficial effect in a few individuals with depression [30,40], perhaps as few as 5-10%. In particular, these

---

[49] Basal ganglia: A group of nuclei located deep in the brain that are involved in processing of commands from the motor cortex before they are sent to the spinal cord.

[50] Rigidity: *one type of increase in muscle tone at rest; characterized by increased resistance to passive stretch, independent of velocity and symmetric about joints; increases with activation of corresponding muscles in the contralateral limb. Two basic types are cogwheel rigidity and lead-pipe rigidity* (Stedman's Electronic Medical Dictionary, Version 7.0).

[51] Tardive dyskinesia: involuntary, repetitive movements manifesting as a side effect from use of medications such as L-Dopamine.

[52] Affective diseases: *a group of mental disorders characterized by a mood disturbance.* (Stedman's Electronic Medical Dictionary, Version 7.0).

medications seem to have little beneficial effect on mild depression [24]. These medications also have severe side effects, some of which may be related to the fact that serotonin is not only used as a transmitter substance in the brain and the spinal cord but serotonin is also found in many other parts of the body. The attempts to treat depression by medications that increase serotonin in the brain because studies have found serotonin to be low in depressed people has similarities to attempts to treat lower back pain by correcting anatomical abnormalities that are evident from MRIs (see page 120). The lack of success in such attempts show that symptoms are not necessarily caused by the abnormalities that can be detected. The causes of diseases are often more complex and factors such as plastic changes in function may be the real cause of the symptoms of many diseases.

While not denying that serotonin is involved in depression, it seems reasonable to suggest that the cause of such diseases are more complex than just an imbalance of a neural transmitter system. The suggestion that neural plasticity and other factors such as the immune system [118] and neurotrophic factors of various kinds may play important roles is likely to change the way these common disorders will be treated in the future.

A change has already begun in that some psychiatrists are beginning to use Omega-3, fatty acids, together with folic acid, a B vitamin and physical exercise for treatment of depression instead of medications that affect serotonin (SSRIs). Physical exercise cause an increase in brain derived neurotrophic factor (BDNF) [55] and that may be one of the beneficial effects of exercise. Some beneficial effects of complementary and alternative medicine (CAM) such as St. John's wart (Hypericum perforatum), S-adenosyl-l-methionine (SAMe), and acupuncture have been used [2] This is a sign of a change in not only how the diseases are treated but also in the perception which recognizes that the brain is malleable in many ways and that this can cause symptoms and signs of diseases including affective disorders.

There are indications of involvements of the dorsal and medial thalamus in affective diseases such as depression. Anatomical (autopsy) studies have shown that individuals with depression have 31% more cells in the dorsal and medial parts of the thalamus [155]. The report by Young and co workers [155] seems to be the first evidence that a psychiatric disease is associated with detectable structural abnormalities which means that there are significant anatomical and functional abnormalities in limbic circuits in a major affective (mood) disease.

The nerve cells in these parts of the thalamus have direct (subcortical) connections to many structures such as the amygdala and other nuclei that are involved in emotional reactions (see Appendix A). Nerve cells in the dorsal and medial thalamus project to secondary sensory cortices and association cortices, bypassing primary sensory cortices. This may be important in many diseases. That there are more nerve cells in these parts of the thalamus in individuals with depression than in those who do not have depression may suggest depression has similarities with disorders such as autistic spectrum diseases (see Appendix C).

Other recent studies have found a relationship between depression and cardiovascular diseases [56], which may indicate that the abnormalities in depression are more widespread and affecting not only a certain neural transmitter system of the brain (the serotonin system). Such wider views on affective disorders may open new possibilities for treatment and it would not be surprising to see further evidence of a role of neural plasticity in some affective diseases such as depression.

11. CHILDHOOD DEVELOPMENT GOING WRONG: DEVELOPMENTAL DISEASES

In other parts of this book, I have discussed the necessity of activation of neural plasticity for the developing organism and I have shown how activation of neural plasticity provides a "midcourse correction" of the organization and function of many parts of the brain that genetics has laid down before birth (see page 42, 62, 67, 86, 92, 111). This mid-course correction provides extensive modifications of the function and organization of the central nervous system. These plastic changes that normally occur in early childhood are in fact necessary for the development of normal functions as was discussed in Chapter III. A fault in the expression of neural plasticity that occurs during early childhood has been implicated in causing developmental diseases such as autistic spectrum diseases [99]. Similar faults in corrections of the function and the organization of the brain after birth may also occur in other developmental neurological disorders.

The symptoms and signs of autism spectrum disorders are described in Appendix C, which also discusses suggestions about the cause of these symptoms and theories of how failure to correctly activate neural plasticity during the first years of life may be the cause of the symptoms and the signs of the disease.

12. ADDICTION

I have earlier in this book postulated that activation of neural plasticity has a wider role regarding both beneficial and harmful effects than what is generally assumed. Addiction to substances of various kinds (including food) is one kind of disease in which neural plasticity may play a role. There is now research in progress that seems to show that certain kinds of addictions can be treated successfully by electrical activation of certain regions of the brain (in animals) [76]. Such treatment is generally assumed to activate neural plasticity or to reverse plastic changes that have already occurred. If such treatment is successful it would support the suggestion that some forms of addiction are plasticity diseases.

13. WHAT CAUSES PLASTICITY DISEASES?

Determining the *cause* of diseases becomes a matter of how one elects to define the word "cause". Intuitively, events such as diseases would have one well-defined cause but in reality this is rarely the case. I have earlier given examples where several factors must be present at the same time to cause a disease. In some diseases, none of these factors alone could cause symptoms. Determining the cause of a disease is therefore often unclear. In many instances, several conditions must be present at the same time to turn neural plasticity on in a way that causes noticeable symptoms and signs of disease.

Spinal dorsal nerve roots have been shown to be sensitive to mechanical manipulation causing pain [60]. Irritation of cranial nerve roots seems to be especially prone to cause changes of central structures. Examples are spasm in the face (hemifacial spasm) that can be cured by moving a blood vessel off the facial nerve where it enters the brainstem. However, as was discussed earlier (page 126), the neural activity that causes the spasm is not generated in the nerve where it is contact with the blood vessel as was believed earlier [50]. Instead it is generated in the brain (in the facial motonucleus) as a results of activation of neural plasticity [91].

The question is then what actually caused the symptoms (spasm and pain). Was it the contact between a blood vessel and the root of a nerve that was necessary for giving the symptoms or was it the changed function of the respective nuclei, or was it some other (unknown) factor that was necessary to produce the these changes in function?

Nevertheless the success of curing hemifacial spasm by moving a blood vessel off the nerve root indicates the close contact between a nerve root and a blood vessel is *necessary* for creating the symptoms [91]. The finding that many people have similar close contact between the facial nerve root and a blood vessel but no symptoms [138] shows that the close contact between a blood vessel and a nerve root is *not sufficient* to cause the symptoms.

The symptoms would only become present if two or more conditions were present, of which one was the close contact between a nerve root and a blood vessel [91]. The other factor is unknown, but since both (or all) factors are necessary it is sufficient to remove just one of the factors to achieve (complete) cure.

For the purpose of treatment it is convenient to regard the contact between a blood vessel and the respective nerve root as the cause of the symptoms because that can be remedied (by the microvascular decompression operation).

If lower back pain was caused by compression or irritation of spinal nerve roots one would expect similar exceptional results from surgical relief of the compression as of cranial nerves to treat hemifacial spasm and trigeminal neuralgia but vast experience shows that surgical treatment is not effective in treating low back pain.

That many diseases have more than one cause is a further complication for obtaining a correct diagnosis and this diminishes the likelihood of successful treatment.

13.1. Making a Diagnosis

A part of making a diagnosis[53] is finding the cause of a disease. There are many reasons why determining the cause of a patient's ailment can be unclear and ambiguous. We now regard all symptoms to have some kind of organic (biologic) cause although we may not be able to detect the organic abnormality, one reason being shortcomings in our arsenal of diagnostic methods. For example, we are well equipped to detect structural abnormalities but poor in detecting functional abnormalities. Some detectable changes may be missed because the tests are misinterpreted or because nobody specifically looks for certain abnormalities. (We tend to see only what we look for). This occurs more often than many would presume. When no cause can be found it has sometimes been regarded that the patient was outright malingering.

The term "functional disease"[54] has often been used to describe diseases caused by changes in function of the brain or spinal cord. Such diseases are sometimes referred to as psychiatric diseases. An example is "Munchausen's Syndrome"[55] (a patient who suffers from a deep seated need to be sick, without any gain) and other diseases that do not exist except in the mind of the patient. Many diseases are labeled "neurosis"[56] when no physical fault can be found for a patient's complaints.

13.2. When Does a Disease Start?

Most people will say that a disease starts when the symptoms appear. However, there are many diseases that do not produce symptoms in their early stages; examples are various forms of cancer. One reason is that there is a threshold regarding the ability of tumors to activate sensory systems necessary to give symptoms such as pain. Many of the diseases that affect the nervous system slowly do not give symptoms in the early stage of the disorder. One reason for that is the existence of *reserves*.

Symptoms do not appear before a disease has progressed to the extent where these reserves are used up. This is the reason why symptoms in many diseases do not become evident before some time after the disease process has started. Most parts of the nervous system (peripheral nerves, the spinal cord and the brain) have reserves, which means that a certain number of nerve fibers or nerve cells can be lost without any noticeable change occurs in function of most structures of the brain, spinal cord and peripheral nerves. If a disease slowly destroys nerve fibers, symptoms will not become apparent before the reserves are used up. For instance, young people have more nerve fibers in their peripheral nerves than

---

[53] Diagnosis: *"The determination of the nature of a disease, injury, or congenital defect.* Stedman's Electronic Medical Dictionary.

[54] The meaning of "functional disorder" is: *a disorder characterized by physical symptoms with no known or detectable organic basis,* according to. Stedman's Electronic Medical Dictionary.

[55] Munchausen's syndrome: *Repeated fabrication of clinically convincing simulations of disease for the purpose of gaining medical attention; a term referring to patients who wander from hospital to hospital feigning acute medical or surgical illness and giving false and fanciful information about their medical and social background for no apparent reason other than to gain attention.* (Stedman's Electronic Medical Dictionary, Version 7.0).

[56] Neurosis:

1. *A psychological or behavioral disorder in which anxiety is the primary characteristic; defense mechanisms or any phobias are the adjustive techniques that a person learns to cope with this underlying anxiety. In contrast to the psychoses, people with a neurosis do not exhibit gross distortion of reality or gross disorganization of personality but in severe cases, those affected may be as disabled as those with a psychosis.*
2. *A functional nervous disease, or one in which there is no evident lesion.*
3. *A peculiar state of tension or irritability of the nervous system; any form of nervousness.* (Stedman's Electronic Medical Dictionary, Version 7.0).

necessary for normal function and therefore some nerve fibers can be lost or injured without causing any symptoms. These reserves are gradually depleted with age and when totally depleted typical signs such as various forms of neuropathy will produce symptoms immediately. The depletion of reserves may be accelerated by various kinds of diseases. Also, age related changes start normally before any symptoms are present because of the natural reserves. Only when the reserves have been depleted will symptoms appear.

This means information about when a disease starts may be incorrect and attempts to find a cause of the disease by relating events that have occurred at the time the disease manifested by symptoms may be misleading.

An example of how the existence of reserves can cause misunderstandings comes from experience with poliomyelitis. Poliomyelitis caused different degrees of damage to peripheral nerves. In some the damage was light and only the reserves were affected. These individuals had no deficits after the end of the acute phase of the disease. When such people later in life acquired symptoms of lost function that were similar to those of more severe forms of poliomyelitis, people began to speculate the polio virus had not left the body. These late occurring symptoms can, however, better be explained by the effect of the loss of reserves that occurred during the acute phase of poliomyelitis that the persons had many years earlier. If that had depleted or reduced the reserves, losses that occurred later such as from normal aging will produce signs of neuropathy much earlier than in persons who have not had poliomyelitis earlier and lost their reserves.

REFERENCES

[1] Alexander GE, Moses H. Carbamazepine for hemifacial spasm. *Neurology*. 1982;32(3):286-7.

[2] Andreescu C, Mulsant BH, Emanuel JE. Complementary and alternative medicine in the treatment of bipolar disorder - A review of the evidence. *J Affect Disord*. 2008;110:16-26.

[3] Arnold LM, Russell IJ, Diri EW, Duan WR, Young JPJ, Sharma U, et al. A 14-week, Randomized, Double-Blinded, Placebo-Controlled Monotherapy Trial of Pregabalin in Patients With Fibromyalgia. *J Pain*. 2008.

[4] Auger RG, Whisnant JP. Hemifacial spasm in Rochester and Olmsted County, Minnesota, 1960 to 1984. *Arch Neurol*. 1990(47):1233-4.

[5] Baguley DM. Hyperacusis. *J R Soc Med*. 2003;96(12):582-5.

[6] Baloh RW, Honrubia V. *Clinical neurophysiology of the vestibular system*. Philadelphia: F.A.Davis Company; 1990.

[7] Barberá J, Albert-Pampló R. Centrocentral anastomosis of the proximal nerve stump in the treatment of painful amputation neuromas of major nerves. *J Neurosurg*. 1993;79(3):331-4.

[8] Barker FG, Jannetta PJ, Bissonette DJ, Larkins MV, Jho HD. The long-term outcome of microvascular decompression for trigeminal neuralgia. *N Eng J Med*. 1996;334:1077-83.

[9]   Barker FG, Jannetta PJ, Bissonette DJ, Shields PT, Larkins MV. Microvascular
        Decompression for Hemifacial Spasm. *J Neurosurg*. 1995;82:201-10.

[10]   Bernhard CG, Bohm E, Hojeberg S. A new treatment of status epilepticus; intravenous
        injections of a local anesthetic (lidocaine). 1955;74(2)::208-14.

[11]   Boden SD, McCowin PR, Davis DO, Dina TS, Mark AS, Wiesel S. Abnormal
        magnetic-resonance scans of the cervical spine in asymptomatic subjects. A prospective
        investigation. *J Bone Joint Surg Am*. 1990;72(8):1178-84.

[12]   Bonica JJ. Introduction: semantic, epidemiologic, and educational issues. In: Casey KL,
        editor. *Pain and central nervous system disease: the central pain syndromes*. New
        York: Raven Press; 1991. p. 13-29.

[13]   Boswell MV, Cole BE. *Weiner's Pain Management. 7nd ed.*: American Academy of
        Pain Management; 2007.

[14]   Brach JS, Van Swearingen JM, Lenert J, Johnson PC. Facial Neuromuscular Retraining
        for Oral Synkinesis. *Plastic and Reconstructive Surgery*. 1997;99(7):1922-31.

[15]   Brattberg G, Parker MG, Thorslund M. The prevalence of pain among the oldest old in
        Sweden. *Pain*. 1996;67(1):29-34.

[16]   Buck LB. Smell and Taste: The Chemical Senses. In: Kandel ER, Schwartz JH, Jessell
        TM, editors. *Principles of Neural Science*. 4th ed. New York: McGraw-Hill; 2000. p.
        625-47.

[17]   Bushnell MC, Apkarian AV. Representation of pain in the brain. In: McMahon SB,
        Koltzenburg M, editors. *Wall and Melzak's Textbook of Pain*. Amsterdam: Elsevier;
        2006. p. 107-24.

[18]   Cacace AT, Cousins JP, Parnes SM, McFarland DJ, Semenoff D, Holmes T, et al.
        Cutaneous-evoked tinnitus. II: Review of neuroanatomical, physiological and
        functional imaging studies. *Audiol Neurotol*. 1999;4(5):258-68.

[19]   Cacace AT, Lovely TJ, McFarland DJ, Parnes SM, Winter DF. Anomalous cross-modal
        plasticity following posterior fossa surgery: Some speculations on gaze-evoked
        tinnitus. *Hear Res*. 1994;81:22-32.

[20]   Campbell CM, Edwards RR, Fillingim RB. Ethnic differences in responses to multiple
        experimental pain stimuli. *Pain*. 2005;113:20-6.

[21]   Carlton S, Willis W, Jasmin L. Peripheral sensitization and inflammation: sensory
        nerves are a two way street. *Program and abstracts of the 25th Annual Scientific
        Meeting of the American Pain Society;*. 2006;May 3-6, 2006; San Antonio, Texas. Oral
        Session 304.

[22]   Cenci MA, Lundblad M. Post- versus presynaptic plasticity in L-DOPA-induced
        dyskinesia. *J Neurochem*. 2006;99(2):381-92.

[23]   Charabi S, Thomsen J, Tos M, Charabi B, Mantoni M, Børgesen SE. Acoustic
        neuroma/vestibular schwannoma growth: past, present and future. *Acta Otolaryngol
        (Stockh)*. 1998;118:327-32.

[24]   Chatwin J, Kendrick T, Group TS. Protocol for the THREAD (THREshold for
        AntiDepressants) study: a randomised controlled trial to determine the clinical and
        cost-effectiveness of antidepressants plus supportive care, versus supportive care alone,
        for mild to moderate depression in UK general practice. *BMC Fam Pract*. 2007;8(2).

[25] Cheetham C, Finnerty G. Plasticity and its Role in Neurological Diseases of the Adult Nervous System. *Adv Clin Neurosci Rehabil.* 2007;7(3):8-9.

[26] Coelho CB, Sanchez TG, Tyler RS. Tinnitus in children and associated risk factors. In: Langguth B, Hajak G, Kleinjung T, Cacace A, Møller AR, editors. *Tinnitus: Pathophysiology and Treatment.* Amsterdam: Elsevier; 2007. p. 169-78.

[27] Craig KD. Emotions and psychobiology. In: McMahon SB, Koltzenburg M, editors. *Wall and Melzak's Textbook of Pain.* Amsterdam: Elsevier; 2006.

[28] Crofford LJ. Pain management in fibromyalgia. *Curr Opin Rheumatol.* 2008;20(3):246-50.

[29] Dancause N. Vicarious function of remote cortex following stroke: recent evidence from human and animal studies. *Neuroscientist.* 2006;12:489-99.

[30] Das UN. Folic acid and polyunsaturated fatty acids improve cognitive function and prevent depression, dementia, and Alzheimer's disease—But how and why? *Prostaglandins Leukot Essent Fatty Acids.* 2008;78:11-9.

[31] De Ridder D, De Mulder G, Menovsky T, Sunaert S, Kovacs S. Electrical stimulation of auditory and somatosensory cortices for treatment of tinnitus and pain. In: Langguth B, Hajak G, Kleinjung T, Cacace AT, Møller AR, editors. *Tinnitus, Pathophysiology and Treatment.* Amsterdam: Elsevier; 2007. p. 377-88.

[32] Densert B, Sass K. Control of symptoms in patients with Ménière's disease using middle ear pressure applications: Two years follow-up. *Acta Otolaryng (Stockh).* 2001;121:616-21.

[33] Densert O. Adrenergic innervation in the rabbit cochlea. *Acta Otolaryngol (Stockh).* 1974;78:345-56.

[34] Doubell TP, Mannion RJ, Woolf CJ. The dorsal horn: state-dependent sensory processing, plasticity and the generation of pain. In: Wall PD, Melzack R, editors. *Handbook of Pain.* 4 ed. Edinburgh: Churchill Livingstone; 1999. p. 165-81.

[35] Eggermont J, J,. *The correlative brain. Theory and Experiment in neural interaction.* Berlin: Springer-Verlag; 1990.

[36] Eggermont JJ. Correlated neural activity as the driving force for functional changes in auditory cortex. *Hear Res.* 2007;229:69-80.

[37] Eggermont JJ. Pathophysiology of tinnitus. In: Langguth B, Hajak G, Kleinjung T, Cacace A, Møller AR, editors. *Tinnitus: Pathophysiology and Treatment.* Amsterdam: Elsevier; 2007. p. 19-35.

[38] Eisenhart-Rothe VR, Rittmeister M. Drug therapy in complex regional pain syndrome type I). *Orthopade.* 2004;33(7):796-803.

[39] Esteban A, Molina-Negro P. Primary hemifacial spasm: a neurophysiological study. *J Neurol Neurosurg Psych.* 1986;49:58-63.

[40] Fava M. Augmentation and combination strategies in treatment-resistant depression. *J Clin Psychiatry.* 2001;62 Suppl 18:4-11.

[41] Ferguson JH. Hemifacial spasm and the facial nucleus. *Ann Neurol.* 1978;4:97 103.

[42] Flor H. Cortical reorganisation and chronic pain: implications for rehabilitation. *J Rehabil Med.* 2003;41 Suppl:55-72.

[43] Forge A, Schacht J. Aminoglycoside antibiotics. *Audiol Neurotol.* 2000;5:3-22.

[44] Fredrikson M, Wik G, Fischer H, Andersson J. Affective and attentive neural networks in humans: a PET study of Pavlovian conditioning. *Neuroreport.* 1995;7(1):97-101.

[45] Fromm G. Medical treatment of patients with trigeminal neuralgia. *Fromm GH and Sessle BJ Trigeminal Neuralgia.* Boston: Butterworth-Heinemann; 1991. p. 133-44.

[46] Fromm GH, Sessle BJ. *Trigeminal Neuralgia.* Boston: Butterworth Heineman; 1991.

[47] Gallagher RM. Primary Headacher Disorders. In: Boswell MV, Cole BE, editors. *Weiner's Pain Management 7nd ed*: American Academy of Pain Management.; 2007.

[48] Gardner W. Crosstalk -- The paradoxical transmission of a nerve impulse. *Arch Neurol.* 1966;14:149-56.

[49] Gardner W, Miklos M. Response of trigeminal neuralgia to "decompression" of sensory root. *JAMA.* 1959(170):1773-6.

[50] Gardner WJ. Concerning the mechanism of trigeminal neuralgia and hemifacial spasm. *J Neurosurg.* 1962(19):947-58.

[51] Gardner WJ, Sava GA. Hemifacial spasm -- a reversible pathophysiologic state. *J Neurosurg.* 1962(19):240-7.

[52] Gerken GM, Hesse PS, Wiorkowski JJ. Auditory evoked responses in control subjects and in patients with problem tinnitus. *Hear Res.* 2001;157:52-64.

[53] Goble TJ, Farmer GE, Møller AR, Thompson LT. Acute corticosteroid administration alters place-field stability in a fixed environment: comparison to physical restraint and noise exposure. 2009.

[54] Goddard GV. Amygdaloid stimulation and learning in the rat. *J Comp Physiol Psychol.* 1964; 58:23-30.

[55] Gómez-Pinilla F, Ying Z, Roy RR, Molteni R, Edgerton VR. Voluntary exercise induces a BDNF-mediated mechanism that promotes neuroplasticity. *J Neurophysiol.* 2002;88(5):2187-95.

[56] Goodwin RD, Davidson KW, Keyes K. Mental disorders and cardiovascular disease among adults in the United States. *J Psychiatr Res.* 2008.

[57] Hitzelberger WE, Witten RM. Abnormal myelograms in asymptomatic patients. *J Neurosurg.* 1968;28:204-6.

[58] Hoffmann HJ, Reed GW. Epidemiology of Tinnitus. In: Snow JB, editor. *Tinnitus: Theory and Management.* Hamilton: BC Decker; 2004. p. 16-41.

[59] House JW, Brackmann DE. Tinnitus: surgical treatment. *Tinnitus (Ciba Foundation Symposium 85).* London: Pitman Books Ltd.; 1981.

[60] Howe JE, Loeser JD, Calvin JH. Mechanosensitivity of dorsal root ganglia and chronically injured axons: a physiologic basis for radically pain of nerve root compression. *Pain.* 1977;3:25-41.

[61] Jannetta P. Cranial rhizopathies. In: Yomans J, editor. *Neurological Surgery.* Philadelphia: W.B. Saunders; 1990. p. 4169-82.

[62] Jannetta PJ. Arterial compression of the trigeminal nerve at the pons in patients with trigeminal neuralgia. *J Neurosurg.* 1967; 26:169-2.

[63] Jannetta PJ. Hemifacial spasm caused by a venule: Case report. *Neurosurgery.* 1984;14:89-92.

[64] Jastreboff PJ. Tinnitus as a phantom perception: Theories and clinical implications. In: Vernon JA, Møller AR, editors. *Mechanisms of Tinnitus*. Boston: Allyn & Bacon; 1995. p. 73-93.

[65] Jastreboff PJ, Sasaki CT. Salicylate-induced changes in spontaneous activity of single units in the inferior colliculus of the guinea pig. *J Acoust Soc Amer*. 1986;80:1384-91.

[66] Jenkins WM, Merzenich MM, Ochs MT, Allard T, Guic-Robles E. Functional reorganization of primary somatosensory cortex in adult owl monkeys after behaviorally controlled tactile stimulation. *J Neurophysiol*. 1990;63(1):82-104.

[67] Johnson PC, Brown H, Kuzon WM, Balliet R, Garrison JL, Campbel J. Simultaneous quantitation of facial movements: the maximal static response assay of facial nerve function. *Ann plastic surg*. 1994;32:171-9.

[68] Katusic S, Beard C, Bergstralh E, Kurland L. Incidence and clinical features of trigeminal neuralgia, Rochester, Minnesota 1945-1984. *Ann Neurol*. 1990(27):89-95.

[69] Kingery WS. A critical review of controlled clinical trials for peripheral neuropathic pain and complex regional pain syndromes. *PAIN*. 1997;73(2):123-39.

[70] Kohama I, Ishikawa K, Kocsis JD. Synaptic reorganization in the substantia gelatinosa after peripheral nerve neuroma formation: aberrant innervation of lamina II neurons by beta afferents. *J Neurosci*. 2000;20:1538-49.

[71] Kreutzberg GW. Neurobiology of regeneration and degeneration the facial nerve. In: May M, editor. *The facial nerve*. New York: Thieme; 1986.

[72] Langguth B, Hajak G, Kleinjung T, Cacace A, Møller A, editors. *Tinnitus, Pathophysiology and Treatment*. Amsterdam: Elsevier; 2007.

[73] Lenz FA, Gracely RH, Romanoski AJ, Hope EJ, Rowland LH, Dougherty PM. Stimulation in the human somatosensory thalamus can reproduce both the affective and sensory dimensions of previously experienced pain. *Nature Medicine*. 1995;1(9):910-3.

[74] Levine RA, Abel M, Cheng H. CNS somatosensory-auditory interactions elicit or modulate tinnitus. *Exp Brain Res*. 2003;153(4):643-8.

[75] Levine RA, Nam EC, Oron Y, Melcher JR. Evidence for a tinnitus subgroup responsive to somatosensory based treatment modalities. In: Langguth B, Hajak G, Kleinjung T, Cacace A, Møller AR, editors. *Tinnitus: Pathophysiology and Treatment*. Amsterdam: Elsevier; 2007. p. 195-207.

[76] Levy D, Shabat-Simon M, Shalev U, Barnea-Ygael N, Cooper A, Zangen A. Repeated electrical stimulation of reward-related brain regions affects cocaine but not "natural" reinforcement. *J Neurosci*. 2007;27(51):14179-89.

[77] Lobarinas, Yang G, Sun W, Ding D, Mirza N, Dalby-Brown W, et al. Salicylate- and quinine-induced tinnitus and effects of memantine. *Acta Otolaryngol Suppl*. 2006;556.

[78] Lockwood A, Salvi R, Coad M, Towsley M, Wack D, Murphy B. The functional neuroanatomy of tinnitus. Evidence for limbic system links and neural plasticity. *Neurology*. 1998;50:114-20.

[79] Long D. Surgical treatment for back and neck pain. In: McMahon SB, Koltzenburg M, editors. *Wall and Melzak's Textbook of Pain*. Amsterdam: Elsevier; 2006. p. 683-97.

[80] Long DM. Chronic back pain. In: Wall PD, Melzack R, editors. *Handbook of Pain*. 4 ed. Edinburgh: Churchill Livingstone; 1999. p. 539-8.

[81] Lowry LD, Eisenman LM, Saunders JC. An absence of tinnitus. *Otol Neurotol.* 2004;25(4):474-8.

[82] Mattox DE, Reichert M. Meniett device for Meniere's Disease: Use an Compliance at 3 and 5 years. *Otology & Neurotology.* 2007;29:29-32.

[83] McCormick DA, Contreras D. On the cellular and network bases of epileptic seizures. *Ann Rev Physiol.* 2001;63:815-46.

[84] McMahon SB, Koltzenburg M, editors. *Wall and Melzak's Textbook of Pain.* 5th ed. Amsterdam: Elsevier, Churchill, Livingstone; 2006.

[85] Melzack R. McGill Pain Questionnaire. *Pain.* 1975;1:277-99.

[86] Melzack R. Phantom limbs. *Sci Am.* 1992;266:120-6.

[87] Merzenich MM, Kaas JH, Wall J, Nelson RJ, Sur M, Felleman D. Topographic reorganization of somatosensory cortical areas 3b and 1 in adult monkeys following restricted deafferentiation. *Neuroscience.* 1983; 8(1):3-55.

[88] Morgan DH. Tinnitus of TMJ origin. *J Craniomandibular practice.* 1992;10(2):124-9.

[89] Møller AR. Pathophysiology of tinnitus. *Ann Otol Rhinol Laryngol.* 1984;93:39 44.

[90] Møller AR. Hemifacial spasm: Ephaptic transmission or hyperexcitability of the facial motor nucleus? *Exp Neurol.* 1987;98:110-9.

[91] Møller AR. Cranial nerve dysfunction syndromes: Pathophysiology of microvascular compression. In: Barrow DL, editor. *Neurosurgical Topics Book 13, 'Surgery of Cranial Nerves of the Posterior Fossa,' Chapter 2.* Park Ridge. IL: American Association of Neurological Surgeons; 1993. p. 105-29.

[92] Møller AR. Vascular compression of cranial nerves. I: History of the microvascular decompression operation. *Neurol Res.* 1998;20:727-31.

[93] Møller AR. Similarities between severe tinnitus and chronic pain. *J Amer Acad Audiol.* 2000;11:115-24.

[94] Møller AR. Pathophysiology of Tinnitus. In: Sismanis A, editor. *Otolaryngol Clin N Am.* Amsterdam: W.B.Saunders; 2003. p. 249-66.

[95] Møller AR. *Hearing: Anatomy, Physiology, and Disorders of the Auditory System, 2nd Ed.* Amsterdam: Academic Press; 2006.

[96] Møller AR. *Neural plasticity and disorders of the nervous system.* Cambridge: Cambridge University Press 2006.

[97] Møller AR. Neural Plasticity in Tinnitus. In: Møller AR, editor. *Reprogramming the Brain.* Amsterdam: Elsevier; 2006. p. 367-74.

[98] Møller AR. *A new epidemic: Harm in Medicine.* Nova Science Publishers; 2007.

[99] Møller AR. Neurophysiologic abnormalities in autism. In: Mesmere BS, editor. *New Autism Research Developments.* New York: Nova Science Publishers; 2007.

[100] Møller AR. The role of neural plasticity. In: Langguth B, Hajak G, Kleinjung T, Cacace A, Møller A, editors. *Tinnitus: Pathophysiology and Treatment.* Amsterdam: Elsevier; 2007. p. 37-45.

[101] Møller AR. Tinnitus and Pain. In: Langguth B, Hajak G, Kleinjung T, Cacace A, Møller AR, editors. *Tinnitus: Pathophysiology and Treatment.* Amsterdam: Elsevier; 2007. p. 47-53.

[102] Møller AR. Tinnitus: Present and Future. In: Langguth B, Hajak G, Kleinjung T, Cacace A, Møller A, editors. *Tinnitus, Pathophysiology and Treatment*. Amsterdam: Elsevier; 2007. p. 3-16.

[103] Møller AR, Jannetta PJ. On the origin of synkinesis in hemifacial spasm: Results of intracranial recordings. *J Neurosurg*. 1984;61:569-76.

[104] Møller AR, Kern JK, Grannemann B. Are the non-classical auditory pathways involved in autism and PDD? *Neurol Res*. 2005;27:625-9.

[105] Møller AR, Møller MB, Yokota M. Some forms of tinnitus may involve the extralemniscal auditory pathway. *Laryngoscope*. 1992; 102: 1165-71.

[106] Møller AR, Pinkerton T. Temporal integration of pain from electrical stimulation of the skin. *Neurol Res*. 1997;19:481-8.

[107] Møller AR, Rollins P. The non-classical auditory system is active in children but not in adults. *Neurosci Lett*. 2002;319:41-4.

[108] Møller MB, Møller AR, Jannetta PJ, Sekhar LN. Diagnosis and surgical treatment of disabling positional vertigo. *J Neurosurg*. 1986;64:21-8.

[109] Mühlnickel W, Elbert T, Taub E, Flor H. Reorganization of auditory cortex in tinnitus. *Proc Nat Acad Sci USA*. 1998;95(17):10340-3.

[110] Myers EN, Bernstein JM. Salicylate ototoxicity. *Arch Otolaryngol*. 1965;82:483-93.

[111] Nielsen V. Pathophysiological aspects of hemifacial spasm. Part I. Evidence of ectopic excitation and ephaptic transmission. *Neurology*. 1984;34:418-26.

[112] Nikolajsen L, Jensen TS. Phantom Limb. In: McMahon SB, Koltzenburg M, editors. *Wall and Melzak's Textbook of Pain*. Amsterdam: Elsevier; 2006. p. 961-71.

[113] Norena AJ, Eggermont JJ. Changes in spontaneous neural activity immidiately after an acoustic trauma: Implications for neural correlates of tinnitus. *Hear Res*. 2003;183:137-53.

[114] Norena AJ, Eggermont JJ. Enriched acoustic environment after noise trauma reduces hearing loss and prevents cortical map reorganization. *J Neurosci* 2005;25(3):699-705.

[115] Österberg A, Boive J, Thuomas KÅ. Central pain and multiple sclerosis - prevalence and clinical characteristics. *Eur J Pain*. 2005;9(5):531-42.

[116] Price DD. Psychological and neural mechanisms of the affective dimension of pain. *Science*. 2000;288:1769-72.

[117] Price DD, Long S, Huitt C. Sensory testing of pathophysiological mechanisms of pain in patients with reflex sympathetic dystrophy. *Pain*. 1992;49:163-73.

[118] Rajkowska G, O'Dwyer G, Teleki Z, Stockmeier CA, Miguel-Hidalgo JJ. GABAergic neurons immunoreactive for calcium binding proteins are reduced in the prefrontal cortex in major depression. *Neuropsychopharmacology*. 2007;32(2):471-82.

[119] Ramachandran VS. Behavioral and magnetoencephalographic correclates of plasticity in the adult brain. *Proc Natl Acad Sci*. 1993;90:10413-20.

[120] Ramachandran VS, Hirstein W. The perception of phantom limbs. The D. O. Hebb lecture. *Brain*. 1998;121 (Pt 9)(Pt 9):1603-30.

[121] Rasminsky M. Ephaptic transmission between single nerve fibers in the spinal nerve roots of dystrophic mice. *J Physiol (Lond)*. 1980;305:151-69.

[122] Rauschecker JP. Auditory cortical plasticity: a comparison with other sensory systems. *Trends Neurosci*. 1999;22:74-80.

[123] Reed GF. An audiometric study of 200 cases of subjective tinnitus. *Arch Otolaryngol.* 1960;71:94-104.

[124] Robertson D, Irvine DR. Plasticity of frequency organization in auditory cortex of guinea pigs with partial unilateral deafness. *J Comp Neurol.* 1989;282(3):456-71.

[125] Rubinstein B. Tinnitus and craniomandibular disorders - is there a link? *Swed Dental J Suppl* 2003;95:1-46.

[126] Russell IJ, Bieber CS. Myofacial pain and fibromyalgia syndrome. In: McMahon SB, Koltzenburg M, editors. *Wall and Melzak's Textbook of Pain 5th ed* Amsterdam: Elsevier, Churchill, Livingstone; 2006.

[127] Saadah ES, Melzack R. Phantom limb experiences in congenital limb-deficient adults. *Cortex.* 1994;30(3):479-85.

[128] Saito S, Møller AR. Chronic electrical stimulation of the facial nerve causes signs of facial nucleus hyperactivity. *Neurol Res.* 1993;15:225-31.

[129] Saito S, Møller AR, Jannetta PJ, Jho HD. Abnormal response from the sternocleidomastoid muscle in patients with spasmodic torticollis: Observations during microvascular decompression operations. *Acta Neurochir (Wien).* 1993;124:92-8.

[130] Salt AN. Regulation of endolymphatic fluid volume. *Ann N Y Acad Sci.* 2001;942:306-12.

[131] Sandkühler J. Learning and memory in pain pathways. *Pain.* 2000;88:113-8.

[132] Sen CN, Møller AR. Signs of hemifacial spasm created by chronic periodic stimulation of the facial nerve in the rat. *Exp Neurol.* 1987;98:336-49.

[133] Sherman RA, Sherman CJ, Parker L. Chronic phantom and stump pain among American veterans: results of a survey. *Pain.* 1984;18:83-95.

[134] Shore S, Zhou J, Koehler S. Neural mechanisms underlying somatic tinnitus. In: Langguth B, Hajak G, Kleinjung T, Cacace A, Møller AR, editors. *Tinnitus: Pathophysiology and Treatment.* Amsterdam: Elsevier; 2007. p. 107-23.

[135] Simpson A, K,, Cholewicki J, Grauer J. Chronic low back pain. *Curr Pain Headache.* 2006;10(6):431-6.

[136] Snow JB, editor. *Tinnitus: Theory and Mangement.* Hamilton: BD Decker Inc.; 2004.

[137] Stangerup S-E, Caye-Thomasen P, Tos M, Thomsen J. The natural history of vestibular Schwannoma. *Otol Neurotol.* 2006;27:547-52.

[138] Sunderland S. Microvascular relations and anomalies at the base of the brain. *J Neurol Neurosurg Psychiatry.* 1948;11:243-57.

[139] Syka J, Rybalko N. Threshold shifts and enhancement of cortical evoked responses after noise exposure in rats. *Hear Res.* 2000;139:59-68.

[140] Szczepaniak WS, Møller AR. Evidence of neuronal plasticity within the inferior colliculus after noise exposure: A study of evoked potentials in the rat. *Electroenceph Clin Neurophysiol.* 1996;100:158-64.

[141] Taddio A, Katz J. The effects of early pain experience in neonates on pain responses in infancy and childhood. *Paediatr Drugs.* 2005;7(4):245-57.

[142] Tang NK, Crane C. Suicidality in chronic pain: a review of the prevalence, risk factors and psychological links. *Psychol Med.* 2006;36(5):575-86.

[143] Taub E, Uswatte G, Elbert T. New treatments in neurorehabilitation founded on basic research. *Nature Rev Neurosci.* 2002;3(3):228-36.

[144] Tetzlaff W, Graeber MB, Kreutzberg GW. Reaction on motoneurons and their microenvironment to axotomy. *Exp Brain Res*. 1986;3(Suppl,13):3-8.

[145] Tinazzi M, Zanette G, Volpato D, Testoni R, Bonato C, Manganotti P, et al. Neurophysiological evidence of neuroplasticity at multiple levels of the somatosensory system in patients with carpal tunnel syndrome. *Brain*. 1998;121(9):1785-94.

[146] Tyler RS. *Tinnitus Handbook*. Clifton Park, NJ: Delmar Cengage Learning; 2000.

[147] Valls-Sole J, Tolosa ES. Blink reflex excitability cycle in hemifacial spasm. *Neurology*. 1989;39:1061-6.

[148] Wall JT, Kaas JH, Sur M, Nelson RJ, Felleman DJ, Merzenich MM. Functional reorganization in somatosensory cortical areas 3b and 1 of adult monkeys after median nerve repair: possible relationships to sensory recovery in humans. *J Neurosci*. 1986;6(1):218-33.

[149] Wall P. *Pain: The Science of suffering*. Rose S, editor. New York: Columbia University Press; 2000.

[150] Weber H. The natural history of disc herniation and the influence of intervention. *Spine*. 1994;19:2234-8.

[151] Wolfe F, Ross K, Anderson J, et al. The prevalence and characteristics of fibromyalgia. *Arthritis and Rheumatism*. 1995;38:19-28.

[152] Wolff BB, Langley S. Cultural Factors and the Response to Pain: A Review. *American Anthropologist, New Series,*. 1968;70:494-501.

[153] Woolf CJ, Salter MW. Plasticity and pain: role of the dorsal horn. In: McMahon SB, Koltzenburg M, editors. *Wall and Melzak's Textbook of Pain*. Amsterdam: Elsevier; 2006. p. 91-105.

[154] Wu WJ, Sha SH, Schacht J. Recent advances in understanding aminoglycoside ototoxicity and its prevention. *Audiol Neurootol*. 2002;7(171-4).

[155] Young KA, Holcomb LA, Yazdani U, Hicks PB, German DC. Elevated neuron number in the limbic thalamus in major depression. *Am J Psychiatry*. 2004;161(7):1270-7.

Chapter V

TREATMENT OF PLASTICITY DISEASES

ABSTRACT

Correct diagnosis is necessary for success in treatment, but plasticity diseases are often difficult to diagnose. Few of the common plasticity disorders can be diagnosed by means of diagnostic tests currently available. Patient history is often the most important factor for obtaining a correct diagnosis. Another obstacle in obtaining a correct diagnosis of plasticity disorders is related to the fact that many physicians and surgeons are unfamiliar with neural plasticity as being a cause of symptoms. This is especially the case in connection with common diseases such as many forms of pain and tinnitus. Common diseases where activation of neural plasticity plays an important role, such as lower back pain, also have anatomical abnormalities such as broken spinal discs that are shown on MRI. However, these signs are often not causing the pain but are just common abnormalities occurring simultaneously.

Treatment options for plasticity diseases are often unconventional. Using medications that are used for treatment of epilepsy does not seem logical but has been found to be effective in treatment of many pain conditions. Moving blood vessels off cranial nerve roots for facial pain and spasm are among the most effective treatments known. Electrical stimulation of nerves (TENS) and more recently stimulation of the spinal cord and various parts of the brain have been found useful in treatment of some forms of pain and tinnitus. Stimulation of the vagus nerve is studied now and may become a valid alternative. Some of the treatments currently used for treating some forms of pain are also promising for treatment of depression and addiction.

Assessment of treatment progress is difficult because of a lack of objective measures. Testing of prospective treatments is hampered by the placebo effect, which is often misunderstood. It is evident that the placebo effect experienced in testing new drugs is a real effect but it lasts only a short time. Therefore, comparison of a treatment with a placebo for determining the usefulness of a drug is not a valid method for selecting a functional treatment.

In assessing the effect of a treatment, it is important to ask the patient the right questions. A patient may feel that pain or tinnitus is unaffected by a treatment but when asked the patient may admit that he/she now can sleep and do intellectual work again.

1. INTRODUCTION

Knowledge is important for having a good life. This is applicable when it comes to one's own body and its ailments. Understanding what is known about the function of the human body can help a person live better, and living a longer life. Knowledge and understanding is especially important when it comes to ailments and how to reduce the risk of acquiring ailments. A patient's understanding of his/her disease can often help to select the treatment that provides the most benefit or avoid treatments that have no benefit. The role of health care providers, be it physicians, surgeons, physician's assistants or nurses, should be that of consultants to the patient. The patient provides, of course, information about symptoms and observations regarding his/her medical problems. Nevertheless, the patients should also be knowledgeable about their own ailment so they can discuss treatment and give suggestions to their physicians and surgeons about which treatment (if any) would provide the greatest benefits with the lowest risks of complications. The incentives by the health care system to provide such insight are not great, and often factors such as hospitals' profit and physicians and surgeons' income play a role in the treatment advice given to patients. The risk of law suits is often used to promote tests of various kinds that may not be medically justified or providing benefits to the patient [63].

Many people expect their doctor to cure them either by prescribing a medication of by performing an operation. Only in the best of situations may a treatment completely cure a disease. On the other end of the scale are diseases where available treatments do not change the way the disease progresses. In the middle of this scale are treatments that can "manage" a disease and ameliorate the symptoms and signs of the disease and we will call that "managing" a disease. An important part of managing diseases such as central pain and severe tinnitus regards giving relief from suffering and helping patients cope with their diseases. As is common for most forms of treatment, we know very little about why some work in some patients and why the same treatment has no beneficial effect on a similar disease in other patients. The difficulties in affecting how a disease would have progressed without treatment are just a reminder that it is difficult to interfere with biological systems.

The wonders of medications are promoted by the pharmaceutical industry and supported by physicians and surgeons, often in agreement with economic interests of the health care system [63]. In the real world, medications (and surgery) have much less beneficial effects than believed and what is promised by the pharmaceutical industry in their slick advertisements. Physicians and surgeons often give their patients an overly optimistic outlook regarding the ability of medications and surgery to provide benefits, let alone cure diseases. The side effects of both medications and surgical operations are often much more severe than expected by the patients and what is disclosed by physicians and surgeons, and in particular, by the pharmaceutical industry.

People who are ill unquestionably ask: What made me sick? When a person is healthy knowing the risk of being sick is important– it is said that for example one in one thousand get the flu; getting the flu or not is a game of chance. When disease strikes an individual person it is no longer chance that rules, it is reality. If a person does not know the chance of getting a disease and gets it, then it is a surprise. And the next question to be expected would be: How can I get cured?

If one would ask what *could* cause illnesses a long list will appear; bacterial and viral infections, cancer of various kinds, bodily injuries, strokes, heart attacks etc. All these diseases have some clear physical signs; bacteria or virus are present, occlusion of blood vessels, cells that grow wild in cancer, or damage to various body parts.

There is one kind of diseases that are unlikely to show up in people's lists of diseases and their causes, and perhaps not even in most physicians' list of diseases. This is *plasticity diseases*. Plasticity diseases are caused by changes in the function of the nervous system. Changes in the function of the nervous system can occur because the brain and the spinal cord are *malleable*, which means that the brain and the spinal cord can change the way they function.

Activation of neural plasticity is involved in creation of the symptoms of many diseases that are now regarded to be of an unknown cause. Examples are some forms of common diseases such as chronic pain, tinnitus and various forms of muscle spasm. Activation of neural plasticity is also involved in rare diseases such as hemifacial spasm, spasmodic dysphonia, and spasmodic torticollis among others. Plasticity diseases are often incorrectly assumed to have other causes.

For treatment to be successful it is necessary to have a correct diagnosis – treating a patient for something he/she does not have does not benefit the patient, only cause risks of side effects. It is also helpful to know what caused the disease and what changes in anatomy and functions are associated with the disease. Finally, it is necessary to know how to reverse what caused the disease. This is a series of gigantic requirements that have been fulfilled for only a few diseases.

Poor understanding and lack of awareness of neural plasticity as a cause of symptoms and signs of disease contributes to incorrect diagnoses and inadequate treatments of many patients. Patients with plasticity diseases are often treated for a different disease than the one they have, or not treated at all.

As discussed in Chapter IV, plasticity diseases do not just affect one part of the nervous system but a series of different structures. The first thing to do when it comes to providing a cure for a plasticity disease would be to identify the structure that causes or has caused the problems or find the structure that controls the function that is not operating normally. Many parts of the brain or spinal cord may have abnormal neural activity because they receive faulty signals; it would not help to aim treatment at structures that behave abnormally just because they receive irregular signals from other parts of the brain or spinal cord that are affected by disease.

It is not an understatement that treatment of plasticity diseases implies a challenge to all health care professionals, be it physicians in many specialties of medicine and surgery, psychologists, physical therapists or audiologists. There are several reasons for that. Plasticity diseases, with a few exceptions, do not have objective signs and there are no tests that can help determine if a person has a plasticity disease. Plasticity diseases typically have different forms and very different degrees of severity. There are no tests available to distinguish between such different forms of a disease.

The fact that many individuals with plasticity diseases have symptoms but no signs that can be verified by tests is an obstacle because the practice of medicine is now centered on tests. It is generally assumed if something does not show up on a test it is not there and the patient must have imagined his/her symptoms. This is one reason why the reorganizing of the brain and the spinal cord as occurs in plasticity diseases, has received much less attention than diseases that have detectable structural and chemical abnormalities.

While it is known that change of life style often can be beneficial, medications and surgery are currently the preferred ways of treating diseases. People's, including physicians', seemingly unrestrained belief in medications and surgical operations is a hindrance in adequately treating many diseases especially plasticity diseases. Medications (pills) have been promoted by physicians and pharmaceutical companies but that kind of treatment is often ineffective and can have serious side effects. Patients' blind trust in someone with a medical license and in multinational pharmaceutical companies that bombard us with slick advertising hinders the use of simple and effective treatments.

Many diseases resolve without any treatment and symptoms of many diseases can be alleviated by change in life style - exercise and eating right and moderately. Plasticity diseases are not different in these respects. Unfortunately, many people find it much easier to take some medications than attain a healthy life style. Likewise, many people believe that an operation will solve all their problems but it often leads to great disappointment. Surgery is a brutal way of treatment that often has serious side effects and complications.

2. DIAGNOSIS OF PLASTICITY DISEASES

Earlier, physicians mostly relied on physical examination of the patient and in particular asked them pertinent questions. Physicians then also let the patient describe in detail what their problems were. This technique is now disappearing and the reliance on tests for diagnosing ailments of all kinds has increased dramatically.

Some diseases such a cancer, strokes, bacterial and viral infections, allergies, etc. have obvious signs which can be verified by known clinical tests. Many kinds of heart diseases also belong to this group. Many plasticity diseases such as central neuropathic pain and severe tinnitus that are caused by change in the function of the spinal cord and the brain have no signs that can be detected by the diagnostic methods currently available. This makes it difficult to diagnose plasticity diseases.

Plastic changes cannot be seen on imagining tests such as MRIs, and the changes cannot be evaluated by any commonly used clinical tests. Plasticity diseases often have ambiguous symptoms and signs and are often diagnosed incorrectly. Often different physicians arrive at a different diagnosis.

Pain and tinnitus have no visible signs and there are no medical tests that can reveal their severity or even confirm their existence. The first step in diagnosis of plasticity diseases is to listen to what the patient says. It is important that the physician understand that symptoms and signs can be caused by changes in the function of the brain or spinal cord that are not accompanied with structural changes that can be seen on MRIs or detected by other "objective" tests.

The fact that there are no tests that can show where the problem is located makes treatment difficult. Tinnitus is intuitively associated with the ear and is therefore assumed that there must be something wrong with the ear. This may be so for some forms of tinnitus but the more severe forms are caused by something going wrong in the nervous system. Central neuropathic pain is often referred to a certain location on the body although there is nothing wrong there. Instead, the pain is caused by something being wrong in the brain or the spinal cord. Treatment of the place where the symptoms are felt therefore has no benefit.

It seems natural to direct tests and treatment to the symptoms but it would be better to direct the treatment to what caused the symptoms. In diseases of neural plasticity this would mean first finding out what had caused the problems and then designing a treatment that could reverse what had caused the activation of neural plasticity. Such treatment would involve, for example, electrical stimulation of pain nerves in the case of pain and sound stimulation in the case of tinnitus. The results may likely not come immediately but when the treatment is repeated many times positive results are often achieved.

Incorrect diagnoses are often made and enormous expenses imposed for tests that cannot detect the cause of diseases that are brought on by activation of neural plasticity.

The imaging tests that are available cannot provide information about the ability of the connections between nerve cells to forward messages that arrive from other nerve cells. MRIs show coarse structure of the nervous system but do not show its fine structure. Trying to detect changes in function of the nervous system using MRIs is almost like trying to find out what a factory manufactures from looking at a picture of the building. (One can get some hints but no definite information from what is known as functional MRI (FMRI[57]).

Electrophysiological tests such as sensory evoked potentials[58] can provide some information about altered functions of some neural systems. These techniques are much better in assessing functions than MRIs, but electrophysiological tests also have many shortcomings. Electrophysiological measures such as evoked potentials that can be recorded in humans reflect the neural activity of many millions of nerve cells and therefore only indirectly reflect abnormalities in the function of individual nerve cells. Event related potentials (ERP[59]) are a kind of evoked potentials that are assumed to reflect perception of sensory signals. The different components of ERPs occur later than what is known as sensory evoked potentials.

This means that whoever is to evaluate the character, intensity and mere existence of such sensory perceptions as central pain and central tinnitus must rely on the patient's description. A physician will assess such symptoms by asking the patient to describe them. A person's description of experiences such as tinnitus and pain is not always objective and it may depend on other factors than the nature and character of the tinnitus or pain; the person's vocabulary and ability to express him or herself the person's current state of mind – happy or sad, etc. are all factors that affect how a patient describe his/her symptoms. This means a physician will get very different descriptions of symptoms that may have similar causes. Some have tried to circumvent these obstacles by having patients fill out written

---

[57] Functional MRI: Measure change in blood flow or blood oxygenation (BOLD)-fMRI, Blood-Oxygen-Level-Dependent fMRI). Its use in studies of function of different brain structures is based on the assumption that increased neural activity causes increased blood flow.

[58] Sensory evoked potentials: Electrical potentials that are elicited by sensory stimuli (sounds, light or electrical stimulation of nerves) to activate sensory regions of the brain.

[59] Event related potentials: Evoked potentials with long latencies.

questionnaires but this may add another uncertainty, namely the patient's ability to understand written questions and express him/herself in writing.

Nowadays, the patients' descriptions are often given to a nurse who then communicates it to the physician after editing and sorting the information from the patient. This "filter" of information the nurse provides many times leaves out important details and it cannot communicate nuances in a patient's description.

It is often said that the physician does not have time to listen to the patients – when it actually means the physicians do not take the time to do this very important part of a diagnostic workup. I have discussed these and other common problems in modern health care in a recent book [63].

Nowadays physicians tend to focus on the results of tests for making a diagnosis, less on symptoms and much less on the cause of the symptoms. Abnormal MRIs get more attention than symptoms although the abnormalities shown on the MRI may not be the "cause" of the symptoms. An example is abnormal vertebral discs, which are often found in patients with lower back pain, but individuals who have no symptoms whatsoever have similar abnormalities as discussed in Chapter IV, page 102). That means that the abnormal MRI findings may not be the cause of a patients' symptoms – just a coincidence, which is also supported by the fact that surgical treatment of the common lower back pain is often unsuccessful [53].

Frenetic search for objective signs of plasticity diseases such as pain and tinnitus can lead to harm and incorrect diagnosis because of misinterpretation of diagnostic tests and because most diagnostic tests have false positive results (signs of diseases when there is no disease).

The symptoms of some diseases that have been regarded as being caused by structural abnormalities are in fact caused by functional changes, which means that the diseases are plasticity diseases. One example is synkinesis[60] which often occurs when peripheral nerves have regenerated after injuries. When studies showed that the synkinesis could be successfully treated by exercise of facial muscles [9] it became clear that the synkinesis must have been caused by changes in function and not because of changes in structure.

Until recently, synkinesis after regeneration of nerves following injury to peripheral nerves was assumed to be caused by outgrowing nerve fibers (after injury) that did not find their correct (muscle) targets.

The abnormality that causes such symptoms as tinnitus and central neuropathic pain may not come from the place where the patient feels it comes from – instead the abnormal neural activity that causes the symptoms are generated in the brain without help from signals from the body. Think of pain in the foot. People would immediately think that there is something wrong with the foot, but the problem may be in the spinal cord or the brain.

Pain in an amputated limb [58] (phantom pain) and tinnitus [41] in deaf people including individuals with a severed hearing nerve are perhaps the most convincing evidence that symptoms such as pain and tinnitus may be referred to a different location than where the abnormal neural activity that causes the sensation is generated. Tinnitus is referred to the ear

---

[60] Synkinesis: *Involuntary movement accompanying a voluntary one, as the movement of a closed eye following that of the uncovered one, or the movement occurring in a paralyzed muscle accompanying motion in another part* (Stedman's Electronic Medical Dictionary, Version 7.0).

even in individuals whose hearing nerve has been severed, disconnecting the ear from the brain so that information from the ear cannot reach the brain. The tinnitus that such individuals experience can therefore not possibly be caused by something being wrong with the ear but instead it is caused by something going wrong in the brain.

Directing attention to the wrong anatomical structures is an obstacle in treatment because patients, their physicians and surgeons alike are tempted to direct their treatment to the location where the pain is felt, or in the case of tinnitus, to the ear. Such treatment can of course not benefit the patient; just cause aggravations and risks of side effects.

Symptoms that are felt at a different place than where the abnormality that caused the symptoms is located are more common than people normally believe and it is the cause of many incorrect diagnoses and unsuccessful treatments of many forms of pain and tinnitus.

Symptoms of plasticity diseases may occur a long time after the disease process has started. Symptoms of a disease that slowly destroys nerve fibers will not occur when the disease begins because destruction of the first few nerve fibers most likely does not cause any symptoms. Only after the *reserve* has been used up will symptoms appear (see page 94). The same is the case for nerve cells in the brain and the spinal cord. This all means that a patient's answer to "when did you first notice your problem" which most physicians will ask often does not tell when the disease really began.

3. TREATMENT OF PAIN

Despite being the most common cause for visiting the emergency room in the US, treatment of pain is generally inadequate. There are several reasons for that. Little is taught in medical schools about pain and its treatment. Consequently, the medical profession is poorly equipped to take care of patients with pain in general. Inadequate use of existing and effective medications to treat different forms of pain is common. Physicians may refrain from prescribing the most effective pain medication because of (often misunderstood and exaggerated) risks of addiction. Legislation makes it difficult to use effective pain medications such as opioids (synthetic substances that have morphine-like action) in adequate amounts [63].

There are many other reasons why so many people suffer unnecessarily from pain. Incorrect diagnosis prevents a correction of what causes the pain. If the cause cannot be reversed then the symptoms should be treated to relieve the person's suffering.

Albert Schweitzer said 1953:

To the millions of people in every country who live and die in needless pain:

"We must all die. But if I can save him from days of torture, that is what I feel is my great and ever new privilege. Pain is a more terrible lord of mankind than even death itself." from: Sacramento-el dorado medical society. Ad hoc committee on the treatment of pain - 1990

3.1. Medications for Treatment of Acute Pain

There are several medications available for treatment of acute pain. Depending on the severity of the pain, medications such as aspirin, ibuprofen, naprosyn and acetaminophen (also known as paracetamol, Tylenol) are effective and relatively safe medications. Nevertheless aspirin, ibuprofen and naprosyn have side effects such as a risk of stomach bleeding, best known from aspirin, which may also cause bleeding in other part of the body. (Aspirin should not be given to children under the age of 10 because of the risk of Rye's disease). Some individuals are allergic to any one or more of these medications. Paracetamol (Tylenol) has a serious risk of a side effect known as hepatoxicity (damaging to the liver), which is regarded to occur almost in everybody who ingests more than 4,000 mg per day [36,51].

Aspirin stops synthesis of a substance called prostaglandin, which is important for causing the typical signs of inflammation -- swelling, redness, etc. -- that is part of the body's reaction to harmful stimuli. Ibuprofen and naprosyn are so-called non-steroidal anti-inflammatory drugs (NSAID Aspirin, ibuprofen, naprosyn, etc.) because they also reduce inflammatory reactions. The NSAIDs above inhibit two enzymes known as cyclo-oxygenase 1 and 2 (COX1 and COX2). Only one of these (COX2) is important for inflammatory reactions while it is believed that COX1 is of value in protecting the lining of the stomach. Some time ago, so-called selective COX2 inhibitors became available (celecixib (Celebrex) and rofecixib (Vioxx). Experience did not support the assumption they were better and had less risk of stomach bleeding than older medications such as ibuprofen. In addition, these new medications turned out to have serious side effects in the form of increased risk of cardiovascular diseases, and they also gave allergic reactions in some individuals. New medications, etoricoxib and Arcoxia, (not approved in the US) that are the second generation of selective COX2 inhibitors have recently been developed. These are supposed to be more selective COX2 inhibitors than the older kinds.

3.2. Treatment of Chronic Pain

Chronic pain such as arthritis can be treated by similar medications as used for acute pain. In addition to these medications opioids such as Fentanyl and oxycodone (hydrocodone) are often used. Fentanyl is administered as a patch on the skin and oxycodone can be given as a pill. Opioids can create addictions, which makes prescription of these medications heavily regulated by law and physicians are often restrictive in prescribing them. The risk of addiction is often overstated and depends on how addiction is defined [63,82,94].

Use of opioids over a long period of time can cause hyperalgesia (increased sensitivity to painful stimuli) [2], which seems paradoxical that a pain reliever can cause hyperalgesia. This means that people who have used opioids type of pain relievers such as Fentanyl may acquire an increased sensitivity to pain. This is poorly known and people including physicians seem to focus on the addictive effect of opioids, which, as we have discussed earlier is very unlikely to occur [63]. These drugs also often cause tolerance, which means that their effect decreases with time and the dosage had to be increased to maintain a beneficial effect.

Many forms of pain have unknown causes and the treatment is inadequate. An example is the common low back pain. Even pain that has a known cause, such as pain from traumatic injuries, may still be difficult to manage. Little is known about the cause of such pain conditions as fibromyalgia and myofascial pain, and available treatments are only partly effective for curing the diseases or for reducing the symptoms. Tension headaches and migraines are in a similar group. A new kind of treatments using electrical stimulation of the skin that is innervated by the first spinal nerve (C2 dorsal root) by electrodes placed under the skin on the back of the head can decrease the pain from migraine and tension headache [19,85]. Electrical stimulation of the vagus nerve may offer benefits in pain management.

A particular form of pain, trigeminal neuralgia is unique in that it has several and rather effective treatments that last a long time (see page 179).

3.3. Treatment of Central Neuropathic Pain

Central neuropathic pain was discussed in Chapter IV. The pain in this disease is a phantom sensation similar to the phantom limb symptoms. Pain from any location and from any cause can develop into central neuropathic pain. The start is often an injury to peripheral nerves but often no cause can be found. Central neuropathic pain is a challenge both regarding diagnosis and treatment.

It is often not possible to eliminate central pain completely with the treatments that are currently available. However, the pain can almost always be reduced, often to a level where the person can have a reasonable quality of life. This is why it is more appropriate to aim at *management* of pain than at cure of pain. If that is clearly explained to patients it makes their expectations realistic. If, on the other hand, patients are given the impression that a cure is possible (freedom of pain) many will be disappointed and repeatedly be looking for other treatments.

3.3.1. Treatment with Medications

Different members of the opioid family of medications are common choices for treating central pain [74]. Side-effects, tolerance and possibly addiction are obstacles in long-time use of opioids but these are often exaggerated. Usually several other medications are used together with pain relievers such as opioids and paracetamol (Tylenol).

Medications that are not directly pain relievers such as tricyclic antidepressants and anti epileptic medications are effective in ameliorating central pain. Tricyclic antidepressants such as nortriptyline and antiepileptic medications such as gabapentin (Neurontin) and pregabalin (Lyrica) are now in general use to treat central pain (and neuralgia (page 118) and pain such as diabetes neuropathy page 95, 112, 117, 119).

Recently, several other medications have emerged as having beneficial effects on central pain. Ketamine, Tryptophan and Omega-3 fatty acids are examples of medications that were developed for other purposes but are now tried for treating central pain. Different kinds of NMDA (N-methyl-D-aspartate) receptor antagonists are also being tried.

It is known that a certain receptor for the transmitter substance glutamate, the NMDA receptor, is involved in neural plasticity and thereby in central pain. Using medications that are antagonists to the NMDA receptor would therefore theoretically be excellent candidates for treatment of central pain, but so far practical medications have not been developed. The best known attempt in this direction is probably the experimental medication, MK801 or Dizocilpine, which was developed a long time ago as an antiepileptic medication. It at first looked promising for use in treatment of diseases such as central pain, but it was later found that it had serious side effects such as being neurotoxic (damaging to nervous structures) and hepatoxic (damaging to the liver). The company that developed MK 801 has stopped further development of this substance.

Ketamine has similarities with the street drug Phencyclidine (PCP) and is also an NMDA receptor antagonist. Ketamine is used as an anesthetic in surgical operations. In lower dosages it has found use for treating central pain, used especially for treatment of Complex Regional Pain Syndrome (CRPS) type I and II (see page 123). It is available under the name of Ketanest.

Ketamine has a host of effects such as antidepressant, decreased central sensitization and by its NMDA antagonistic effects it increases the sensitivity of another glutamate receptor, the AMPA receptor, which may be what causes its beneficial effect on depression. The side effects of Ketamine naturally depend on the dosage in which it is given the most serious ones are hallucinations that may last for a long time. Ketamine and other NMDA antagonists are used as pharmacological models of schizophrenia.

Tryptophan is used as an adjunct to medications to treat central pain [77]. It decreases the tolerance that often develops when opioids are used to treat pain for a long time [37]. It also decreases tolerance to the antitussive (suppression of coughing) effects of opioids [45].

L-tryptophan is a precursor to serotonin (5-hydroxytryptamine). It is an essential amino acid (that cannot be synthesized in the body); it is readily available in most protein based foods and it is commercially available as a food supplement. People take tryptophan because it seems to induce sleep [38].

Omega-3 fatty acids (alpha-linolenic acid (ALA), eicosapentaenoic acid (EPA), and docosahexaenoic acid (DHA)) may be beneficial in treatment of central pain, although it has been difficult to find an effect when tried in population. Omega 3 has been shown to have a beneficial effect in other forms of pain such as inflammatory joint pain [30]. These substances have many functions; they regulate signal transduction and gene expression and protect nerve cells from death.

A study using rats [92] has shown that omega-3 enriched dietary supplements can protect against reduced plasticity and the impaired learning ability that occurs after traumatic brain injury.

3.4. Treatment of Neuralgia

Neuralgia are disorders of nerves that typically give sharp pain that is localized to particular regions of the body. Trigeminal neuralgia (typical face pain) is often used as an example of neuralgia but it differs in many ways from other kinds of neuralgias such as those caused by viral infections. Face pain has two forms, typical and atypical, both kinds have no known cause (but one of them, typical face pain, has effective treatments). Typical face pain is characterized by neuralgia symptoms, such as shooting pain in a certain region of the face on one side. Atypical face pain is characterized by constant burning throbbing pain in one side of the face.

3.4.1. Trigeminal Neuralgia

Although it has not been directly proven that trigeminal neuralgia (typical face pain) is a plasticity disease, there is strong evidence that the pain in this disease is caused by plastic changes in the trigeminal nucleus or other places in the brain. Before effective treatments were available, trigeminal neuralgia caused people to commit suicide, which tells something about the intensity of the pain. There are at least three treatments in general use for trigeminal neuralgia. The first choice is often medications (carbamazepine (Tegretol), phenytoin (Dilantin) and baclofen (Lioresal) [27]). The second kind of treatment consists of making a small lesion in the trigeminal nerve (rhizotomy) either surgically or by heat (from application of radiofrequencies) [83]. A variant of this kind of injury to the trigeminal nerve is injection of glycerol around the trigeminal ganglion [33]. A third kind of treatment consists of moving a blood vessel off the root of the trigeminal nerve (microvascular decompression operation, see page 179) [28,39,61] (for a review of the history of this operation see [62]).

The medications, namely carbamazepine (Tegretol) and phenytoin (Dilantin), are sodium channel blockers [27] and they are also effective in treating epilepsy. Other antiepileptic medications such as gabapentin (Neurontin) and pregabalin (Lyrica) are now in general use to treat trigeminal neuralgia and other forms of neuralgia such as from diabetes neuropathy. That these medications are effective treatments for trigeminal neuralgia support the assumption that the disease is a plasticity disease. Baclofen (Lioresal) is another medication that has beneficial effects on trigeminal neuralgia [27].

All three treatments aimed at the trigeminal nerve are very effective. Microvascular decompression operations completely cure the disease in as many as 85% of the patients [6]. The other treatments are about as effective.

There are no known effective treatments for atypical face pain, but medical treatment used for typical face pain can have some beneficial effect. Deep brain stimulation (electrical impulses applied to certain structures in the brain) is beginning to come into use also for treating trigeminal neuralgia that has failed other treatments [26]. Stimulation of the upper part of the spinal cord at the level of the second vertebrae (which has the first dorsal root where sensory information enters the spinal cord) is also effective in reducing the pain in atypical face pain and also in anesthesia dolorosa[61])

3.4.2. Diabetes Neuropathy

Diabetes neuropathy is associated with pain and tingling sensations together with reduced sensation of touch and also weakness. Diabetes neuropathy can be treated with some success by medications used to treat people with epilepsy, such as gabapentin (Neurontin) or its newer variations (pregabalin, Lyrica). This medication may be assumed to work on diabetes neuropathy by interrupting plastic changes somewhere in the chain of structures that behave pathologically. The medication does not cure the underlying disease, diabetes, which is the cause of diabetes neuropathy.

3.5. Treatment of Lower Back Pain

Lower back pain deserves a special mention because it is so common and because commonly used treatments are so ineffective -- in many cases they make the symptoms worse. Lower back pain is not normally regarded as a plasticity disease but as was discussed earlier in this book (page 102), it has many properties of a plasticity disease.

Lower back pain is often treated by surgical operations. However, it has been concluded that surgical indications for lower-back pain are in general ill defined [71]. In fact, many have worse pain after such operations and the problems often persist. This is in addition to complications that are always a risk in surgical operations.

The lack of success from common back operations often spurs new operations. It is not uncommon that patients have 3-5 operations only to find that their situation is just becoming worse. Only in well-selected patients, and after failure of conservative treatment, is surgery regarded to be justified [53]. Conservative treatment using medications and rest after an acute attack followed by increasing levels of exercise is far more effective and can often relieve the symptoms within 2-3 months [54,71]. Effective medications are pain relievers of the non-steroidal anti-inflammatory medications (NSAID). In more severe situations opioids such as oxycodone have a beneficial effect. Tricyclic anti-depressive medications such as nortriptyline and those used to treat people with epileptic seizures such as pregabalin (Lyrica) are effective in treating many forms of lower back pain (as well as many other forms of pain). The most effective remedy to bring people with lower back pain back to productive and enjoyable lives is to use several treatment procedures that work in concert with each other: medications, rest and exercise.

It has been questioned whether the routine of using MRI examinations of patients with low back pain is justified [89]. The structural defects that can be seen from examining MRIs may steer treatment in a wrong direction. That there are detectable abnormalities does not mean that these abnormalities cause the pain.

---

[61] Anesthesia dolorosa: an especially debilitating pain condition that consists of constant burning pain and numbness in the face.

3.6. Local Treatment

3.6.1. Electrical Stimulation of Nerves in the Skin

Transderm electric nerve stimulation (TENS) has been in use for many years for treatment of different pain conditions [90]. It is effective to treat many forms of lower back pain. The use of TENS is not beneficial to all individuals with pain and its use requires cooperation from the patient and proper adjustment of the strength and frequency of the impulses.

A device similar to a pager is connected to two or more electrodes placed on the skin and delivers electrical impulses. Electrical impulses applied to the skin activate nerves of the sensory system of the body (somatosensory system). The patient adjusts the strength to get a strong tingling sensation but not so strong that it becomes painful. Such electrical stimulation has an immediate effect in that it can provide inhibitory influence on pain cells in the dorsal horn of the spinal cord (see page 228). It also has a long term effect by promoting activation of neural plasticity that can counteract the changes in the function of the nervous system that cause plasticity induced pain such as central neuropathic pain.

3.6.2. Electrical Stimulation of the Spinal Cord and the Brain

Electrical stimulation of certain structures (the dorsal column) in the spinal cord has been used for some time in treatment of chronic and severe pain such as lower back pain [60]. More recently the repertoire of such stimulations has been extended to many different parts of the brain using different ways of applying the stimulation. The targets of such stimulation have been the thalamus [1] and regions of the cerebral cortex (premotor cortex) [59]. It has also recently been shown that electrical stimulation of the part of the cerebral cortex that receives signals from the skin and other parts of the body (somatosensory cortex) can relieve pain [17,19]. Some of these methods are also effective in treating pain that occurs after amputations (part of phantom limb syndrome) and other forms of pain that is caused by nerves that have been disrupted (de-afferentation pain). Electrical stimulation of the vagus nerve (the tenths cranial nerve) has also been shown to relieve pain in some individuals [49].

Electrical stimulation of the spinal cord and the brain has been done by implanting electrodes on the structure that are to be activated. Electrical currents can also be induced in the brain by strong impulses of magnetic fields applied outside the head. This provides a non-invasive way to activate structures in the brain. For that, a coil of wires through which a strong electrical current is passed is placed close to the scalp over the region of the brain that is to be activated (for a review see: [34]) (Figure 5.1).

The brain is not sensitive to magnetic fields but magnetic fields induce electrical currents in the brain. These currents can activate neural tissue in a similar way as applying electrical impulses through electrodes placed on the surface of the structures of the brain. Because magnetic stimulation is non-invasive, it can be used to test if electrical stimulation would be effective before electrodes are implanted [20]. Magnetic stimulation that induces electrical currents in the outer layer of the brain is one newly introduced method that has been used successfully to treat some forms of central neuropathic pain [17]. Similar methods are used for treatment of tinnitus [50].

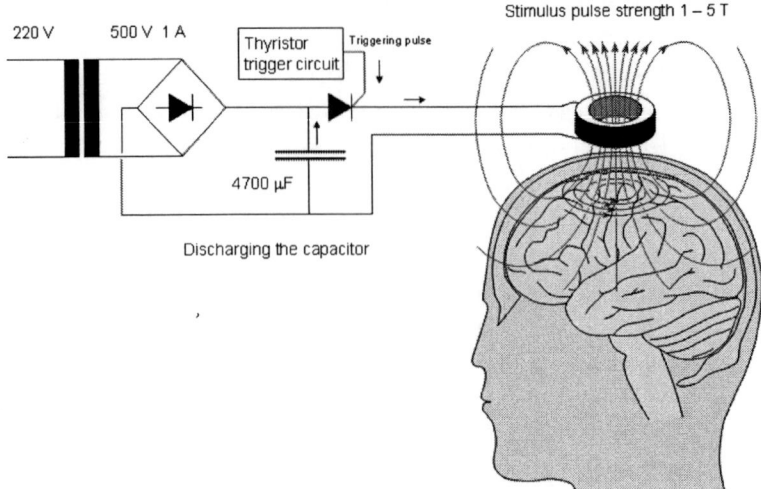

Figure 5.1. Description of how impulses of a strong magnetic field are produced. A capacitor is charged and then suddenly discharged through a coil of wire. This generates an impulse of a strong magnetic field. When the coil is placed close to the scalp, the magnetic impulse generates an electrical impulse inside the skull and that can activate structures in the brain. From Kleinjung, T., Steffens, A., Londero, A., Langguth, B. 2007. Transcranial magnetic stimulation (TMS) for treatment of chronic tinnitus: Clinical effects. In: Langguth, B., Hajak, G., Kleinjung, T., Cacace, A., Møller, A.R., (Eds.), *Tinnitus: Pathophysiology and Treatment, Progress in Brain Research* Vol. 166. Elsevier, Amsterdam. pp. 359-367 [50], reproduced with permission from Elsevier).

3.7. Treatment of Sympathetic Maintained Pain (SMP)

As discussed in Chapter IV, some forms of pain are increased by involvement of the autonomic nervous system. A certain kind of sympathetic maintained pain, (SMP), is now known as "complex regional pain syndrome" (CRPS type I and Type II). These kinds of pain were earlier known as "reflex sympathetic dystrophy" (RSD) and "causalgia", respectively. Treatment of complex regional pain syndromes is a challenge. It is often difficult to get a correct diagnosis because such diseases are complex. Not only is there involvement of the sympathetic nervous system but neural plasticity is also involved in creating the symptoms. Treatment with tricyclic antidepressants (amitriptyline or nortriptyline) and antiepileptic medications such as gabapentin (Neurontin) and pregabalin (Lyrica) are beneficial [14]. There are also indications that many pain conditions that are not regarded as SMP are worsened when the sympathetic nervous system becomes activated. Therefore, medications such as clonidine[62] can often decrease pain at the same time it reduces the elevation in blood pressure that may or may not be caused by the pain. This medication has remarkably few side effects and it has been in use for a long time so it effects are well-known. It is usually prescribed for reduction of excessive perspiration, such as in postmenopausal syndrome, and for high blood pressure, all symptoms of increased sympathetic activity.

---

[62] Clonidine: an α_2 adrenergic agonist.

3.8. Treatment of Fibromyalgia and Myofascial Pain

The relatively recent introduction of pregabalin (Lyrica) in treatment of fibromyalgia seems promising [3]. A combination of several medications has also been reported to have a beneficial effect. Pain relievers such as the non-steroidal anti-inflammatory drugs (NSAIDs), acetaminophen (Tylenol); tricyclic antidepressants (nortriptyline etc.) and other antidepressants (SSRIs) are also used. Only one medication (pregabalin, Lyrica) is FDA approved for treatment for fibromyalgia.

Some individuals with myofascial pain can get relief from local treatment of the trigger points [35]. Careful diagnosis of pain conditions such as myofascial pain is essential for successful treatment.

3.9. Prevention

Prevention is far more effective than treatment for many diseases. In order to prevent a disease from occurring (or rather more realistically, reduce the risk of its occurrence) it is necessary to know how a disease is induced and what internal factors are involved.

3.9.1 Treatment and Prevention of Phantom Limb Sensations

Some studies have indicated that the risk of phantom limb symptoms [70] can be decreased if neural conduction in the nerve that is to be severed is blocked by a local anesthetic before the limb is amputated [44], or by lumbar epidural blockade before the amputation [4]. Other studies have indicated that physical therapy can decrease the abnormal sensation of a phantom limb, including pain.

4. TREATMENT OF MOVEMENT DISEASES

Activation of neural plasticity is involved in some movement disorders, and that should be taken into consideration when treating such diseases. For example, there are indications that synkinesis that often occurs after injuries to peripheral nerves (see page 81, 99, 102) are caused by abnormal connections in the motonuclei, created through activation of neural plasticity. Earlier it was assumed that synkinesis that occurs after injury to peripheral nerves when nerve fibers (axons) have regenerated was caused by outgrowing nerve fibers not finding their correct (muscle) targets and connecting to other muscles instead. The finding that synkinesis can be treated by exercise [9] changed these concepts and provided strong evidence that the cause of the symptoms is activation of neural plasticity. These investigators showed that the unpleasant phenomenon of synkinesis of facial muscles after recovery from paralysis can be reduced or made to go away with by adequate training [9].

Rehabilitation from spasticity[63] that often occurs after spinal cord injuries has been difficult and various methods that have been used have had serious side effects. Some neurosurgeons, such as Dr. Marc Sindou, France, promote cutting parts of spinal nerve roots [79], which provide permanent relief of spasticity. This procedure requires experience and skill and many surgeons do not promote the method because it is technically demanding and it can have adverse effects. Since spasticity is caused by plastic changes in the function of the spinal cord medical treatments with medications such as baclofen (Lioresal) are also used to treat spasticity but the disadvantage is that the drug must always be taken and it has side effects.

Phantom limb syndromes may include symptoms of movement diseases. Some people with phantom limb syndrome may feel that an amputated limb is stuck in the wrong position. A study has shown that viewing an intact limb in a mirror help relieving the phantom limb symptoms [12]. The phantom limb syndrome also includes pain and odd sensations as discussed earlier in this book.

4.1. Physiotherapy

What we usually understand as physical therapy is active exercise. General physical training is beneficial for regaining physical strength and for maintaining physical fitness. Physical fitness enhances well-being in general, something that is needed during recovery from diseases and trauma more than anything else. It is indeed effective to regain strength and use of movement abilities that have been lost or reduced through diseases and trauma. There are a few situations where different techniques for rehabilitation are beneficial. For example, when one arm has weakness after a stroke or other injuries to the brain, it is beneficial to restrict the movement of the arm that is normal while training the arm that has weakness [84].

Electrical stimulation of the cortex may enhance neural plasticity during retraining of movement functions in stroke victims [10].

5. TREATMENT OF SEVERE TINNITUS

Progress in understanding how the hearing nervous system works has helped us better understand the forms of tinnitus that are plasticity diseases. However, still we do not know exactly how best to treat the many forms of tinnitus. It seems clear now that treatment of tinnitus must involve many different approaches and involve several specialties of medicine [32].

To illustrate some common problems in diagnosing and treating a person with severe tinnitus I will use a description of a fictive patient who is seeking medical help for her tinnitus.

---

[63] Spasticity: Increased muscle tension, involuntary contractions, exaggerated muscle reflexes, caused by problems in the spinal cord and the brain.

Mrs. Jones consults her general practitioner for ringing in one ear. She has had it for some time and it seems to be getting worse. The doctor looks in the ear but can see nothing abnormal and therefore refers Mrs. Jones to an ear nose throat (ENT) specialist who also looks in the ear and notes that the tympanic membranes are clear (which means they are normal). He orders a series of test such as an audiogram, acoustic middle ear reflexes, an MRI and some tests of the balance system at a cost of about $5,000. He also asks if she has worked around loud noise, which she has not, and he ask if she is on certain medication, also negative. The nurse who took Mrs. Jones into the examining room measured Mrs. Jones's blood pressure. Before the tests results were available the ENT specialist told Mrs. Jones that he had ordered these tests because tinnitus could be a sign of a vestibular schwannoma (a benign tumor on the balance or hearing nerve), which he explained was a kind of brain tumor. The doctor took no notice of her slightly elevated blood pressure. He knows that the test is not reliable because as always, the nurse measured her blood pressure immediately after Mrs. Jones sat down in the examining room instead of waiting 5 minutes, as should be the rule.

The MRI came back normal and Mrs. Jones was relieved after having lived through days of fear thinking she may have a "brain tumor". The ENT doctor tells Mrs. Jones that there is nothing wrong with her ear and her brain; he has seen her audiogram and looked at the MRI. The doctor also tells Mrs. Jones not to drink coffee and alcohol and have no salt in her food. Mrs. Jones follows his advice but it has no effect on her tinnitus, but continues with these restrictions because the doctor has told her so. Again, Mrs. Jones thinks it over. Is she really hearing anything or is she perhaps crazy? She decided to go to another specialist, a neurologist. The neurologist did the tests a neurologist normally does, independent of the patient's symptoms, namely reflexes, looks in the bottom of her eye for signs of increased pressure in the head. The neurologist also ordered an MRI, again, at a substantial cost. These tests also came out normal and the neurologist told Mrs. Jones that there was nothing wrong with her. She should just go home and enjoy her life. Mrs. Jones had difficultly sleeping because of her tinnitus and she could not concentrate on intellectual tasks. Now the question again arose for Mrs. Jones: Was she crazy, or did she perhaps have a psychiatric disease? She had heard that people with schizophrenia hear voices, so maybe that was what she had. She made an appointment with a psychiatrist, who talked with her but did not order any tests because that is not what psychiatrists do. However, the psychiatrist asked her to come back for several more office visits. After several often lengthy consultations, the psychiatrist came to the conclusion that Mrs. Jones did not have schizophrenia or any other psychiatric disease. The psychiatrist did not know why she had tinnitus.

So what was causing Mrs. Jones' tinnitus? She did not have a vestibular schwannoma[64], which is a benign growth on the balance nerve (and sometimes on the hearing nerve). Instead, she had a disease that was caused by plastic changes in the function of some parts of the brain; we call it central tinnitus. This is a plasticity disease that has many similarities with other plasticity diseases such as central neuropathic pain.

---

[64] Vestibular schwannoma is not cancer and therefore should not deserve to be called a brain tumor -- it grows very slowly but if it gets too big it must be removed. Here is the root of a common misunderstanding: Almost all individuals who have a vestibular schwannoma have tinnitus, but that does not imply that a person with tinnitus has a vestibular schwannoma. In fact, very few people with tinnitus have a vestibular schwannoma.

Mrs. Jones' symptoms and attempts to get a diagnosis were hypothetical, but it is a typical example of what often happens not only to people with tinnitus but also to people with other plasticity diseases. During a time when Ms. Jones' tinnitus just gets worse she had four different specialists' testimonies that there was nothing wrong with her. None of her physicians mentioned neural plasticity. The only one who had any suggestions about how to alleviate her tinnitus was the one who thought she should not drink coffee or alcohol and not eat salt. It did not have any beneficial effect, but the physician had not told her stop the "treatment" if it had no effect on her tinnitus so she continued to deprive herself of some things she enjoyed.

5.1. Why Did Mrs. Jones Not Find Help for her Tinnitus?

So why did these specialists not find anything wrong with Ms. Jones? There should have been no doubt that something was not right with her. There are at least two reasons why these physicians did not identify the problem. One is that at least one of them (the ENT specialist) looked in the wrong place for the problem. While Mrs. Jones referred her problems to the ear (she heard sounds) the abnormality was not in the ear but in her brain. Why did the other two specialists not find anything wrong despite their specialties were diseases of the nervous system? One of the tests they used was the MRI, but that only shows certain abnormalities in the structure of the brain – it does not detect abnormalities in the function of the nervous system. The tool (the MRI) used both by the ENT surgeon and the neurologist produces beautiful pictures that are truly seductive and give a great impression of confidence. There are many serious abnormalities that do not show up in these beautiful pictures of the brain.

The neurologist who looked for abnormalities in reflexes, etc. searched in the wrong parts of the nervous system. The psychiatrist examined high brain functions, again the wrong part of the brain, and in these parts of the brain everything was functioning normally. Therefore, examining the wrong part of the brain was one of reasons these two specialists did not find out what was the cause of Ms Jones' tinnitus.

Despite not finding out what was wrong, one of these specialists anyhow prescribed a treatment, namely refraining from coffee, alcohol and salt. The treatment does not reverse the plastic changes that cause the kind of tinnitus Mrs. Jones had and therefore had no beneficial effect -- just deprived the good lady from the pleasure of things she enjoyed.

Looking at the wrong place of the body, looking for the wrong things and using the wrong tools to diagnose Mrs. Jones' tinnitus made these specialists miss both where in the body the problems were located and what was wrong.

It should be obvious from this example that one has to know where to look and what to look for in order to see something is wrong. These specialists did neither. If they had listened carefully to Mrs. Jones's description of her problems instead of using expensive tools such as MRI they would most likely have arrived at the correct diagnosis and it would have been much less expensive. Prescribing treatment (refraining from coffee and alcohol) without having a diagnosis is not likely to benefit any patient.

Unfortunately, this is rather common in todays medicine: Many expensive tests but no treatment, and often not even a diagnosis [63].

5.2. Medications

Many different medications have been tried for treatment of tinnitus but only in a few individuals have medications had any noticeable beneficial effect [15]. Since most forms of tinnitus are assumed to be caused by hyperactivity (more activity than normal) in the nervous system, medications that would increase inhibition in the nervous systems have been tried. Consequently medications such as benzodiazepines (Xanex, Valium, Klonopin etc.), that are $GABA_A$ receptor agonists and therefore increase inhibition, have been tried, but unfortunately only a few tinnitus patients have experienced any benefit from taking such medications.

The only medication that has shown a beneficial effect in many patients with tinnitus is Lidocain [57], a local anesthetic medication that can only be administrated intravenously and therefore does not offer a practical treatment option. A medication, Tocainide [22], which can be taken as a pill was supposed to have similar effect as Lidocain but it was a failure for treatment of tinnitus. Its beneficial effect was limited and its side effects could not be tolerated.

5.3. Surgery

Some individuals have so severe tinnitus that seems to stem from one ear that they would rather be deaf in that ear than have the tinnitus. A few such individuals have had their hearing nerve cut, which naturally caused deafness in the ear and it has given some individuals relief from the tinnitus [73] indicating that the cause has been in the ear in these individuals. In most people with tinnitus, however, cutting the hearing nerve causes tinnitus in itself and therefore, cutting the hearing nerve is rarely if ever done anymore as a form of treatment.

5.4. Electrical Stimulation of the Skin

The obvious treatment for plasticity diseases is to reverse the changes that have occurred by activation of neural plasticity. Several investigators have shown that electrical stimulation of the skin can change the way tinnitus is perceived. Some investigators have placed electrodes on the skin behind the ears [76] for electrical stimulation. Others have placed electrodes on the wrist to stimulate a nerve (the median nerve) that carry signals from receptors in the skin [65]. In some individuals such stimulation decreases the intensity of the tinnitus and in some it increases the tinnitus. In others electrical stimulation changes the character of the tinnitus and in some it does not affect the tinnitus at all [65]. This is again an indication that tinnitus can be several different diseases.

5.5. Sound

Certain sound stimulation in connection with counseling (Tinnitus Retraining Therapy (TRT) [42,43] can have beneficial effects on tinnitus. Similar treatments were described by Dr. Richard Tyler [86,87]. This is a further example of how appropriate sensory stimulation can alleviate some symptoms of a plasticity disease. Since deprivation of sensory signals can activate neural plasticity, silence can cause tinnitus or make tinnitus worse in people who have the disease. People with tinnitus should avoid silence even if exposure to sounds is unpleasant.

5.6. Hearing Aids and Cochlear Implants

That silence is a strong promoter of tinnitus may explain why hearing loss can cause tinnitus. Hearing aids can therefore be beneficial in some individuals with hearing loss who have tinnitus [21], because hearing aids compensate for the decrease in signals from the ear to the hearing nervous system caused by hearing loss. In a similar way, some deaf individuals who have tinnitus benefit from cochlear implants, which stimulate hearing nerve fibers electrically and thereby provide activation of the hearing nervous system [5].

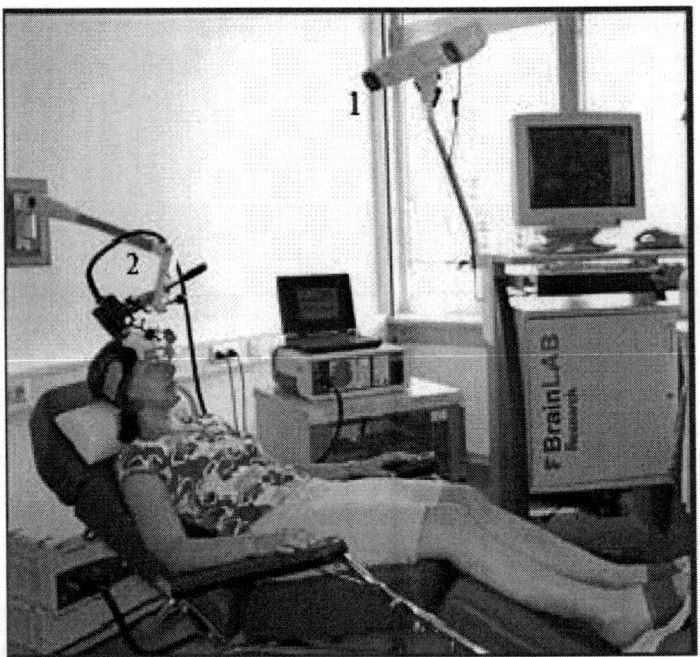

Figure 5.2. Setup used for stimulating regions of the brain with electrical impulses that are induced by impulses of a strong magnetic field (see Figure 5.1). (Reproduced from Kleinjung, T., Steffens, A., Londero, A., Langguth, B. 2007. Transcranial magnetic stimulation (TMS) for treatment of chronic tinnitus: Clinical effects. In: Langguth, B., Hajak, G., Kleinjung, T., Cacace, A., Møller, A.R., (Eds.), *Tinnitus: Pathophysiology and Treatment, Progress in Brain Research* Vol. 166. Elsevier, Amsterdam. pp. 359-367, reproduced with permission from Elsevier [50]).

5.7. Electrical Stimulation of the Brain

Like in treatment of central pain, electrical stimulation of certain regions of the brain is beginning to be used for treatment of tinnitus [18]. Not all individuals with tinnitus benefit from such electrical stimulation; therefore, before implantation of electrodes on the brain for magnetic stimulation, a noninvasive method (see page 181) is used to test if electrical stimulation will benefit the patient [18]. Other investigators have used similar impulses of a strong magnetic field applied through the intact scalp to induce electrical currents in the brain for treatment of tinnitus [50] (see Figure 5.2).

5.8. Prevention of Tinnitus

Since many people get tinnitus (and hearing loss) after exposure to loud sound, one way of reducing the risk of tinnitus is to avoid exposure to loud sounds. Not everybody who is exposed to loud sounds gets tinnitus, but it is not possible to know who will get it and who will not. Medications such as certain antibiotics and cytostatics used in treatment of cancer can also cause tinnitus and hearing loss [25].

Silence and exposure to strong sounds can cause changes in the connections in the brain through activation of neural plasticity and some such changes may cause (central) tinnitus. It is therefore important to avoid silence; studies have shown the benefit of an "augmented acoustic environment" [72,91]. The finding that exposure to sounds of moderate intensity can reduce the risk of hearing loss from exposure to loud noise [72] should further encourage people to avoid silence.

6. TREATMENT OF CRANIAL NERVE DISORDERS

There is a group of diseases that can be cured by moving a blood vessel off the root of cranial nerves. Especially three disorders have very effective treatment in that way. They were mentioned in Chapter IV and are first of all hemifacial spasm and trigeminal neuralgia, but also glossopharyngeal neuralgia and some forms of balance disorders (dizziness), known as disabling positional vertigo (DPV) and some forms of tinnitus. These diseases, except hemifacial spasm can also be treated with some success by medical treatment.

6.1. Surgical Treatment

Microvascular decompression operations consists of moving a blood vessel (often an artery but it can also be a vein) off the root of the respective cranial nerve, cranial nerve V, the trigeminal nerve, for trigeminal neuralgia (typical face pain), the seventh cranial nerve, the facial nerve for hemifacial spasm (face spasm), the ninth cranial nerve for glossopharyngeal neuralgia and the eighth cranial nerve for disabling positional vertigo (balance disorder) and for tinnitus (hearing disorders). All these four cranial nerves are located in the angle between the cerebellum and the part of the brainstem known as the pons, a part of the brainstem.

The rate of cure from microvascular decompression operations is high, for trigeminal neuralgia and hemifacial spasm it is about 85% as documented in larger studies [6,7].

Moving a blood vessel off the intracranial portion of the balance nerve can effectively cure individuals with disabling positional vertigo (DPV) [40,66,67] (Figure 5.3).

In a study of 207 patients with disabling positional vertigo who underwent microvascular decompression operations of their balance nerve [68] 79% were free of symptoms or markedly improved after the operation. This is a similar cure rate as that of face pain and face spasm.

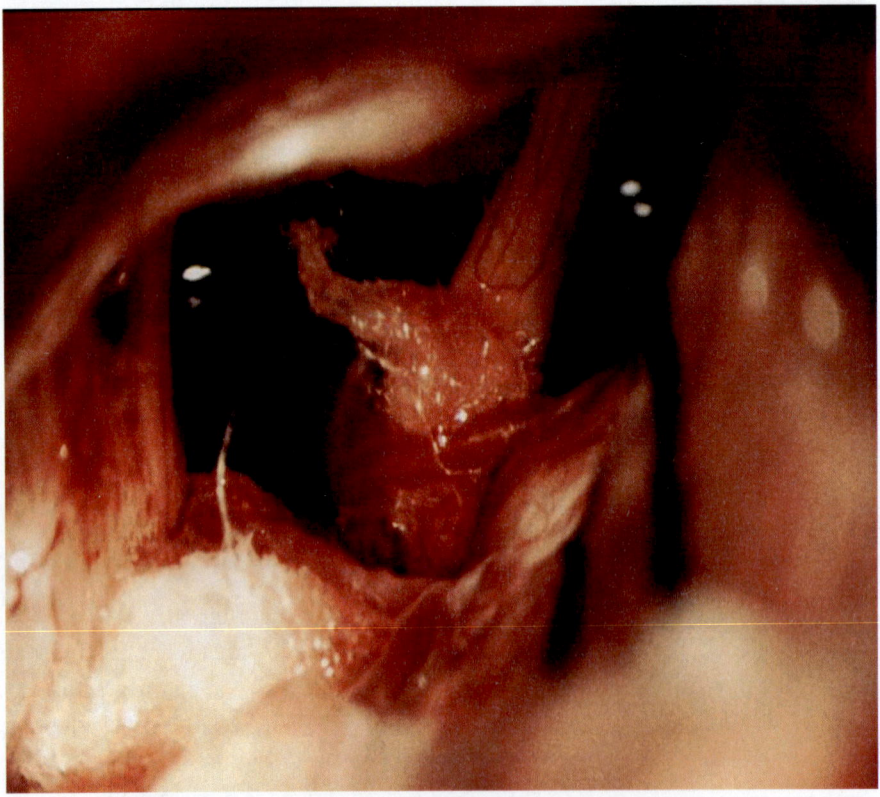

Figure 5.3. The hearing and balance nerve photographed in an operation to treat disabling positional vertigo, showing the hearing and balance nerve with blood vessels in contact and with an implant of shredded Teflon felt to hold the vessel off the nerve.

Microvascular decompression operations of the hearing nerve are also in use for treating some forms of tinnitus but the results are not as good as for treating the balance nerve [64,67]. Only individuals with certain forms of tinnitus can benefit from microvascular decompression of the hearing nerve, and having the correct diagnosis is therefore very important. Individuals who have had their tinnitus for a long time is less likely to benefit from the operation.

A study of 72 patients [67] with severe tinnitus showed that 18.2% had total relief of their tinnitus, 22.2% marked improvement, 8% slight improvement, and 45.8% had no improvement. The results were best for patients who had had their tinnitus in less than 3 years. There was a large difference in the success of this operation for men and women. For women 55% had total or partial relief from their tinnitus while only 29% of men. The operation involving the hearing nerve has a high risk of being damaged in such operations and the surgical damage can cause both hearing loss and tinnitus, which means that the operation can even make the patient's situation worse than it was before the operation.

6.2. Medical Treatment

Trigeminal neuralgia can be treated successfully at least in its early stages, by carbamacepine (Tegretol), a sodium channel blocker that is also used for treatment of epilepsy [27]. There is no known medical treatment for hemifacial spasm. Some patients with disabling positional vertigo can be treated successfully by a small dosage of diazepam (Valium).

7. TREATMENT OF DEPRESSION AND DEMENTIA

Medications that manipulate neural transmitters or change the sensitivity of their receptors are commonly used for treatment of diseases of the brain such as depression, anxiety, and schizophrenia. The belief is that these diseases are caused by fault in certain neural transmitters or their receptors. However, the faults could also be in the connections between nerve cells -- the efficacy of synapses or lack of pruning of connections and programmed cell death. There are indications that activation of neural plasticity is involved in some forms of depression and at least in some forms of dementia. Plastic changes in the brain may explain some of the memory loss which is a typical symptom of dementia.

7.1. Depression

Excess of nerve cells in certain parts of the brain is believed to be involved in causing the symptoms of autism (see Appendix C) and it has recently been found that depression is also associated with more nerve cells than normal in a certain part of the brain [93]. The abundance of cells may be caused by lack of normal pruning and lack of programmed cell deaths. It is possible that these abnormalities may be involved in causing depression or the abnormalities may be a result of other abnormalities. It is difficult to distinguish between cause and effect of observed abnormalities.

The assumption that activation of neural plasticity is involved in depression is supported by the recent experience of treatment of depression using strong magnetic impulses applied to the brain [24]. Such impulses induce electrical currents in the brain that activate nerve cells (see page 182). It is known from other studies that electrical impulses when applied to certain regions of the brain can affect neural plasticity. It has also been shown recently that electrical impulses applied to one of the twelve cranial nerves, the vagus nerve, has beneficial effect on depression [24].

The traditional concept regarding the cause of depression has been that something was wrong with a chemical transmitters system in the brain, especially the serotonin system, and to some extent the noradrenalin system. The common treatment has therefore been directed to correct such imbalance in especially the serotonin system. The common medication for that have been the so-called selective serotonin re-uptake inhibitors (SSRIs) (Prozac, Paxil etc.). It has, however, become evident that these medications are only beneficial in a few individuals. They especially seem to have little or no beneficial effect on less severe incidences of depression [13]. This is why there are now efforts to find other ways to treat depression. The use of magnetic stimulation of certain regions of the brain and electrical impulses applied to the vagus nerve are examples of such new treatments [24].

People with depression seem to have a greater risk of diseases that affect the heart and blood vessels. It has therefore been assumed that these two kinds of diseases may have common factors (see Chapter IV) and may possibly be treated with similar medications. That individuals with depression have an increased risk of cardiovascular disorders has been associated with a omega 3 fatty acid deficiency and elevated homocystein levels [78]. These observations have inspired development of new ways to treat depression. For example, some physicians now prescribe Omega-3 fatty acids for patients with depression, together with folic acid [23], which is important for the body's use of Omega-3 fatty acids. Administration of omega-3 fatty acids and folic acid in treatment of depression also reduce the risk of cardiovascular disorders and age related disorders such as Alzheimer's disease [56].

The balance between Omega-3 and Omega-6 fatty acids is important because these two fatty acids interact and compete for the same enzymes. The eicosanoids produced by Omega-6 fatty acids promote inflammation, platelet clotting and the productions of prostaglandins – all factors that are regarded to increase the risk of not only heart diseases and other vascular diseases but potentially some disorders of the nervous system as well. The eicosanoids produced by Omega-3 fatty acids have the opposite effect, namely acting against inflammation and decreasing the ability of platelets to stick together, which means lowering the risks of cardiovascular diseases and some diseases of the nervous system. The dosage of Omega-3 recommended for people with high triglycerides is now 2-4 grams per day [81].

Both statins and Omega-3 reduces the risks of some diseases of the heart and blood vessels (artherosclerosis) but combined they have better effects than either one alone. High consumption of fish also reduced deaths in cardiac arrhythmia [78].

These fatty acids do not have any known side effects but it is a concern that some of the available preparations may be contaminated with varying amounts of environmental substances. Organic mercury compounds such as methyl mercury, MeHg and polychlorinated biphenyls (PCB) are now present in many fishes and most likely also in fish oil supplements available in capsules [56]. (PCB has multiple effects, including effects on development of the nervous system, before birth [47], see page 245). It might therefore be better to use purified fish oil (capsules) although there is an intuitive preference for "natural" products instead of supplements. The intuition that natural products are better than artificial or synthetic ones is often wrong. It is frequently stated that it is permissible to eat whatever is "natural" but as soon it is packaged in a capsule and sold in health stores or pharmacies, it must be cautioned. This is far from the truth; many "natural" products contain environmental substances that can have serious effects on the nervous system when ingested.

7.2. Dementia

The most obvious signs of dementia are a decline in cognitive functions including memory. Some of these deficits are caused by degeneration of nerve cells but there are signs that some parts of the symptoms are caused by activation of neural plasticity. This assumption is supported by evidence that show that people who are physically and intellectually active have less risk of getting these age related disorders. Such activities can at least postpone the incidence of the symptoms of dementia and even some of the symptoms of Alzheimer's disease [88]. Naturally, physical exercise and intellectual activity also changes things other than what is associated with neural plasticity. For example, physical and perhaps also intellectual activities slow the age related deterioration of the heart and the blood vessels and thereby preserve good blood supply to the brain. It has also been shown that brain derived neurotrophic factor (BDNF) increases through physical exercise [31] (see Chapter IV).

Inflammation of various kinds and altered function of the immune system have been implicated in age related diseases of the brain such as dementia of various kind and Alzheimer's disease. Treatments that boost the immune system and decrease inflammation would therefore seem to be beneficial in treatment of dementia. It has been suggested that medications such as non-steroidal anti-inflammatory drugs (NSAIDs) -- Aspirin, ibuprofen, naprosyn, etc. -- would be beneficial but so far the evidence has been sparse. More recently it has been reported that increased intake of certain fatty acids, Omega 3 and folic acid, has beneficial effect on dementia (as it has on depression, see page 156) [16,56]. Studies have shown that Omega 3 and folic acid can improve cognitive functions in individuals with dementia [16]. Many of the risk factors for dementia are similar to those for cardiovascular diseases.

The commonly used medications to treat dementia are directed to the acetylcholine system of the brain, which in addition to affecting memory is also necessary for activation of neural plasticity.

Electrical stimulation of certain regions of the brain or the vagus nerve may be a way to reduce the effect of dementia and improve memory functions [80].

8. Factors to Consider when Treating Plasticity Diseases

Plasticity diseases are complex and the fact that there are no objective tests that can assess the severity of many of the most common plasticity diseases makes not only the diagnosis difficult but it is also an obstacle in treatment where it would have been valuable to have ways to monitor the efficacy of the treatments used.

8.1. Plasticity Diseases Affect a String of Structures

Plasticity diseases normally involve abnormal neural activity in a series of structures in the brain and spinal cord as discussed earlier in this book (Chapter II and IV, see figure 4.1). Not only do the structures that are pathologic ("sick") have abnormal neural activity, but also the ones that receive abnormal signals from these sick structures simply because they receive faulty signals and not because there is anything wrong with these structures.

The symptoms that a patient with a plasticity disease experience are caused when abnormal neural activity reaches a certain part of the brain, namely the part from where sensations or awareness are elicited. This structure is not necessarily malfunctioning; it may just receive abnormal neural activity from some other structures and therefore acting abnormally.

To complicate matters further, programs or rules that are genetic and epigenetic in origin and modified by external or environmental factors may control the abnormalities caused by activation of neural plasticity. Activity in other groups of nerve cells may cause other reactions such as affective (emotional) reactions.

Aiming treatment at such programs would be an effective way to treat many forms of plasticity diseases. While we know something about the expression of neural plasticity, we know little about the programs that may control the execution of plastic changes. Programs that control normal childhood development may be at fault (page 157). Little is known about the precise location in the brain of nerve cells responsible for the different kinds of reactions to plasticity diseases, such as pain and tinnitus.

8.2. At which Structures should Treatment of Plasticity Diseases be Aimed?

Aiming at the pathologic structures may cure a disease if the treatment can reverse the pathology. Treatment aimed at structures that receive pathologic signals and therefore behave abnormally may ameliorate the symptoms of plasticity diseases as long as the treatment is done. However, it will not cure the disease.

When treating diseases it is therefore important to identify the structure that is "sick". For many disorders this is not difficult but for plasticity diseases it offers a challenge that is greater than it is in many other diseases.

8.3. Similarities with other Diseases

Plasticity diseases are not the only diseases that involve a series of different structures. An example of a common disease that also involves a sequence of structures is diabetes type 2. One of the complications of diabetes is (peripheral nerve) neuropathy, which means that nerves are diseased with pain, tingling sensations and reduced function as a result. One of the more pronounced signs of diabetes is abnormally high level of blood sugar. One would therefore think that it would be beneficial to lower the blood sugar level. A common treatment given to individuals with diabetes type 2 is medications that lower the blood sugar level. It is often recommended that patients with diabetes type 2 take as much medication as needed to lower their blood sugar to a level that is close to normal.

Diabetes neuropathy is at the end of a chain of events affecting a series of different structures and organs (Figure 5.4). The first steps in this chain are genetics in combination with the metabolic syndrome. These pathologies are the subsequent events that, via obesity, cause diabetes neuropathy (and several other pathologic changes). This series of events that occur before diabetic neuropathy becomes manifest is therefore similar to what was discussed above regarding plasticity diseases.

The common treatment (lowering the blood sugar levels with medications) is an example of aiming treatments at fault that are induced by other structures. In the case of diabetes, the increased sugar in the blood is caused by a decreased inability of cells to utilize glucose (sugar) normally. In turn, this is caused by resistance of cells to respond to insulin which is necessary for cells to utilize sugar. This inability is caused by different factors associated with obesity and a group of abnormalities known as the metabolic syndrome, which together with genetic predisposition starts the process of developing diabetes. Attempts to control blood sugar levels by medication means attacking the problems of hyperglycemia (increased blood sugar level), which is a late state of the chain of events that in diabetes 2 leads to diabetes neuropathy (Figure 5.4).

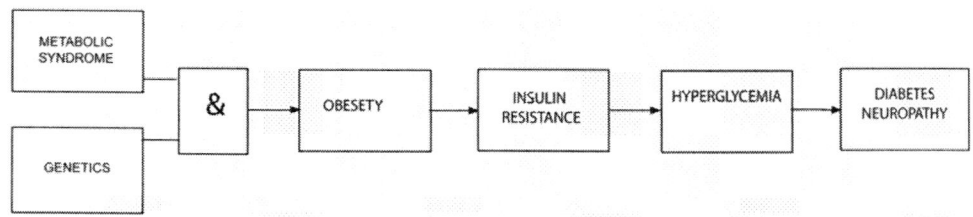

Figure 5.4. Hypothetical flowchart of events that occur in development of type 2 diabetes neuropathy.

A large population study has shown that aggressively treating the elevated blood sugar (hyperglycemia) and bringing it down to normal levels is not beneficial to individuals with diabetes type 2 [29]. The reason seems obvious: treating diabetes by reducing the blood sugar level is not curing the disease.

8.4. Treatment of Diseases Caused by Errors in "Midcourse Correction"

Treatment of developmental diseases such as autism has included medications such as SSRIs that affect the neural transmitter serotonin and strong psychoactive medications used in treatment of schizophrenia. These different medical treatments may affect the symptoms of autism but there is no evidence that they affect the disease and its progression. Various cognitive training programs are also in current use. For example, speech therapy can have some beneficial effects on the disease.

There are many reasons for the failures in treatment of autism with medications. Autism is not a single disease as has been recognized by the introduction of the term "autistic spectrum diseases" (see Appendix C). The symptoms of individuals with what is called autism spectrum diseases range from those causing severe handicap to mild deficits causing mainly difficulty in social interaction. It seems unlikely that a single treatment can be found that would be effective for all individuals with autistic spectrum diseases. There are no tests that can distinguish between the different members of this group of diseases and that contributes to the problems of diagnosing them. Without adequate ways to diagnose the diseases it is difficult to find effective treatments and difficult to monitor the effectiveness of treatments.

As discussed earlier (Chapter IV, Appendix C), diseases such as autism spectrum diseases may be caused by reorganization of the nervous system that normally occurs in the years immediately after birth ("midcourse correction", see page 88) is carried out incorrectly. This reorganization that includes pruning of connections and establishment of new synapses may be controlled by programs that have been laid down before birth.

When the midcourse correction goes awry it is most likely the program (or rules) that fails in one way or another and it would be natural to direct treatment here. These rules are presumably guided by genetics including epigenetic that can change gene expression. The creation of rules is also likely to be affected by environmental factors Errors in these programs may therefore have been caused by environmental factors affecting the mother therefore causing damage before birth (see Appendix C) [47]. If the symptoms are caused by errors in a certain program and if the program is laid down before birth, it would be difficult to find which environmental factors are to blame. It would likewise be difficult to find effective treatments or preventive means that could reduce the likelihood of acquiring the diseases caused by such faults.

The (unsupported) belief that autism might be caused by mercury poisoning (from thimerosal, a preservative containing mercury used in vaccines for measles, mumps and rubella (MMR)) is still alive [69] despite compelling evidence that there is no relationship between autism and childhood vaccinations. In fact, the relationship between mercury and autism has convincingly been disproved in large population studies [55]. This misconception has led to treatment normally used for acute heavy metal poisoning (lead, mercury, etc.) referred to as chelating[65] in children with autism. This technique makes it

---

[65] Chelating: A procedure making it possible for the body to get rid of substances such as heavy metals, by binding the metal atoms to organic substance.

possible to eliminate heavy metals such as lead and mercury from the body. However, the treatment has severe side effects (such as causing dangerously low calcium in the blood [11]). Despite the fact that individuals with autism do not have any signs of poisoning with mercury, these treatments are still practiced (see Appendix C).

This may explain why medical treatments used so far for diseases such as autism have been unsuccessful in affecting the symptoms. The current praxis of treating autism spectrum diseases with psychoactive drugs would not be able to correct the faults in the program that control childhood development of the nervous system.

8.5. Placebo Effect

The gold standard for testing new medications is to compare its effect on a certain disease with that of an inactive substance (often in the form of a sugar pill or another inert substance). In such "double blind" studies, the participants nor the person who administers the test know which pill is real and which is an inactive substance. Double blind studies were introduced many years ago to avoid the subjective bias on the evaluation of new treatments from the participants and the experimenter. If the participants in the studies have any beneficial effect from the administration of such "sugar" pills it is called a "placebo effect" and the medication that is being tested is only regarded to be effective when the effect of the medication is larger than that of the inactive pills.

The word placebo is Latin meaning "I will please". The word was already cited in the editions of the Oxford English Dictionary from 1811. Kaptchuk mentioned that the name "placebo" has been used for at least 200 years in clinical practice by a well meaning doctor who did not have any effective remedy to treat a patient's disease. It was also given to patients who were either hard to please or hard to cure. In modern medicine the meaning of the term placebo is a medication with no medical effect ("sugar pills"). It means an inert harmless substance. After World War II, it became required to include a placebo when testing the effectiveness of new medications. Placebo is an important part of the randomized controlled trials that became the methodological gold standard for testing the efficacy of medications and other methods aimed at treatment of diseases already fifty years ago.

The placebo effect depends on many factors and it is different for each disease for which a medication is tested. In an article published in 1955 by Beecher [8], it was shown that a placebo effect of approximately 35% occurred in many studies of efficacy of medications. The Beecher study showed the effect in 15 experiments comprising of 1082 patients. Other investigators [46,48] found no evidence of placebo effects in studies of the efficacy of medications. Evaluations of treatments for diseases such as central neuropathic pain has a high degree of placebo effect and the beneficial outcomes of administrating an inert substance may occur in as many as 40% of participants.

Many causes have been given for the placebo effect by different investigators: Spontaneous improvement, fluctuation of symptoms, regression to the mean, additional treatment, conditional switching of placebo treatment, scaling bias, irrelevant response variables, answers of politeness, experimental subordination, conditioned answers, neurotic or psychotic misjudgment, psychosomatic phenomena, misquotation, etc. All these factors would produce what would be interpreted as a placebo effect. A list of other reasons for the placebo effects also include experimental subordination, conditioned answers, neurotic or psychotic misjudgment, misquotation, etc. [48]. Many people want to be polite and when given medication they may report an improvement when they may not feel it because they believed they were given an active substance.

Diseases that heal themselves during the evaluation period naturally appear to have a large placebo effect. If a study was started when symptoms were worst and ended when the symptoms had abated any treatment would look as having improved the disease. The severity of many diseases, for example depression, indeed goes up and down during time. A patient's belief they are being treated with an effective substance for his/her disease is also an important cause of placebo effects.

Only recently has it become accepted knowledge that the effect of believing to be treated by an active medication is in fact beneficial to some patients with plasticity diseases.

Regression to the mean[66] has been suggested as causing placebo effects. Because of the regression to the mean a person with very strong symptoms when first asked is likely to have less strong symptoms when asked again. Likewise, a person with weak symptoms is likely to have stronger symptoms when asked later.

When it was discovered that the body has its own production of chemicals that are very similar to opioids used for pain management, it was thought that the observed placebo effect in pain medication studies was simply caused by an increased production of the body's own pain relievers. This suggestion was supported by a study by Levine and Fields [52] who found that sensation of pain increased after an injection of a chemical called naloxone. Naloxone is an antagonist to opioids and eliminates the pain relieving effect of substances such as morphine.

Intuitively there is something wrong in having a beneficial effect on the pain from administration of a sugar pill, but the explanations mentioned above gave the placebo effect some respect. However, it is still not known exactly how anticipation can increase the internal production of these opioids.

8.5.1. Can the Placebo Effect be Used for Treatment?

For treating tinnitus and some forms of pain the placebo effect is large, sometimes as much as 40%. If this is so, why do we not start using placebo treatments? Ethical concerns have been raised regarding treatment with inactive substances. Telling a patient that he/she is being treated by a medication that is known by the physicians to have no beneficial effect has been used for many years. Is it ethically acceptable to use placebo therapy as a part of empathy (the ability to recognize, perceive and feel directly the emotion of another person), not to be confused with compassion (understanding of the emotional state of another and a desire to alleviate suffering), from health care personnel is another question. It is very likely and there is indeed evidence that a physician who shows interest in the patient's condition and comfort a placebo may in fact reduce the patient's suffering from diseases such as chronic pain or tinnitus.

8.5.2. Disadvantages of the Placebo Effect

It is now known that the placebo effect does not last very long. If a test is repeated, the placebo effect declines rapidly. It could very well be that the medications or other forms of treatment would in fact have a long-term effect. A medication that is found to be only equally effective as a placebo when tested using the conventional double blind method would be much better than the placebo effect when used over long time. This all means that we have probably discarded some valuable treatments because their effects on the symptom were not much better than placebo at the time tested.

There is no doubt that the double blind studies are not a magic method of identifying effective treatments from ineffective ones. It may even be directly misleading. One reason is that it is not a comparison between treatment and no treatment, because for many diseases placebo is a highly effective treatment; at least during the time it is used. So why do we cling to double blind studies as the only way of testing the efficacy of treatments? Because everybody does it is probably the best answer.

8.6. Testing Patients with Different Forms of a Disease

There are other reasons why useful remedies to treat plasticity diseases may have been abandoned. This may occur when a new treatment is tested in a group of individuals with different forms of tinnitus. If the group includes individuals with three different forms of tinnitus and the new treatment is only effective for treating one kind, perhaps only 20-30% of the participants may have any beneficial effect because they are the only ones in the group that have the disease for which the treatment is effective. There is a risk that this will not be enough for the new treatment to be accepted, although it may be very effective in a small group of patients. This is one reason why it is important to be able to distinguish different forms of a disease such as tinnitus. Another disease with great variations is autism.

8.7. Assessing the Results of Treatment

A patient who has been treated for a plasticity disease such as pain or tinnitus may report the strength of the pain or tinnitus was not affected by the treatment. Upon closer examination, the patient may reveal that he/she feels better after the treatment and that he/she is able to do intellectual work he/she could not do before. This is just an indication that the saturation (the level where the worsening of the disease does not have any effect on the measure used to assess the severity of the disease in question) has been reached earlier for sensation than for these other effects, such as "feeling bad" or the ability to concentrate on

---

[66] Regression to the mean is a theory that states that when a person who is tested for something has an extreme value, that person will have a less extreme value the next time he/she is tested.

intellectual work. This may mean that different signs of pain such as the perceived strength and the effect on daily life may saturate at different levels (figure 5.5).

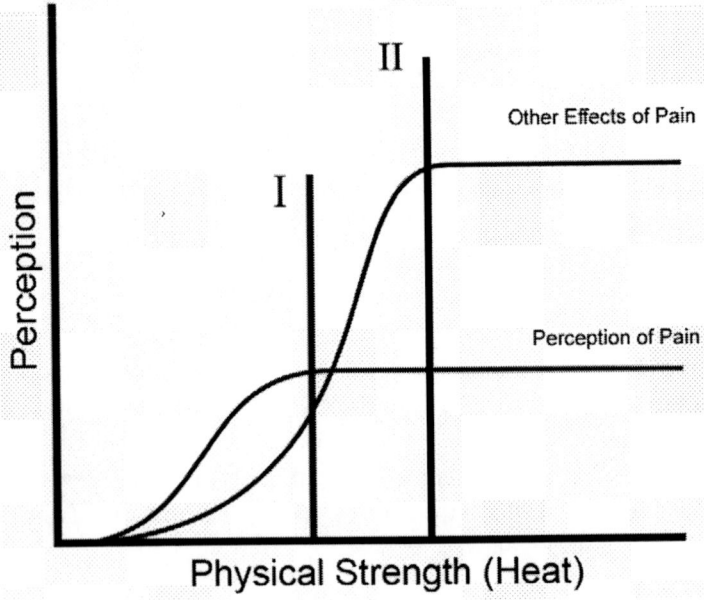

Figure 5.5. Illustration of different saturation levels for sensation and other signs of heat induced pain.

When what cause the pain increases above a certain strength the perception of how strong the pain is will not increase (above I in Figure 5.5) but the other effects such as the emotional reaction may still increase. This reasoning is also valid regarding treatment. Improvement (reduction) of pain between I and II in Figure 5.5 will not give the impression that the pain has improved when the patient is asked if the strength of the pain has changed but these other effects, being able to sleep, work etc may very well have improved.

8.8. How Can Better Treatments be Developed?

Progress often comes when someone thinks "outside the box". Defying conventional thinking has brought revolutionary results to many areas of medicine and science, but it has also brought failures. To name a few successes, the discovery of penicillin (Alexander Fleming), cure of stomach ulcer with antibiotics (Robin Warren and Barry Marshall), and the introduction of administration of antibiotics before surgical operations ("Malis' cocktail"), which reduced the risk of wound infections (by the neurosurgeon, Leonid Malis) [75]. Such inventions always met resistance and it took years before these revolutionary discoveries became accepted in medical praxis. Treatments may already have been developed for the treatment of some plasticity diseases but the treatments may have been discarded for various reasons.

A few suggestions about improvements of treatments would include better ways of testing new treatments. As pointed out above, the double blind method may have caused discarding of some useful treatments.

8.9. How to Get Rid of Assumptions about Cause of Diseases?

Almost as important as discovering new treatments is the ability to abandon treatments that are not beneficial to the patient. Many treatments that are in general use are ineffective and it is a mystery why such treatments are still used. Surgical operations for lower back pain, SSRIs for depression are examples where many individuals are being subjected to treatments that offer little or no benefit to the patient but have risks of side effects of various kinds [63].

The assumed cause of many diseases is incorrect because we do not know enough. When knowledge has accumulated and the invalid assumption has been corrected one would think that the obsolete assumptions about cause would be ignored. We find, perhaps to our surprise, that many such obsolete assumptions are still used by many people including physicians and other health care professionals.

There are many examples of how difficult it is to get rid of something that was learned once. We are often concerned about how to teach people facts but little attention has been paid to how to erase erroneous facts and hypotheses such as about the cause of diseases.

REFERENCES

[1]   Anderson WS, O'Hara SO, Lawson HC, Treede R-D, Lenz FA. Plasticity of pain-related neuronal activity in the human thalamus. In: Møller AR, editor. *Reprogramming the brain*. Amsterdam: Elsevier; 2006. p. 353-64.

[2]   Angst MS, Clark DJ. Opioid-induced hyperalgesia: A qualitative systematic review. *Anesthesiology*. 2006;104:570–87.

[3]   Arnold LM, Russell IJ, Diri EW, Duan WR, Young JPJ, Sharma U, et al. A 14-week, Randomized, Double-Blinded, Placebo-Controlled Monotherapy Trial of Pregabalin in Patients With Fibromyalgia. *J Pain*. 2008.

[4]   Bach S, Noreng MF, Tjellden NU. Phantom limb pain in amputees during the first 12 months following limb amputation, after preoperative lumbar epidural blockade. *Pain*. 1988;33:297-301.

[5]   Baguley DM, Atlas MD. Cochlear Implants and Tinnitus. In: Langguth B, Hajak G, Kleinjung T, Cacace A, Møller AR, editors. *Tinnitus, Pathophysiology and Treatment*. Amsterdam: Elsevier; 2007. p. 347-55.

[6]   Barker FG, Jannetta PJ, Bissonette DJ, Larkins MV, Jho HD. The long-term outcome of microvascular decompression for trigeminal neuralgia. *N Eng J Med*. 1996;334:1077-83.

[7]   Barker FG, Jannetta PJ, Bissonette DJ, Shields PT, Larkins MV. Microvascular Decompression for Hemifacial Spasm. *J Neurosurg*. 1995;82:201-10.

[8]   Beecher HK. The powerful placebo. *J Am Med Assoc.* 1955;159(17):1602-6.

[9]   Brach JS, Van Swearingen JM, Lenert J, Johnson PC. Facial Neuromuscular Retraining for Oral Synkinesis. *Plastic and Reconstructive Surgery.* 1997;99(7):1922-31.

[10] Brown JA, Lutsep HL, Cramer SC, Weinand M. Motor cortex stimulation for enhancement of recovery after stroke: Case report. *Neurol Res.* 2003;25:815-8.

[11] Brown MJ, Willis T, Omalu B, Leiker R. Deaths resulting from hypocalcemia after administration of edetate disodium: 2003-2005. *Pediatrics.* 2006 118(2):534-6.

[12] Chan BL, Witt R, Charrow AP, Magee A, Howard R, Pasquina PF, et al. Mirror therapy for phantom limb pain. *N Engl J Med* 2007;357(21):2206-7.

[13] Chatwin J, Kendrick T, Group TS. Protocol for the THREAD (THREshold for AntiDepressants) study: a randomised controlled trial to determine the clinical and cost-effectiveness of antidepressants plus supportive care, versus supportive care alone, for mild to moderate depression in UK general practice. *BMC Fam Pract.* 2007;8(2).

[14] Chung YO, Bruehl SP. Complex Regional Pain Syndrome. *Curr Treat Options Neurol.* 2003;5:499-511.

[15] Darlington CL, Smith PF. Drug treatments for tinnitus. In: Langguth B, Hajak G, Kleinjung T, Cacace A, Møller AR, editors. *Tinnitus, Pathophysiology and Treatment.* Amsterdam: Elsevier; 2007. p. 249-62.

[16] Das UN. Folic acid and polyunsaturated fatty acids improve cognitive function and prevent depression, dementia, and Alzheimer's disease—But how and why? *Prostaglandins Leukot Essent Fatty Acids.* 2008;78:11-9.

[17] De Ridder D, De Mulder G, Menovsky T, Sunaert S, Kovacs S. Electrical stimulation of auditory and somatosensory cortices for treatment of tinnitus and pain. In: Langguth B, Hajak G, Kleinjung T, Cacace AT, Møller AR, editors. *Tinnitus, Pathophysiology and Treatment.* Amsterdam: Elsevier; 2007. p. 377-88.

[18] De Ridder D, De Mulder G, Verstraeten E, Seidman M, Elisevich K, Sunaert S, et al. Auditory cortex stimulation for tinnitus. *Acta Neurochir Suppl.* 2007;97(2):451-62.

[19] De Ridder D, De Mulder G, Verstraeten E, Sunaert S, Moller A. Somatosensory cortex stimulation for deafferentation pain. *Acta Neurochir.* 2007;97(Suppl. Pt. 2):67-74.

[20] De Ridder D, De Mulder G, Walsh V, Muggleton N, Sunaert S, Møller A. Magnetic and electrical stimulation of the auditory cortex for intractable tinnitus. *J Neurosurg.* 2004;100(3):560-4.

[21] Del Bo L, Ambrosetti U. Hearing aids and the treatment of tinnitus. In: Langguth B, Hajak G, Kleinjung T, Cacace AT, Møller AR, editors. *Tinnitus, Pathophysiology and Treatment.* Amsterdam: Elsevier; 2007. p. 341-55.

[22] Emmett JR, Shea JJ. Treatment of tinnitus with tocainide hydrochloride. *Otolaryngol Head Neck Surg.* 1980;88:442-6.

[23] Fava M. Augmentation and combination strategies in treatment-resistant depression. *J Clin Psychiatry.* 2001;62 Suppl 18:4-11.

[24] Fitzgerald PB, Daskalakis ZJ. The use of repetitive transcranial magnetic stimulation and vagal nerve stimulation in the treatment of depression. *Curr Opin Psychiatry.* 2008;21(1):25-9.

[25] Forge A, Schacht J. Aminoglycoside antibiotics. *Audiol Neurotol.* 2000;5:3-22.

[26] Franzini A, Leone M, Messina G, Cordella R, Marras C, Bussone G, et al. Neuromodulation in treatment of refractory headaches. *Neurol Sci 2008 May;29 Suppl 1:S65-8.* 2008 Suppl 1:S65-8.

[27] Fromm G. Medical treatment of patients with trigeminal neuralgia. In: Fromm GH and Sessle BJ *Trigeminal Neuralgia.* Boston: Butterworth-Heinemann; 1991. p. 133-44.

[28] Gardner W, Miklos M. Response of trigeminal neuralgia to "decompression" of sensory root. *JAMA.* 1959(170):1773-6.

[29] Gerstein HC, et a. Action to Control Cardiovascular Risk in Diabetes Study Group: Effects of intensive glucose lowering in type 2 diabetes. *N Engl J Med.* 2008;358(24):2545-59.

[30] Goldberg RJ, Katz J. A meta-analysis of the analgesic effects of omega-3 polyunsaturated fatty acid supplementation for inflammatory joint pain. *Pain.* 2007;129:210-23.

[31] Gómez-Pinilla F, Ying Z, Roy RR, Molteni R, Edgerton VR. Voluntary exercise induces a BDNF-mediated mechanism that promotes neuroplasticity. *J Neurophysiol.* 2002;88(5):2187-95.

[32] Goodey R. Tinnitus treatment: state of the art. In: Langguth B, Hajak G, Kleinjung T, Cacace AT, Møller AR, editors. *Tinnitus, Pathophysiology and Treatment.* Amsterdam: Elsevier; 2007. p. 237-46.

[33] Hakanson S. Trigeminal neuralgia treated by injection of glycerol into the trigeminal cistern. *Neurosurgery.* 1981(9):638-46.

[34] Hallett M. Transcranial magnetic stimulation and the human brain. *Nature.* 2000;406:147-50.

[35] Han SC, Harrison P. Myofascial pain syndrome and trigger-point management. *Regional Anesthesia.* 1997;95(2):89-101.

[36] Heubi JE, Barbacci MB, Zimmerman HJ. Therapeutic misadventures with acetaminophen: hepatoxicity after multiple doses in children. *J Pediatr.* 1998;132(1):22-7.

[37] Ho IK, Brase DA, Loh HH, Way EL. Influence of L-tryptophan on morphine analgesia, tolerance and physical dependence. *Pharmacol Exp Ther.* 1975;193(1):35-43.

[38] Hudson C, Hudson SP, Hecht T, MacKenzie J. Protein source tryptophan versus pharmaceutical grade tryptophan as an efficacious treatment for chronic insomnia. *Nutr Neurosci.* 2005;8(2):121-7.

[39] Jannetta PJ. Trigeminal neuralgia and hemifacial spasm ? etiology and definitive treatment. *Trans Am Neurol Assoc.* 1975(100):53-5.

[40] Jannetta PJ, Møller MB, Møller AR. Disabling positional vertigo. *New Engl J Med.* 1984(310):1700-5.

[41] Jastreboff PJ. Phantom auditory perception (tinnitus): Mechanisms of generation and perception. *Neurosci Res.* 1990;8:221-54.

[42] Jastreboff PJ. Tinnitus as a phantom perception: Theories and clinical implications. In: Vernon JA, Møller AR, editors. *Mechanisms of Tinnitus.* Boston: Allyn & Bacon; 1995. p. 73-93.

[43] Jastreboff PJ. Tinnitus retraining therapy. In: Langguth B, Hajak G, Kleinjung T, Cacace AT, Møller AR, editors. *Tinnitus, Pathophysiology and Treatment*. Amsterdam: Elsevier; 2007. p. 415-23.

[44] Jensen TS, Nikolajsen L. Pre-emptive analgesia in postamputation pain: an update. In: Sandkühler J, Bromm B, Gebhart GF, editors. *Nervous system plasticity and chronic pain*. Amsterdam: Elsevier; 2000. p. 493-503.

[45] Kamei J, Mori T, Kasuya Y. Effects of L-tryptophan on the development of tolerance to the antitussive effects of dihydrocodeine. *Jpn-J-Pharmacol* 1991;55(3):403-6.

[46] Kaptchuk T. Bulletin of the History of Medicine. *Lancet*. 1998;351:1722-5.

[47] Kenet T, Froemke RC, Schreiner CE, Pessah IN, Merzenich MM. Perinatal exposure to a noncoplanar polychlorinated biphenyl alters tonotopy, receptive fields, and plasticity in rat primary auditory cortex. *Proc Natl Acad Sci U S A*. 2007;104(18):7646-51.

[48] Kienle GS, Kiene H. J Clin Epidemiol. 1997;50(12):1311-8.

[49] Kirchner A, Birklein F, Stefan H, Handwerker HO. Left vagus nerve stimulation suppresses experimentally induced pain. *Neurology*. 2000;55(8):1167-71.

[50] Kleinjung T, Steffens A, Londero A, Langguth B. Transcranial magnetic stimulation (TMS) for treatment of chronic tinnitus: Clinical effects. In: Langguth B, Hajak G, Kleinjung T, Cacace A, Møller AR, editors. *Tinnitus, Pathophysiology and Treatment*. Amsterdam: Elsevier; 2007. p. 359-67.

[51] Lee WM. Acetaminophen and the U.S. Acute Liver Failure Study Group: lowering the risks of hepatic failure. *Hepatology*. 2004;40(1):6-9.

[52] Levine JD, Gordon NC, Fields HL. The mechanism of placebo analgesia. *Lancet*. 1978;23:654-7.

[53] Long D. Surgical treatment for back and neck pain. In: McMahon SB, Koltzenburg M, editors. *Wall and Melzak's Textbook of Pain*. Amsterdam: Elsevier; 2006. p. 683-97.

[54] Long DM. Chronic back pain. In: Wall PD, Melzack R, editors. *Handbook of Pain*. 4 ed. Edinburgh: Churchill Livingstone; 1999. p. 539-8.

[55] Madsen KM, Hviid A, Vestergaard M, Schendel D, Wohlfahrt J, Thorsen P, et al. A population-based study of measles, mumps, and rubella vaccination and autism. *N Engl J Med*. 2002;347(19):1477-82.

[56] Martin CM. Omega-3 fatty acids: proven benefit or just a "fish story"? *Consult Pharm*. 2008;23(3):210-2; 4; 7-21.

[57] Melding PS, Goodey RJ, Thorne PR. The use of lignocaine in the diagnosis and treatment of tinnitus. *J Laryngol Otol*. 1978;92:115-21.

[58] Melzack R. Phantom limbs. *Sci Am*. 1992;266:120-6.

[59] Meyerson BA, Lindblom U, Linderoth B, Lind G. Motor cortex stimulation as treatment of trigeminal neuropathic pain. *Acta Neurochir - Supplementum*. 1993;58:105-3.

[60] Meyerson BA, Linderoth B. Mechanism of spinal cord stimulation in neuropathic pain. *Neurol Res*. 2000;22:285-92.

[61] Møller AR. Cranial nerve dysfunction syndromes: Pathophysiology of microvascular compression. In: Barrow DL, editor. *Neurosurgical Topics Book 13, 'Surgery of Cranial Nerves of the Posterior Fossa,' Chapter 2*. Park Ridge. IL: American Association of Neurological Surgeons; 1993. p. 105-29.

[62] Møller AR. Vascular compression of cranial nerves. I: History of the microvascular decompression operation. *Neurol Res.* 1998;20:727-31.

[63] Møller AR. *A new epidemic: Harm in Medicine.* Nova Science Publishers; 2007.

[64] Møller AR, Møller MB. Microvascular decompression operations In: Langguth B, Hajak G, Kleinjung T, Cacace A, Møller AR, editors. *Tinnitus: Pathophysiology and Treatment.* Amsterdam: Elsevier; 2007. p. 397-400.

[65] Møller AR, Møller MB, Yokota M. Some forms of tinnitus may involve the extralemniscal auditory pathway. *Laryngoscope.* 1992; 102: 1165-71.

[66] Møller MB. Results of microvascular decompression of the eighth nerve as treatment for disabling positional vertigo. *Ann Otol Rhinol Laryngol.* 1990;99:724-29.

[67] Møller MB, Møller AR, Jannetta PJ, Jho HD. Vascular decompression surgery for severe tinnitus: Selection criteria and results. *Laryngoscope.* 1993;103:421-7.

[68] Møller MB, Møller AR, Jannetta PJ, Jho HD, Sekhar LN. Microvascular decompression of the eighth nerve in patients with disabling positional vertigo: Selection criteria and operative results in 207 patients. *Acta Neurochir (Wien).* 1993;125:75-82.

[69] Mutter J, Naumann J, Schneider R, Walach H, Haley B. Mercury and autism: accelerating evidence? *Neuro Endocrinol Lett.* 2005;26(5):439-46.

[70] Nikolajsen L, Jensen TS. Phantom Limb. In: McMahon SB, Koltzenburg M, editors. *Wall and Melzak's Textbook of Pain.* Amsterdam: Elsevier; 2006. p. 961-71.

[71] Nordin M, Balague F, Cedraschi C. Nonspecific lower-back pain: surgical versus nonsurgical treatment. *Clin Orthop Relat Res.* 2006;443:156-67.

[72] Norena AJ, Eggermont JJ. Enriched acoustic environment after noise trauma reduces hearing loss and prevents cortical map reorganization. *J Neurosci* 2005;25(3):699-705.

[73] Pulec JL. Cochlear nerve section for intractable tinnitus. *ENT Journal.* 1995;74(7):469-76.

[74] Rowbotham MC, Twilling L, Davies PS, Reisner L, Taylor K, Mohr D. Oral opioid therapy for chronic peripheral and central neuropathic pain. *N Engl J Med* 2003;348(13):1223-32.

[75] Savitz SL. Leonard I. Malis and prophylactic antibiotics. *Mt Sinai J Med.* 1997;64(3):187-8.

[76] Schulman A, Tonndorf J, Goldstein B. Electrical tinnitus control. *Acta Otolaryngol (Stockh).* 1985;99:318-25.

[77] Seltzer S, Dewart D, Pollack RL, Jackson E. The effects of dietary tryptophan on chronic maxillofacial pain and experimental pain tolerance. *J Psychiatr Res.* 1982;17(2):181-6.

[78] Severus WE, Littman AB, Stoll AL. Omega-3 fatty acids, homocysteine, and the increased risk of cardiovascular mortality in major depressive disorder. *Harv Rev Psychiatry.* 2001;9(6)::280-93.

[79] Sindou M, Jeanmonod D. Microsurgical-DREZ-otomy for treatment of spasticity and pain in the lower limbs. *Neurosurgery.* 1989;24:655-70.

[80] Sjögren MJ, Hellström PT, Jonsson MA, Runnerstam M, Silander HC, Ben-Menachem E. Cognition-enhancing effect of vagus nerve stimulation in patients with Alzheimer's disease: a pilot study. *J Clin Psychiatry.* 2002;63:972-80.

[81] Skulas-Ray AC, West SG, Davidson MH, Kris-Etherton PM. Omega-3 fatty acid concentrates in the treatment of moderate hypertriglyceridemia. *Expert Opin Pharmacother*. 2008;9:1237-48.

[82] Sullivan P. OxyContin-abuse problem appears limited to US. *CMAJ Canadian Medical Association Journal*. 2001;165(5).

[83] Sweet WH. Percutaneous methods for the treatment of trigeminal neuralgia and other faciocephalic pain: Comparison with microvascular decompression. *Semin Neurol*. 1988;8:272-9.

[84] Taub E, Uswatte G, Elbert T. New treatments in neurorehabilitation founded on basic research. *Nature Rev Neurosci*. 2002;3(3):228-36.

[85] Thimineur M, De Ridder D. C2 area neurostimulation: a surgical treatment for fibromyalgia. *Pain Med* 2007;8(8):639-46.

[86] Tyler R, Babin RW. Tinnitus. In: Cummings CW, Fredickson J-M, Harker L, Krause CJ, Schuller DE, editors. *Otolaryngology, Head and Neck Surgery*. St. Louis, MO: Mosby; 1986. p. 3201-17.

[87] Tyler RS, Gogel SA, Gehringer AK. Tinnitus Activities Treatment. In: Langguth B, Hajak G, Kleinjung T, Cacace AT, Møller AR, editors. *Tinnitus, Pathophysiology and Treatment*. Amsterdam: Elsevier; 2007. p. 425-34.

[88] Verghese J, et al. . Leisure Activities and the Risk of Dementia in the Elderly. *New Eng J Med*. 2003;348:2508-16.

[89] Weiner DK, Kim YS, Bonino P, Wang T. Low back pain in older adults: are we utilizing healthcare resources wisely? *Pain Med*. 2006 7(2):101-2.

[90] Willer JC. Relieving effect of TENS on painful muscle contraction produced by an impairment of reciprocal innervation: An electrophysiological analysis. *Pain*. 1988;32:271-4.

[91] Willott JF, Turner JG, Sundin VS. Effects of exposure to an augmented acoustic environment on auditory function in mice: roles of hearing loss and age during treatment. *Hear Res*. 2000;142:79–88.

[92] Wu A, Ying Z, Gomez-Pinilla F. Dietary omega-3 fatty acids normalize BDNF levels, reduce oxidative damage, and counteract learning disability after traumatic brain injury in rats. *J Neurotrauma*. 2004;21(10):1457-67.

[93] Young KA, Holcomb LA, Yazdani U, Hicks PB, German DC. Elevated neuron number in the limbic thalamus in major depression. *Am J Psychiatry*. 2004;161(7):1270-7.

[94] Ytterberg SR, Mahowald ML, Woods SR. Codeine and oxycodone use in patients with chronic rheumatic disease pain. *Arthritis Rheum*. 1998;41(9):830-1.

Chapter VI

IS NEURAL PLASTICITY PURPOSEFUL AND BENEFICIAL OR NOT?

ABSTRACT

Some kinds of neural plasticity are beneficial to individuals, some kinds are not, and other kinds are directly harmful. Neural plasticity when activated can affect many body functions in different ways some are purposeful and some of which no purpose can be found. From a developmental (Darwinian) view, purpose must serve reproduction and chances of survival during reproductive age. Pain from burns causes an involuntary reaction and serves the purpose of avoiding further damage. However pain from diseases, such as appendicitis, that could not be affected before the advent of modern medicine and surgery must be regarded as purposeless. The plastic changes that shift the functions of damaged portions of the brain and spinal cord to functional areas is an example of purposeful neural plasticity. Things that increase survival beyond reproductive age may not be counted as purposeful because from an evolutionary point of view survival beyond reproductive age does not serve any purpose.

1. INTRODUCTION

Many aspects of neural plasticity were discussed in earlier Chapters of the book, and it was concluded that some plastic changes are beneficial to an individual person - some are not and some are directly harmful. In this Chapter, I will discuss which kind of plastic changes have a purpose, what the purpose is, and how that is related to the benefit or harm to an individual person that may occur from activation of neural plasticity. I will use the term "purposiveness" in the meaning "serving some purpose" without placing value on the purpose.

There are several kinds of benefit. Benefit can be promoting survival; it can be promoting reproduction. Replacement of lost functions by shifting tasks to other regions of the brain is a benefit, adaptation to changing demands are other benefits from activation of neural plasticity. In our industrialized society, other definitions of benefit apply, such as longevity beyond reproductive age. Some functions are purposive but not beneficial to an individual person. Others are both purposive and beneficial.

In this Chapter, I will especially discuss purposiveness and benefit to an individual person from plastic changes in the spinal cord and the brain, and discuss why neural plasticity is important for survival, reproduction, and for the wellbeing of individuals, and how neural plasticity plays a different role when modern health care is available than when it is not. First let's discuss what purposiveness means.

2. PURPOSIVENESS

The word "purposiveness", meaning having a purpose or being purposively, first appeared in a 1943 article by Bigelow, Rosenblueth, and Winer titled, "Behavior, Purpose and Teleology" [1]. Two of the authors of this paper, Arturo Rosenblueth and Norbert Winer, were great thinkers who developed new theories with wide implications and which changed the way we think about many things. (Norbert Winer started the development of Cybernetics, the study of complex systems such as communication system, control systems used, and many aspects of modern life with his book "Cybernetics or Control and Communication in Animal and Machine", published in 1948).

The authors of the article by Bigelow, et al. divided active behavior into groups of functions that are purposeless and groups that are purposeful. Purposeless, the opposite of purposeful, is regarded as being the same as random behavior. A purposeful behavior is a behavior that is directed to the attainment of a goal. Purposeless behavior is not directed to a goal. Purposiveness also involves intent. Design through natural selection can therefore not be purposive because it is done without intent.

Darwinism is the term usually used to describe evolution of species on the basis of the ideas of Charles Darwin (1809-1882), natural selection ("selection of the fittest" originating by Herbert Spencer, 1820-1903). Jean-Baptiste Lamarck (1744-1829), another contributor of ideas about evolution, proposed at an early time (1802-1809) that evolution proceeded in accordance with natural laws. Darwin's theory states that the different species have evolved because offspring have small natural variations (mutations) and that selection of the fittest over time lead to development of better members of individual species. The individuals with larger changes would lead to the evolution of different species or, more often, disappear because they had disadvantages.

Lamarck is credited for the theory of inherence of acquired characters, which means that he believed that acquired properties could be passed on to offspring. Lamarck's theories were published long before those by Darwin. Darwin published his "On the Origin of Species by Means of Natural Selection" in 1859 [2]. Lamarck was the first to propose a comprehensive theory about how forces that made organisms more complex drew organisms up a ladder of complexity, but the term 'Darwinism' became the common term for many different suggestions about the evolution of species.

Darwin's theory describes a way to create design out of chaos without the use of any intelligent mind [4]. In other words, evolution of species according to the theory of Darwin is based on natural selection, and therefore a design without the influence of a designer.

2.1. Purposefulness and Benefit from Activation of Neural Plasticity

According to the theory of Darwin, one would assume that all bodily functions have developed because they would serve a purpose that would promote reproduction and promote survival until reproduction was completed. Ragnar Granit, a prominent Swedish neuroscientist, concluded in his 1977 book, "The purposive brain" The MIT Press, Cambridge, MA, [5], that the brain (in general) must be assumed to be purposive.

Activation of neural plasticity is not always purposive and not always beneficial to an individual person. As we will see below, there are many functions that do not promote survival.

2.2. Purposive and Beneficial Plasticity

Adaptation to changing demands is both purposeful and beneficial to an individual person. Replacing the function of damaged parts of the brain and the spinal cord is another example of a function that is both purposive and beneficial to an individual person.

The re-organization that occurs in childhood ("midcourse correction", page 87) through activation of neural plasticity is both purposive and beneficial when performed in the way it is normally executed. This kind of neural plasticity may be regarded to occur in accordance with Darwinian evolution [3] in that it serves survival until reproduction.

This form of plastic changes are therefore purposive and beneficial in that it increases the individual's ability to compete for reproduction, and it thereby may serve the purpose of selecting beneficial properties in offspring. This would benefit not the target individual, but future generations.

An example of genetically related changes that highly promote survival comes from insects. One is industrial melanism, which means that the darkness in color of some species of moths increased in sooty districts of Manchester and Birmingham in England during the time of industrialism where pollution was strong. The increased darkness made it easier for the moths to hide against dark trees. This was a rapid evolution.

Another evolution involving insects regards night moths' defense against flying bats. These moths have 4 cells on their thorax, which are sensitive to the ultrasound that bats use to localize their prey. The moths can determine when a bat is approaching, and determine from which direction so that it can take evasive maneuvers. It can also determine if the bat is far away or close. If the bat is close, the moth folds its wings and falls to the ground as the fastest escape.

The ability of the brain to change its function widely, as occurs during childhood development, is unique for the brain and the spinal cord. The function of some parts of the brain can be taken over by other parts, such as occurs after strokes.

Other parts of the body do not have such flexibilities, although organs such as the liver and the heart can change their size in response to change in demands they do not change their function as radically as the central nervous systems can. For example, it is true that ingestion of substances that make use of a specific enzyme system in the liver (the P450 cytochrome system) makes that system work more and such substances are subsequently metabolized faster.

3. THE DEVELOPMENT OF THE CENTRAL NERVOUS SYSTEM (BRAIN AND SPINAL CORD)

It is not known with any degree of accuracy how many nerve cells there are in the brain. In an adult individual may have at least 100 billion nerve cells. As was discussed in Chapter I Pakkenberg for example, has estimated that the average number of nerve cells in the neocortex is about 20 billion. The total number of synapses in the human cortex has been estimated to $1,500 \times 10^{12}$ (150 trillion). These estimates have a high degree of uncertainty. The organization of the brain and the spinal cord is naturally controlled by genes (heredity), but there are not enough genes to control the development of each nerve cell and each connection. The 30,000 genes that seem to be involved in the development of the brain cannot possibly direct the organization of all the individual nerve cells, their synapses and connections in the brain and the spinal cord. It must therefore instead be assumed that the organization of the brain and the spinal cord is guided by rules, (or programs) the design of which is directed by genes. These programs then control the development of the brain before birth.

When discussing development of the brain and the spinal cord, it may therefore be more appropriate to discuss the development of programs that control the development rather than discussing the development of each nerve cell and its connections. This concept is also applicable to understanding of some developmental diseases such as autism.

Studies of the development of the nervous system indicate that genetic factors first control the gross organization of the brain, and then after birth the organization is completed through activation of neural plasticity ("midcourse correction") that is most likely rule controlled. After that, the organization of the nervous system is "fine tuned" through activation of neural plasticity, guided by sensory signals and by use. This fine tuning requires signals from the environment (sensory signals) but probably also signals from the body, and it may be guided by programs in a similar way as the childhood development discussed above.

Similar programs or rules as controlled the development of the brain before birth is likely to direct the modifications of the brain that occur after birth ("midcourse correction", page 87).

4. PAIN

Pain can be protective and some forms of pain are life-saving bodily functions with a clear purpose. The sensation of pain from traumatic injuries is purposeful and important for survival at all ages, and therefore it is important for reproduction. The withdrawal reflex is often mentioned as an example of a purposeful and beneficial function that is important for survival. It is elicited by activation of pain receptors in the limbs (hands and feet) and can prevent burning and other forms of trauma by rapid withdrawal of the limb without "asking" the brain.

Pain signals from structures that have been injured by trauma are purposeful and beneficial to an individual person because it may prevent manipulation of wounds that could impair healing. Tenderness of wounds is purposeful because it defines an area of trauma. It is beneficial because it promotes leaving the wound and its surroundings alone without manipulations that could impair the healing process, and that may have survival benefit. These are examples of functions that may serve the purpose of survival and reproduction.

Pain from worn joints is purposive because it provides information about joints being worn. Knowing about that may benefit the individual person by reducing the use, thus, decreasing further wearing on already damaged joints.

Pain from ischemia of the heart muscle (angina) is purposeful because it warns about danger to the heart. It is beneficial because it causes reduced physical activity, reducing the work load on the heart. One can also ask why about half of myocardial infarctions do not have pain. Is that just a fault in the signaling ischemia or are there differences in the disorders that give these two reactions?

Many forms of headache are purposeless and provide no benefit to the individual. Headache caused by trauma, including chemical trauma such as occurs after ingestion of poisons (including alcohol), are purposeful and can be beneficial to an individual person as a signal to avoid repeating what caused the headache. Headache caused by strokes or tumors may be purposive, but of little benefit before modern medicine was developed.

Abdominal pain caused by appendicitis is purposeful because it warns about a danger (death), but it was not beneficial until modern surgery and medicine had evolved. Appendicitis as many other diseases of internal organs was almost always deadly before antibiotics became available and surgery became possible. Before the advent of medical treatments, such warning would not provide any benefit to a person because there were no interventions available that could prevent death from appendicitis. Other forms of pain from organs in the abdomen also signal disorders that do not have any natural remedies and were therefore these warnings were not beneficial before medical and surgical remedies became available. It would therefore not seem as such functions could have developed in the Darwinian sense because they were of no benefit to the individual person. This is a reminder that much of what we now believe is beneficial would not have been beneficial before the advent of modern medicine.

Pain caused by activation of neural plasticity does not seem to have a purpose.

5. MISTAKES BY NATURE

Darwinian theories and the suggestion about the survival of the fittest can explain the development of beneficial and purposive plasticity but cannot explain the development of purposeless and harmful plasticity (plasticity diseases). One may therefore ask if the development of the plastic changes that cause plasticity diseases was a mistake of nature. Was it an example of nature rolling the dice in biological developments? Was the game lost?

A similar question, whether "God rolled the dice" in the development of the Universe has been extensively discussed among theoretical physicists. Quantum mechanics, which is an important area of theoretical physics, is not accurate and may resemble a game. For example, only the likelihood of an electron being in a certain place can be determined. Einstein, who was against the theory of randomness in physics, said: "Anyway, I am sure he (God) does not play dice". Could this have similarities the central nervous system (the spinal cord and the brain), where it is not possible to predict the location of a single synapse or a nerve cell?

Central pain is probably the largest group of plasticity diseases that are purposeless with no known benefit. Development of the central neuropathic pain would therefore not seem to be favored by evolution. Tinnitus is equally purposeless and without benefit.

Since plasticity diseases are purposeless, they may be regarded as a mistake in evolution. If so, does nature try to correct its mistakes, and will harmful plasticity (plasticity diseases) vanish as evolution goes forth?

Plasticity diseases such as chronic pain and tinnitus may not impair the ability to reproduce noticeably because these diseases mostly occur late in life. If the goal is increased survival by natural selection to improve reproduction, the improvement must occur before the end of the period of reproduction, which for women now is around the age of 40 years and much higher for men.

There may therefore be little evolutionary pressure to eliminate such diseases by natural selection. What is more important is a historical prospective, where people did not outlive their ability to reproduce. If plasticity diseases had occurred to our ancestors during their reproductive life, one would have assumed that they would have been eliminated by natural selection, because they would have impaired the ability to reproduce.

Events that occur late in life (probably just later than 40 years) may not have had any influence on (Darwinian) development. It would take many thousands of years before what occurs after 40 years of age could in any way influence development.

REFERENCES

[1]   Bigelow J, Rosenblueth A, Wiener N. Behavior, Purpose and Teleology. *Philosophy of Science*. 1943;10:18-24.

[2]   Darwin C. *The Origin of Species*. Wordsworth: Ware; 1998.

[3]   De Ridder D, Van de Heyning P. The Darwinian plasticity hypothesis for tinnitus and pain. In: Langguth B, Hajak G, Kleinjung T, Cacace A, Møller A, editors. *Tinnitus, Pathophysiology and Treatment*. Amsterdam: Elsevier; 2007. p. 55-60.

[4]   Dennet D. *Darwin's dangerous idea. Evolution and the meanings of life*. New York: Simon and Schuster.; 1995.

[5]   Granit R. *The purposive brain*. Cambridge, MA: The MIT Press; 1977.

APPENDIX A

1. ANATOMY AND PHYSIOLOGY OF ACUTE PAIN

Neural plasticity is involved in many forms of chronic pain, such as central neuropathic pain and neuralgias of various kinds. In order to understand the role of neural plasticity in the various kinds of pain, it is necessary to understand the anatomical and functional basis for acute pain. We will therefore first discuss acute pain and describe the neural circuits in the spinal cord and in the brain that are engaged. After that we will discuss how signals from receptors in the body are processed in the nervous system to finally cause the sensation of pain.

1.1. Pain Receptors

Pain receptors convert heat, cold, pressure from injury, and certain chemicals into nerve signals that are conducted to the spinal cord by nerve fibers that are part of peripheral nerves. Two kinds of nerve fibers, Aδ and C fibers, innervate pain receptors and enter the spinal cord where they make synaptic contact with special nerve cells. In Aδ fibers, the axons are covered by myelin; C-fibers, have no such coverage. The C-fibers conduct nerve impulses very slowly (0.2-1 meter/sec), and Aδ fibers conduct impulses much faster (5-30 meter/sec; 0.5-3 cm per millisecond).

Pain is generally unpleasant, which is a difference from sensory perceptions, and has been used as punishment. The pain signals that these two kinds of nerve fibers carry activate different parts of the brain, and this is why they cause different kinds of sensation. We will discuss this more later.

There are many ways that pain receptors are stimulated under normal conditions and during diseases. Pain receptors can be activated by injury to the body (from accidents, surgery etc.), by illnesses of various kinds, or they can be activated without any known causes. Surgery always causes injury and that causes pain. Many diagnostic tests are painful. Lack of oxygen to tissue (causing ischemia) normally causes pain. Inflammation is a common cause of pain, such as is in worn out joints that become inflamed (osteoarthritis). Chemicals from inflammation activate nerve fibers that signal pain to the brain. Over-stimulation of receptors that normally signal touch and vibration can also cause pain.

Substances such as capsaicin (from red pepper) can activate pain receptors, which is why it gives a burning sensation when applied to the skin.

1.1.1. What Happens when Pain Receptors are Stimulated?

Let us start at the beginning of the events that eventually give rise to sensations of acute pain and cause many different bodily reactions. The first step is stimulation of special receptors, known as nociceptors because they respond to harmful stimuli.

What happens when stepping on a hard object illustrates some aspects of acute pain. First, pain receptors are activated and they send signals to the spinal cord. A very short time after pain receptors have been stimulated a stinging pain sensation is felt and the pain sensation points distinctly to the point under the foot where it hit the sharp object. After a short time a burning sensation appears. The stinging pain that is felt immediately is caused by signals that are carried in the faster conducting pain fibers (Aδ) and this give information about the precise location where the injury occurred. The signals that cause the burning sensation travel in slower conducting nerve fibers. The burning pain sensation is less precisely located (Figure A.1).

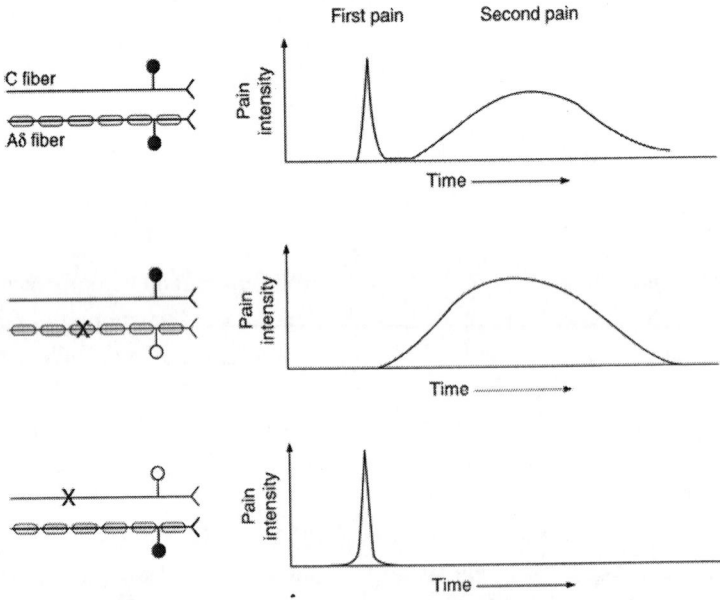

Figure A.1. Two kinds of pain are carried in two kinds of nerve fibers; myelinated (Aδ) and unmyelinated (C) fibers. The signals that are carried in Aδ fibers produce a fast pain and those carried in C fibers produce a later and more prolonged slow burning pain sensation. Severing or blocking Aδ fibers (middle part) eliminates the fast pain, and blocking C fibers eliminates the slow pain (lower part of the figure). (Reproduced from Møller, A.R. 2003. *Sensory Systems: Anatomy and Physiology* Academic Press, Amsterdam with permission from Elsevier [6].

1.2. Anatomy of the Pain Nervous System

The anatomy of the pain pathways from the skin, muscles, tendons and joints involves peripheral nerves that communicate the information to the spinal cord and the brain. Pain sensations from the internal organs (visceral pain) are communicated to the spinal cord through nerves that mainly follows the sympathetic nerves. Pain from the head is transmitted by cranial nerves to the trigeminal nucleus that is located in the brainstem.

The pain pathways (the anterior-lateral system) have many similarities with the non-classical pathways of other sensory systems. Classical literature on the anatomy and physiology of the somatosensory system does not include a description of a non-classical somatosensory pathway. I have therefore previously proposed that the pain pathways be regarded as the non-classical pathways of the somatosensory system [6,8]. Like the non-classical pathways of sensory systems such as hearing, vision and taste, the anteriorlateral pain pathways use the dorsal-medial parts of the thalamus. The nerve cells in that part of the thalamus project to the secondary somatosensory cortex and the association cortices, therefore, by-passing the primary somatosensory cortex. There are direct (subcortical) connections from that part of the thalamus to the amygdala (a part of the "emotional brain").

1.2.1. The Spinal Cord
In the middle of the spinal cord are clusters of nerve cells in horn-shaped formations, known as the spinal horns (Figure A.2). The spinal cord has many functions; it processes information from the body before it is sent to the brain and it processes movement commands from the brain before it is sent to muscles.

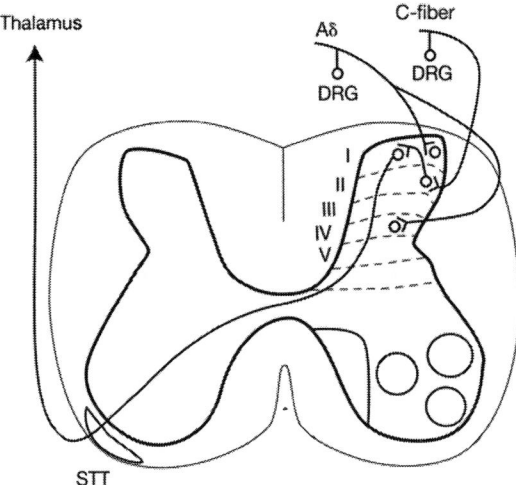

Figure A.2. Illustration of the termination of Aδ fibers and C fibers in the dorsal horn. DRG: Dorsal root ganglia, Lamina I and II are also known as substantia gelantinosa, STT: Spinothalamic tract (Reproduced from: Møller, A.R. 2006. *Neural plasticity and disorders of the nervous system* Cambridge University Press Cambridge [8] Copyright Cambridge University Press 2006. Reprinted with the permission of Cambridge University Press.)

The nerve fibers from pain receptors terminate on cells in the dorsal horn of the spinal cord (Figure A.2).

The dorsal horns have cells that are engaged in processing pain signals and cells that are engaged in processing harmless (innocuous) signals from receptors that respond to touch, etc. There are also cells that process signals from receptors in muscles, joints, and tendons, known as the proprioceptive system. These cells all send signals to the brain through several different *fiber tracts*.

The nerve fibers from pain receptors travel in peripheral nerves that enter the spinal cord as dorsal roots together with nerve fibers that carry sensation of harmless stimuli. Those nerve fibers that carry signals from the spinal cord to make muscles contract exit the spinal cord as ventral roots (Figure A3).

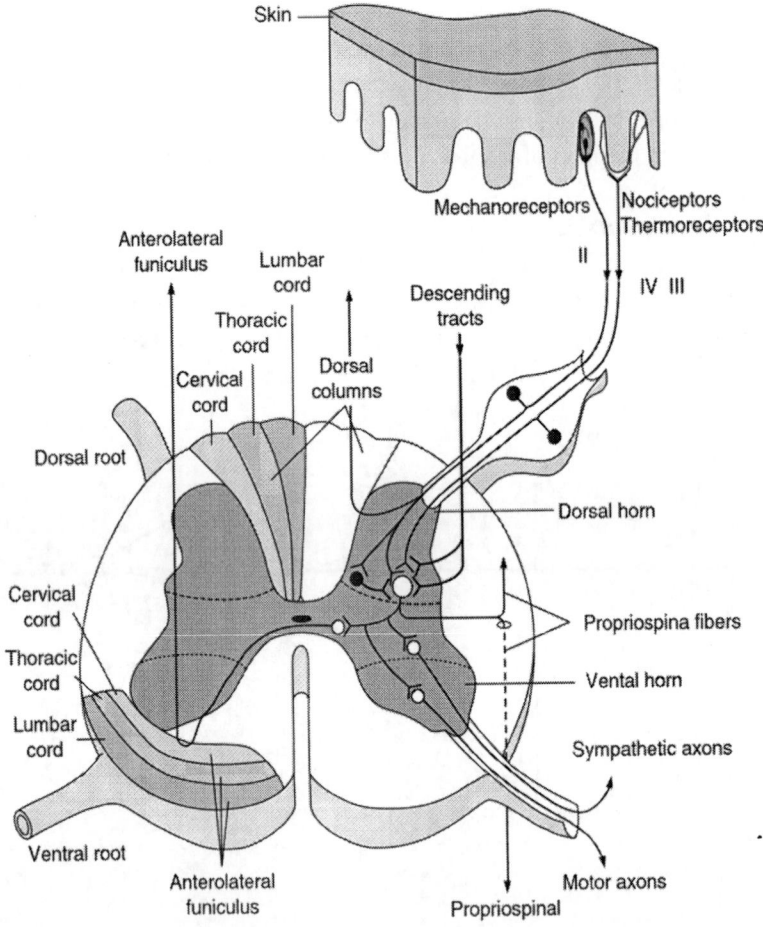

Figure A.3. A more detailed drawing of the connections to nerve cells in the dorsal horn showing the anatomical locations from receptors sensitive to harmful stimuli and those sensitive to harmless stimuli. Connections from the cells in the dorsal horn to the brain and connections from the brain are also shown. (Reproduced from Møller, A.R. 2003. *Sensory Systems: Anatomy and Physiology* Academic Press, Amsterdam, reprinted with permission from Elsevier).

Nerve cells in the parts of the horns located towards the back, the dorsal horns, process sensory information and those parts that are located forward (ventral parts) process movement commands and that is where the nerve cells that directly control the muscles are located.

The nerve fibers from receptors that are sensitive to stimulation that is harmless (innocuous) travel in peripheral nerves and enter the spinal cord in the dorsal roots. Unlike the nerve fibers that carry pain signals, the nerve fibers that carry harmless signals travel uninterrupted as the *dorsal column tracts* (Figure A.3) on the same side of the spinal cord as they entered before the nerve fibers terminate on cells in the dorsal column nuclei located in the upper neck.

The dorsal horns have clusters of nerve cells that contact with each other and process pain signals in a complex but poorly understood manner. The signals that reach these nerve cells from receptors in the skin can activate other nerve cells in the dorsal horn before the information is sent to the brain in certain bundles of nerve fibers (tracts) (Figure A.3).

Each nerve fiber's axon does not only terminate on one cell in the dorsal horn of the spinal cord, but nerve fibers branch (bifurcates) into two fibers, which may terminate on two different cells. One of the branches is likely to branch again, and this can be repeated several times [1,8].

The different branches may terminate on different cells not only in the segment of the spinal cord where they have entered but some branches may terminate on cells in the dorsal horn of other segments of the spinal cord (Figure A.4). In fact, most of the pain fibers branch several times, and the branches terminate in as many as 10 segments from their entry point. Not all the synapses that connect these branches to nerve cells normally conduct nerve impulses. Synapses that do not normally conduct (are dormant) can be brought to conduct nerve impulses through activation of neural plasticity.

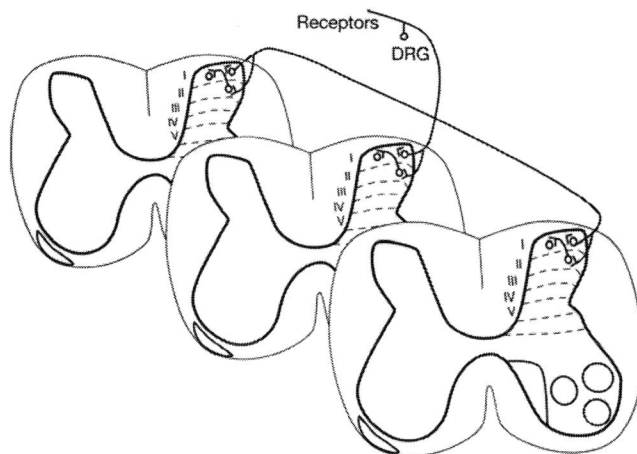

Figure A.4. Illustration of how branches of nerve fibers in the spinal cord terminate nerve cells in segments of the spinal cord that are below and above the segment where the nerve fibers enter the spinal cord. (Reproduced from Møller, A.R. 2006. *Neural plasticity and disorders of the nervous system* Cambridge University Press, Cambridge [8], Copyright © Cambridge University Press 2006. Reprinted with the permission of Cambridge University Press.

In addition to signaling pain sensations to the spinal cord and brain, pain receptors can also cause local effects on the skin (Figure A.5). Nerve impulses in fibers that originate in pain receptors not only lead to the spinal cord, but branches of these axons lead back to the skin [5] where they cause a release of chemicals (neuropathies). These chemicals can stimulate cells in the skin that produce various substances, and may lead to reactions such as dilation of vessels and contractions of small (smooth) muscles in the skin.

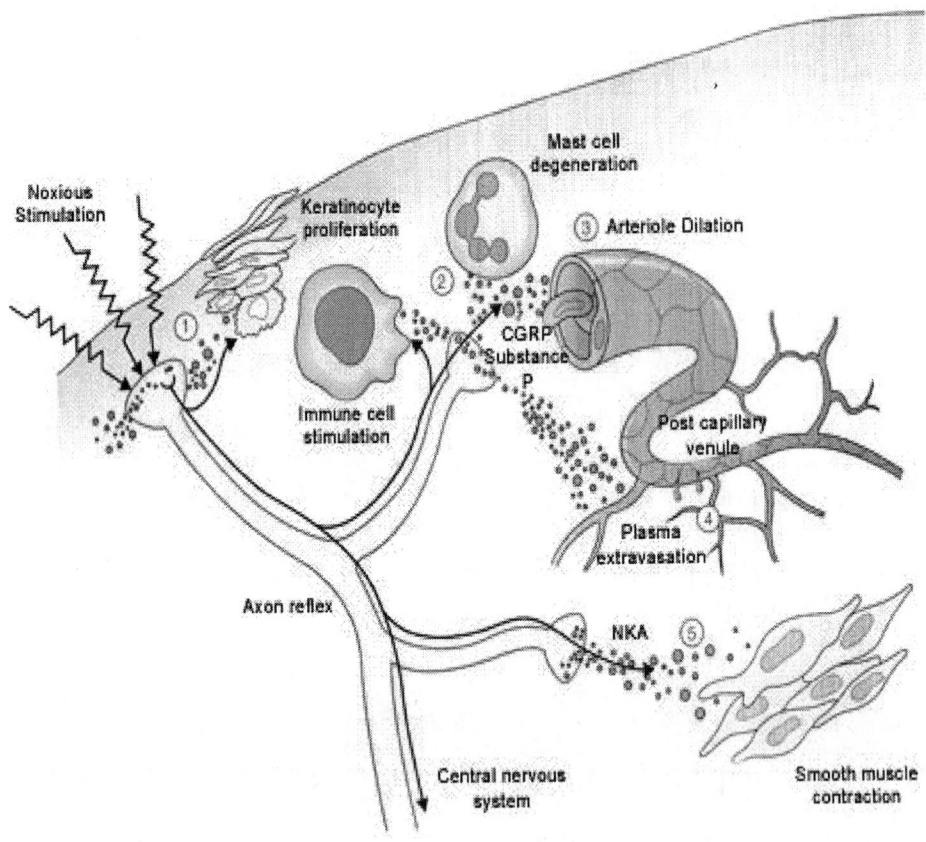

Figure A.5. Stimulation of pain receptors can have local effects without involving the spinal cord. Modified from McMahon, S.B., Koltzenburg, M., (Eds.) 2006. *Wall and Melzak's Textbook of Pain.* Elsevier, Churchill, Livingstone, Amsterdam [4]. Figure 1.21 From Chapter 1, picture by Ian Suk, Johns Hopkins University [5], reprinted with permission from Elsevier).

In the head, nerve fibers that carry pain signals travel to the brainstem in cranial nerves, mostly in the fifth cranial nerve, the trigeminal nerve, and the ninth cranial nerve, the glossopharyngeal nerve (see Figure A.6).

The nerve fibers that carry pain impulses from the face and the mouth (the trigeminal nerve) terminate in the cells of the caudal (caudal meaning 'towards the tail') parts of the trigeminal nucleus in the brainstem (Figure A.6). There are also pain fibers in nerves from the throat (the ninth cranial nerve; the glossopharyngeal nerve). These fibers also terminate in the trigeminal nucleus. The signals from the trigeminal nucleus reach nerve cells in the brain in a similar way as pain signals from the dorsal horn.

The trigeminal nucleus, like the dorsal horn, processes pain signals in a very complex way before the signals are sent higher up in the brain. Nerve cells in the rostral part of the nucleus receive signals from receptors that are sensitive to harmless stimuli such as touch.

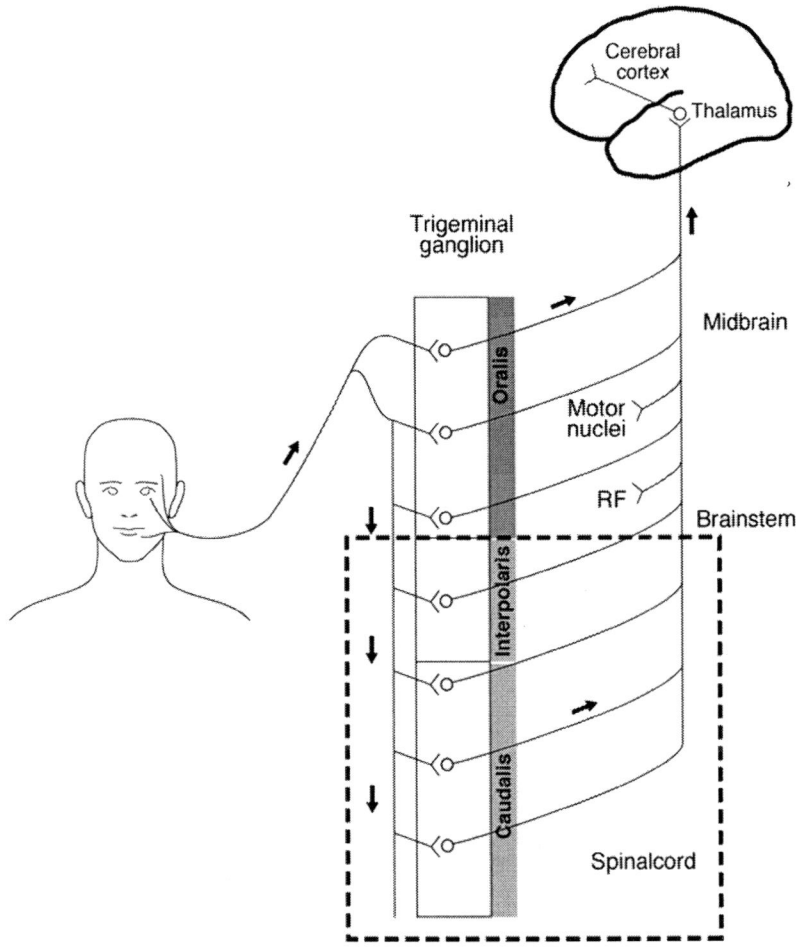

Figure A.6. Schematic drawing of the trigeminal nucleus and its connections from transmitting sensory and pain information from the mouth (Reproduced from: Møller, A.R. 2006. *Neural plasticity and disorders of the nervous system* Cambridge University Press Cambridge. [8] Copyright © Cambridge University Press 2006. Reprinted with the permission of Cambridge University Press).

1.2.2. The Brain

Pain signals from the spinal cord and the trigeminal ganglion ascend in several fiber tracts, together known as the anteriorlateral system. The anteriolateral tracts include the spinothalamic tract, the reticulospinal tract, and mesencephalic tracts. The spinothalamic tract is regarded to be the most important of these.

The axons of the cells in the dorsal column nuclei form the *medial lemnicus,* the fibers of which terminate in the sensory portion of the thalamus (see Figure A.7 and A.8).

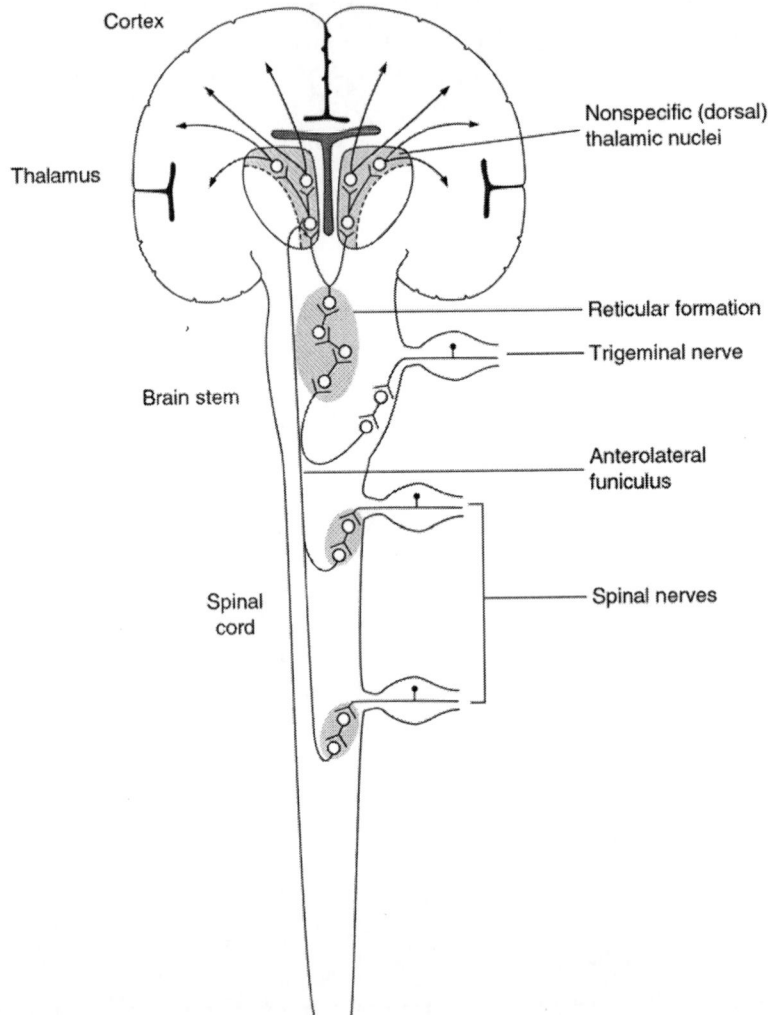

Figure A.7. Anatomical location of the components of the spinothalamic tract (Reproduced from Møller, A.R. 2003. *Sensory Systems: Anatomy and Physiology* Academic Press, Amsterdam, with permission from Elsevier).

Neurologists use the fact that pain and temperature (cold and hot) ascend in the opposite side of the spinal cord to signals from touch receptors to diagnose the location of spinal cord injuries. It should also be noted that the fibers of the anterior lateral tracts have branches, many of which terminate in the reticular formation, which is the system that controls wakefulness. When activated, they wake us up or increase alertness (Figure A.8).

It is a general rule that nerve fibers from all receptors terminate on nerve cells located on the same side of the spinal cord as the receptors. The nerve cells that receive signals from nociceptors are located in the dorsal horn (see figure A.7 and A.8). The axons of these nerve cells cross over to the other side immediately and then form the *anterior lateral tracts*, the nerve fibers of which terminate on cells in the ventral and the dorsal portions of the thalamus.

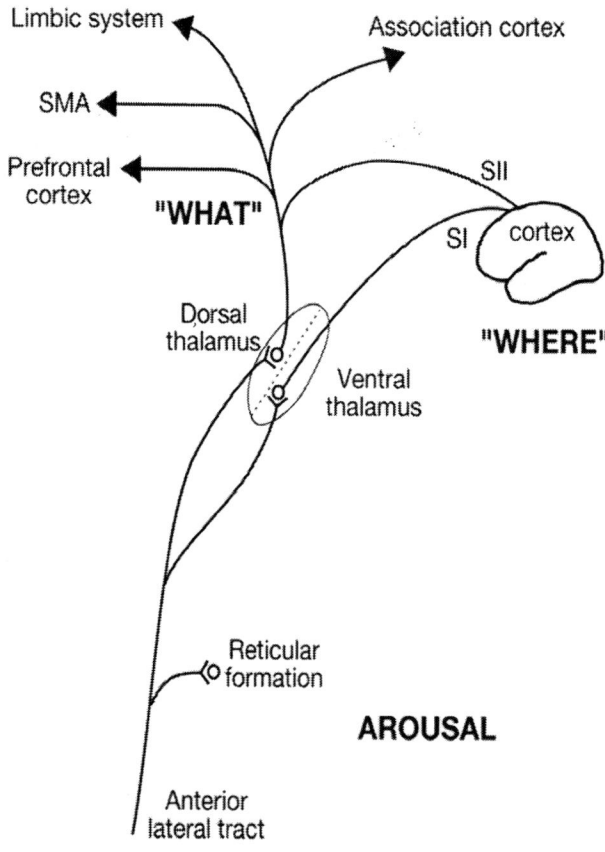

Figure A.8. A schematic drawing of the pain pathways showing that connections from nerve cells in the dorsal horn branches off to the reticular formation before reaching their targets in the dorsal and ventral parts of the thalamus. Nerve cells in the dorsal thalamus project too many different structures, some of which are subcortical. Nerve cells in the ventral portion of the thalamus project mainly to the primary somatosensory cortex. SMA: Supplementary motor area; SI: Primary somatosensory cortex; SII: Secondary somatosensory cortex. (Modified from Møller, A.R. 2006. *Neural plasticity and disorders of the nervous system* Cambridge University Press Cambridge) [8] Copyright © Cambridge University Press 2006. Reprinted with the permission of Cambridge University Press.

The pain pathways that are activated by pain receptors (nociceptors) use both the ventral and the dorsal-medial parts of the thalamus (Figure A.8), and therefore have direct access to limbic structures (the emotional brain) and the somatosensory cortex. That can explain why somatic pain from activation of pain receptors provides both information about where the pain is located and how the pain is felt.

Nerve fibers the trigeminal nuclei join the spinothalamic tract and reach the thalamus in a similar way as fibers from the body. The thalamus plays an important role in all senses except smell (olfaction). The signals that reach the ventral part of the thalamus tell where on the body the pain comes from, and those signal that reach the dorsal part tells something about the pain - mainly burning sensations are caused by activation of nerve cells in the dorsal thalamus (see Figure A.8).

1.3. Pain Signals Reach Many Parts of the Brain

Signals from pain receptors are directed to parts of the "emotional brain", such as the amygdala and the anterior cingulate gyrus to a greater extent than sensory signals. For example, pain signals caused by injury do not only reach the parts of the brain that causes a certain awareness, but it also may activate other parts of the brain that trigger other systems, such as the autonomic nervous system and parts of the brain that give fear and the perception of intrusion and threat (Figure A.9). The region of the brain that causes the sensation of unpleasantness may also be turned on by pain signals. This can explain why pain signals can cause so many different reactions. Of particular interest is the fact that pain signals through the dorsal and medial thalamus can reach some parts of the "emotional brain" through a direct (subcortical) route.

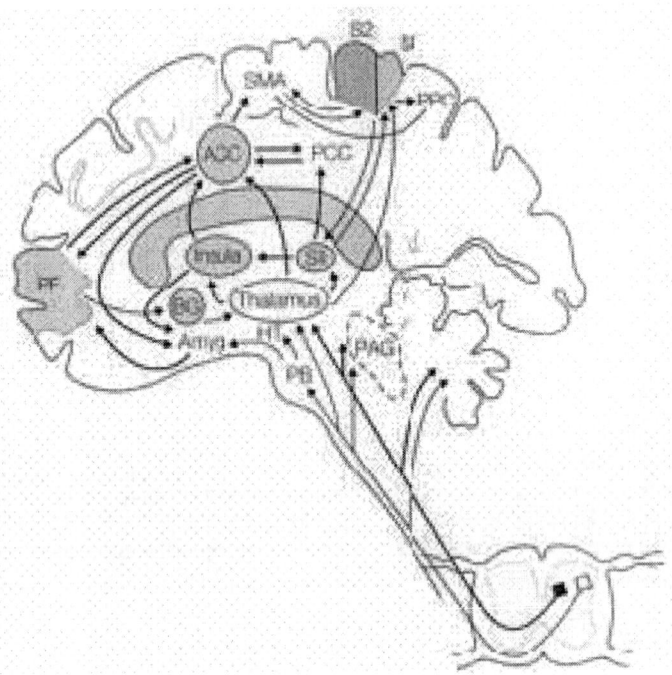

Figure A.9. Illustration of the many different areas of the brain involved in showing how pain signals travel to where they can cause many different reactions. (From McMahon, S.B., Koltzenburg, M., (Eds.) 2006. *Wall and Melzak's Textbook of Pain.* Elsevier, Churchill, Livingstone, Amsterdam. Chapter 6, adapted after Price 2000 [9], Reprinted with permission of Elsevier).

Pain signals engage several parts of the limbic system, including the amygdala and the anterior cingulate gyrus. These structures are known to be involved in pain by the experience that lesions in the cingulum can alleviate pain. The amygdala is mainly known for its role in fear sensations but it is also involved in mood and is believed to be the structures that are faulty in affective (mood) diseases such as depression.

The connections directly from the dorsal and medial nuclei of the thalamus send unprocessed information to the amygdala ("low route") [3], while sensory information normally reaches the amygdala via a long chain of nerve cells in the primary and secondary sensory cortices and association cortices ("high route") [3] (Figure A.10). This subcortical activation of limbic system structures may be responsible for mood related symptoms that accompany central neuropathic pain and also some forms of tinnitus.

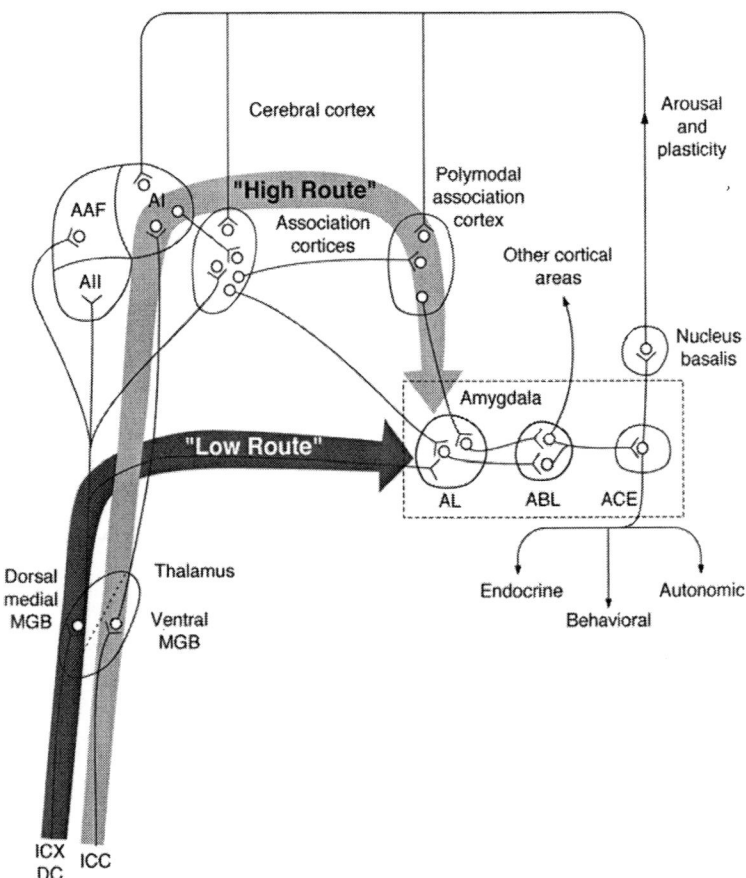

Figure A.10. Schematic illustration of the "high route" and the "low route" from sensory systems to the lateral nucleus of the amygdala. ACE: Central nucleus of the amygdala. AL: Lateral nucleus of the amygdala, ABL: Basolateral nucleus of the amygdala. MGB: Medial geniculate body. (Reproduced from: Møller, A.R. 2006. *Neural plasticity and disorders of the nervous system* Cambridge University Press, Cambridge [8] Copyright © Cambridge University Press 2006. Reprinted with the permission of Cambridge University Press.)

There are connections from the different nuclei of the amygdala to many other parts of the brain (figure A.10), such as those that control secretion of hormones involved in reproduction and secretion of many other hormones that have important roles in running essential functions of the body.

The fact that these non-classical pathways bypass the primary sensory cortices [6] may be why they create emotional symptoms of various kinds.

> The amygdala is the primary target of signals from the olfactory system that mediate information about odors. Perception of sensory information has earlier been associated with the cerebral cortex, but perhaps some of the nuclei in the amygdala can also provide conscious sensory perceptions. The olfactory system has little cortical representations, and the fact that its central projection is mainly to the amygdala may indicate we can perceive sensory signals by the amygdala. It may therefore be suggested that the amygdala plays a role in the perception of pain.

The amygdala also sends signals to the cerebral cortex, which increases alertness of the cortex and promotes neural plasticity in the cerebral cortex (through the cholinergic system of the nucleus basalis) [2,11]. This may have widespread importance but it is so far poorly understood.

Pain signals are only slightly represented in the somatosensory cortices, and this is an important difference from sensory signals such as hearing, vision and touch.

1.4. Modulation of Pain

There are many ways the perception of pain can be modulated. Change in the way pain signals are processed in the neural circuits of the spinal cord and in the brain may increase the sensation of pain. This is known as central sensitization. The perception of the strength of pain, or rather the level of discomfort, can be modulated by high central functions involved in attention. The amount of attention a person places on his or her pain affects how it is perceived ("I have pain, but pain does not have me"). Distraction can decrease the perceived intensity of pain.

Peripheral sensitization of receptors and central sensitization of the neural circuits in the spinal cord and brain play important roles in modulating pain signals, and therefore affect how pain is perceived. The opposite of sensitization, suppression of pain signals, may also occur in the spinal cord and the brain where pain signals can be modulated by signals from other senses and from the brain [10].

Anxiety increases perceived strength of pain sensation, whereas relaxation decreases perceived strength. Relaxing and taking a deep breath can change the perception of many forms of pain. Stress may increase or decrease the sensation of pain.

1.4.1. From Receptors in the Skin

The pain signals that arrive at the nerve cells in the dorsal horn are not transmitted to the brain unaltered. In fact, there are several ways pain signals can be affected before they leave the dorsal horn. As was discussed in Chapter II, both signals from receptors that are sensitive to harmless stimulation, such as touch, can decrease the transmission of pain signals and can also be influenced (decreased or increased) by neural activity that reaches the cells in the dorsal horn from the brain.

The signals from skin receptors are carried in large nerve fibers can inhibit the cells in the spinal cord that process pain signals. Nerve cells in the dorsal horn also receive signals from other nerve cells in the spinal cord and from the brain, which can both decrease and increase the transmission of pain signals. The nerve cells in the dorsal horn can therefore control the way pain signals are going to be forwarded to the brain and thereby alter the way pain is perceived.

Touch of the skin can change the transmission of pain signals in the spinal cord and the trigeminal nucleus and thereby change the sensation of pain (Figure A.11).

The pain cells in the dorsal horn receive signals from other cells located internally in the spinal cord and from various parts of the brain. These signals either increase or decrease the pain signals before they reach the brain and thereby change how intense pain is felt.

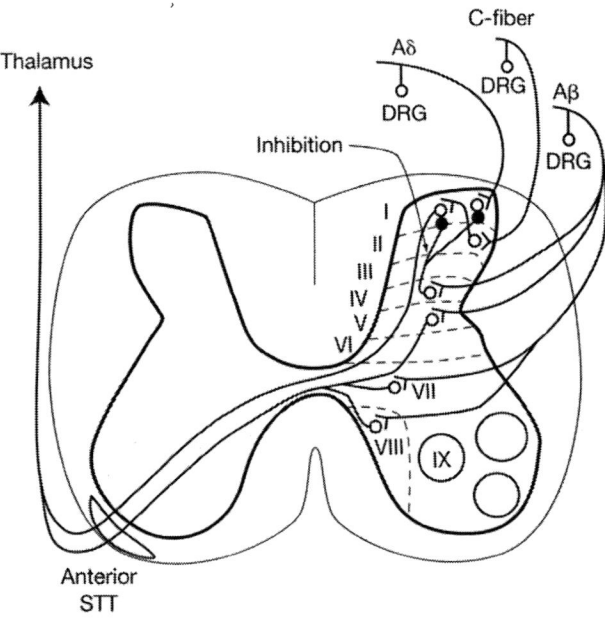

Figure A.11. Schematic drawing of some of the connections to cells in the dorsal horn that are important for pain. The connections to cells in the different parts (lamina) of the dorsal horn from nerve fibers of different types (Aδ Aβ and C fibers) are shown to illustrate how signals from large myelinated fibers (Aβ) can influence the processing of pain signals in the spinal cord. (Reproduced from: Møller, A.R. 2006. *Neural plasticity and disorders of the nervous system* Cambridge University Press Cambridge [8] Copyright © Cambridge University Press 2006. Reprinted with the permission of Cambridge University Press.)

1.4.2. Modulation of Pain by Descending Pathways

There are extensive descending pathways that are part of the pain pathways in the brain. Little is known about the functions of these descending pathways, but they are likely to cause various forms of top-down (from high brain centers to lower ones) influence on the processing of pain signals. It is, of course, known that sensory systems have strong top-down influence (see [7]). The fact that pain sensations can be controlled by hypnosis is a strong sign of such top-down influence. Hypnosis[67] and self-suggestion can prevent or reduce

---

[67] Hypnosis is traditionally regarded as a trance-like condition that can be brought about in a person who accepts suggestions from another person. It is a state of wakefulness in which a person's attention is focused and a state of heightened suggestibility, with diminished awareness of surroundings. Hypnosis is in practical use for management of pain, for treating addictions and phobias, and to some extent for treatment of tinnitus.

perceiving pain such as occurs to fakirs[68]. It is possible for some individuals to induce general freedom of pain (analgesia) for surgical operations through hypnosis, but it is not possible for everybody to get hypnotized in this way. Hypnosis is recognized by medical organizations in the US and in Great Britain for treatment of several disorders. The use of hypnosis in treatment of pain is discussed in Chapter V.

The effects of peripheral and central suppression of pain may explain why pain is perceived differently under different circumstances (such as immediately after a severe injury compared with days later).

This kind of reduced pain perception occurs often in severe injury where the individual does not feel any pain immediately after the injury occurred. This effect is often experienced in accidents and in war induced injuries. It is not known exactly how blockage of pain impulses occurs, but it is believed to occur in the spinal cord. The period of freedom from pain may last 15 minutes or more [10]. Some forms of illness, such as heart attacks, may sometimes be painless, although lack of oxygen (ischemia) normally gives pain.

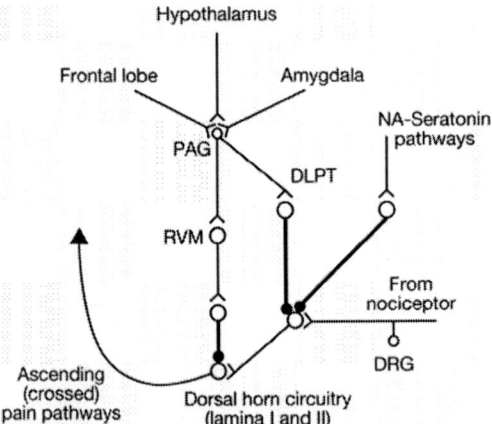

Figure A.12. Sources of signals to the PAG and pathways through which the signals from the PAG can modulate the processing of pain signals in the spinal cord. (Reproduced from: Møller, A.R. 2006. *Neural plasticity and disorders of the nervous system* Cambridge University Press Cambridge [8] Copyright © Cambridge University Press 2006. Reprinted with the permission of Cambridge University Press).

A structure known as the periaquaductal gray (PAG) plays an important role in central control of pain. Nerve cells in the PAG receive input from many parts of the brain, and the PAG influences the processing of pain signals at many stages in the brain as well as in the spinal cord (and the trigeminal nucleus) (Figure A.12). It has been shown that "escapable" pain and "inescapable" pain are processed in different parts of the PAG

There are other descending pathways that can influence how pain signals are processed in the dorsal horn of the spinal cord. One is the dorsolateral pontomesencephalic tegmentum pathway (DLTP) (Figure A.13). Other describing systems originate in the noradrenalin-serotonin system. It has more recently become evident that the vagus nerve (the 10th cranial

---

[68] Fakir: the more extreme picture of a fakir is a near-naked man who walks on burning coals barefooted, or sleeping on a bed of nails during meditation.

nerve) is also involved in modulating pain, and that has had a practical implication in that it is the basis for some forms of treatment (see Chapter V) using electrical stimulation of the vagus nerve.

For an overview of the descending pain pathways, see [8]

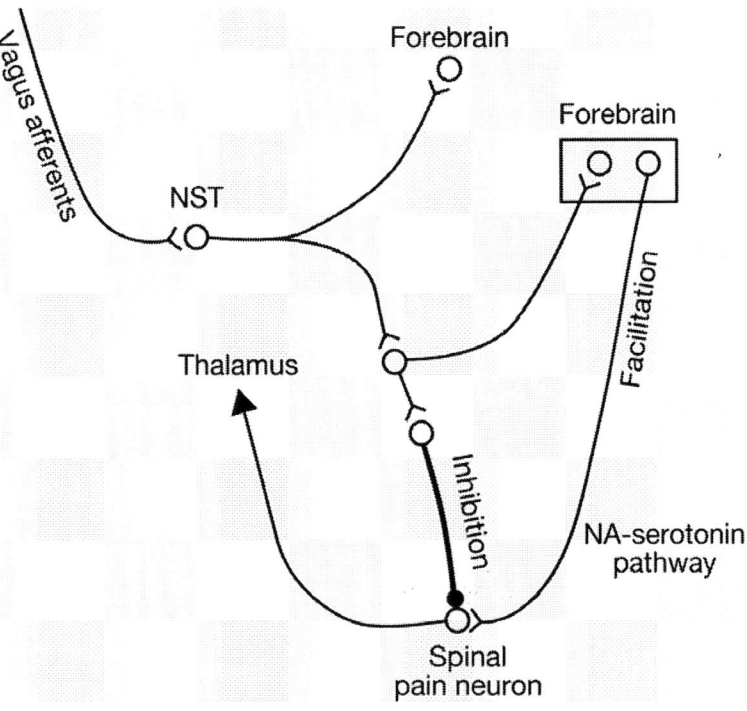

Figure A.13. Schematic illustration of the involvement of the vagus nerve. (Reproduced from: Møller, A.R. 2006. *Neural plasticity and disorders of the nervous system* Cambridge University Press Cambridge [8] Copyright © Cambridge University Press 2006. Reprinted with the permission of Cambridge University Press.)

1.4.3. Modulation of Pain by the Autonomic Nervous System

The autonomic nervous system regulates many functions of the body, and it is absolutely necessary for normal body function. In fact, it is necessary for keeping oneself alive. The autonomic nervous system, as its name suggests, is assumed to function automatically without conscious influence. This is not always true. One of its most important functions is to regulate the flow of blood to different parts of the body so that one does not faint when rising from bed. This occurs without conscious awareness, but there are other functions of the autonomic nervous system that cause conscious awareness.

The sympathetic nervous system is a part of the autonomic nervous system, the other part being the parasympathetic nervous system. The sympathetic nervous system is perhaps best known for its ability to alert the body to dangers and prepare the body for fight and flight. It is often associated with the body's reaction to various kinds of stress, but it has many other functions.

The most visible effect of the sympathetic nervous system is on blood circulation where it regulates the size of arteries and the pumping of the heart. The sympathetic nervous system helps keep enough blood supplied to the head when getting out of bed, increasing blood pressure and the heart's pumping action when using muscles for work, etc. It also causes sweating which cools the body. Another visible effect of increased activity of the sympathetic nervous system is its effect on the eye, where it increases the size of the pupil.

The sympathetic nervous system can be activated by stress of various kinds. Increased body temperature is an example of a danger signal that causes increase in sympathetic activity. The autonomic nervous system plays an important role in regulating how the heart works. In fact, the function of most bodily organs is affected by the sympathetic nervous system. Much of the sympathetic nervous system is mediated by adrenalin secreted from cells in the adrenal medulla. The secretion occurs on command from sympathetic nerve fibers that innervate that organ. Adrenalin indirectly affects the blood circulation and the heart together, with the effect of the sympathetic nerves that terminate on arteries.

The sympathetic nervous system plays an important role in the processing and modulation of pain signals.

The intensity of pain depends on many factors, such as stress, which can both increase and decrease the perceived intensity of pain. These reactions are mediated by the sympathetic nervous system. Activation of the sympathetic nervous system can cause secretion of norepinephrine from sympathetic nerve endings located near pain receptors, and thereby increase their sensitivity. This is known as peripheral sensitization. This may create a vicious circle where increased sympathetic activity increases the pain, which increases the sympathetic activity. This is what is known as sympathetic maintained pain, SMP. Too much peripheral sensitization can cause a pain condition known as reflex sympathetic dystrophy (RSD) (now also known as complex regional pain syndrome type one (CRPS I).

Activation of the sympathetic nervous system can affect (modulate) the transmission of pain signals in the spinal cord and the brain and thereby alter the sensation of pain.

REFERENCES

[1]   Dostrovsky JO, Craig AD. Ascending projection systems. In: McMahon SB, Koltzenburg M, editors. *Wall and Melzak's Textbook of Pain*. Amsterdam: Elsevier; 2006. p. 187-203.

[2]   Kilgard MP, Merzenich MM. Cortical map reorganization enabled by nucleus basalis activity. *Science*. 1998;279:1714-8.

[3]   LeDoux JE. Brain mechanisms of emotion and emotional learning. *Curr Opin Neurobiol.* 1992;2:191-7.

[4]   McMahon SB, Koltzenburg M, editors. *Wall and Melzak's Textbook of Pain.* 5th ed. Amsterdam: Elsevier, Churchill, Livingstone; 2006.

[5]   Meyer RA, Ringkamp M, Campbell JN, Raja SN. Peripheral mechanisms of cutaneous nociception. In: McMahon SB, Koltzenburg M, (Eds.), editors. *Wall and Melzak's Textbook of Pain.* Amsterdam: Elsevier; 2006. p. 3-34.

[6]   Møller AR. *Sensory Systems: Anatomy and Physiology.* Amsterdam: Academic Press; 2003.

[7]   Møller AR. *Hearing: Anatomy, Physiology, and Disorders of the Auditory System, 2nd Ed.* Amsterdam: Academic Press; 2006.

[8]   Møller AR. *Neural plasticity and disorders of the nervous system.* Cambridge: Cambridge University Press 2006.

[9]   Price DD. Psychological and neural mechanisms of the affective dimension of pain. *Science.* 2000;288:1769-72.

[10] Wall P. *Pain: The Science of suffering. Rose S,* editor. New York: Columbia University Press; 2000.

[11] Weinberger NM. Learning-induced physiological memory in adult primary auditory cortex: Receptive field plasticity, model, and mechanisms. *Audiol Neuro-Otol.* 1998;3:145-67.

APPENDIX B

1. ANATOMY AND PHYSIOLOGY OF HEARING

Chapter I gave a general description of how sensory systems work. This Appendix discusses the hearing system in more detail because it is important for understanding of tinnitus and other abnormalities that regard hearing and are related to neural plasticity. The hearing system has three main parts, 1) the ear, 2) the ascending and descending neural pathways and the primary hearing cortex, and 3) higher level cortices (association cortices and their connections to several different brain regions.

It is true that the ear is a sophisticated organ that performs many complex functions. We know much more about how the ear functions than what we know about the function of the hearing nervous system. The nervous system performs complex processing of the signals it receives from the ear, and this processing going awry in one way or another is the basis for symptoms of many forms of tinnitus.

1.1. The Ear

The middle ear makes it possible to effectively conduct airborne sounds to the fluid filled cochlea where the sensory cells that convert sounds into nerve impulses or rather control the impulse traffic in the hearing nerve. The cochlea separate sounds according to their frequencies in such as way that different frequency bands activate different populations of nerve fibers. The cochlea also compresses that intensity range of sounds, which is necessary to code sounds in the impulse pattern of hearing nerve fibers because nerve fibers have a narrow dynamic range. The ear also compresses the intensity of the sounds so sounds they often have a very large range of intensities can be coded in the impulse pattern of the individual nerve fibers in the hearing nerve despite coding of nerve impulses has a narrow dynamic range.

1.2. Hearing Pathways

From the ear, signals of sounds can take two routes to the cerebral cortex. We will call these routes the *classical* and the *non-classical* pathways [9]. They are also known as the lemniscal and the extralemniscal pathways. The targets of these two pathways in the cerebral cortices are different and the processing of sounds is different as well in the nuclei of the respective ascending (climbing) pathways. The classical pathways are much better known than the non-classical ones. Understanding the difference between them is important for understanding some kinds of tinnitus.

In adults, normally only the classical ascending hearing pathway is active but there are indications that also the non-classical pathways are active in children {Møller, 2002 #399}. The non-classical pathway may be turned on abnormally, such as in some individuals with tinnitus [14]. There are also signs of an abnormal use of the non-classical pathways in some autistic individuals [13]. There is evidence that the non-classical pathways are active in young children [15].

There are also extensive descending pathways that follow the ascending pathways from the cerebral cortex all the way down to the ear [9]. The anatomy of these descending pathways is similar to the ascending pathways, and these pathways just travel in the opposite direction, from top down. The anatomy of these descending pathways is well described [18] but we know very little about the function of the descending pathways, which are at least as anatomically extensive as the ascending pathways.

The hearing nervous system is plastic and its organization can be changed through activation of neural plasticity. There is evidence that the frequency tuning in the nervous system requires exposure to sounds, and there is other evidence that the routes that neural activity that is elicited by sounds take can be changed by activation of neural plasticity.

1.2.1. Classical Ascending Hearing Pathways

Most clinical books on hearing have focused on the ear and title space has been devoted to how the hearing nervous system function. The information from the ear about sounds travels along an "information highway" from the ear (the cochlea) to the primary hearing cortex. From there, the information travels to other parts of the cerebral cortex and to other parts of the brain. The signals from the ear enter the brain through the hearing nerve and passes through several nuclei (clusters of nerve cells that function as relay stations) on the way to the cerebral cortex (see Figure B.1). The first such nucleus is the cochlear nucleus, located in the pons (lower or middle part of the brainstem). As the information climbs towards the cerebral cortices, it is interrupted in more nuclei along the way.

From the cochlear nucleus, nerve fibers cross the midline of the brainstem and travel to the next major relay station, the inferior colliculus, in the midbrain on the opposite side of the brain. Before the information reaches the inferior colliculus, some of the nerve fibers are interrupted in nuclei of the superior olivary complex (SOC).

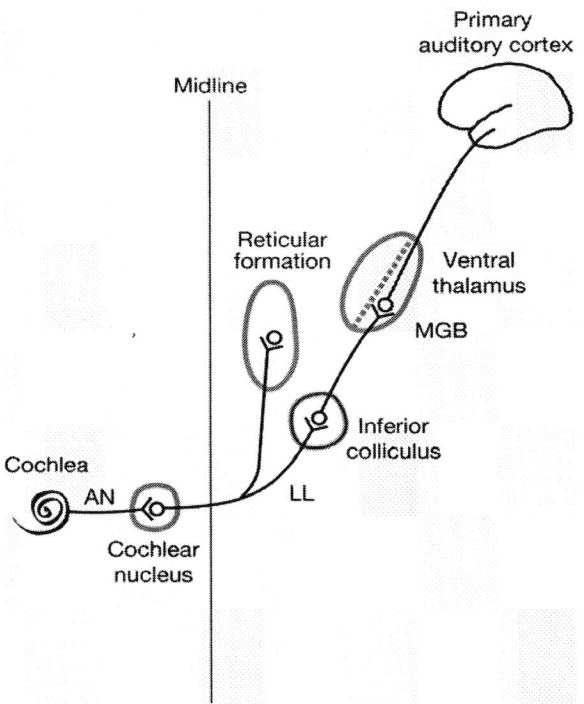

Figure B.1. Simplified schematic drawing of the classical ascending hearing pathway as it proceeds from one ear towards the cerebral cortex on the other side [10]. Reproduced from Møller, A.R. 2006. *Neural plasticity and disorders of the nervous system* Cambridge University Press Cambridge [10] Copyright © Cambridge University Press 2006. Reprinted with the permission of Cambridge University Press.).

A drawing of the classical hearing pathways, laid out on an anatomical picture of the brain, is shown in Figure B.2. There are extensive connections between the two pathways at the midbrain level. Nerve fibers from the nucleus of the lateral lemniscus (LL) and from the inferior colliculus (IC) on one side connect to the inferior colliculus on the other side. These connections ensure that each one of the next relay nuclei of the ascending pathways, the medial geniculate (MG) nuclei (also known as the medial geniculate body, MGB) in the thalamus, receives signals from both ears.

The geniculate bodies on the two sides of the brain have no connections with each other. Large fiber tracts connect the nerve cells in the medical geniculate with nerve cells in the primary hearing cortex, which in humans is located deep in a fissure in the temporal lobe known as Hechel's gyrus.

It is a typical property of the classical pathways that the nerve cells respond only to sounds within a certain narrow frequency range. This means the different nerve cells are "tuned" to a certain frequency. This tuning is important for our ability to distinguish between different sounds. The tuning of nerve cells originates in the cochlea, but is modified in the different nuclei and in the cerebral cortex because nerve cells in these nuclei and cortex receive signals from more than one location along the basilar membrane of the cochlea. The tuning of nerve cells and their organization according to the frequencies to which they respond best in the nuclei of the hearing pathways, including the cerebral cortex, is mostly developed after birth. Correct development requires that the child is exposed to sounds early in life. Animal studies have shown that without exposure to sounds, only a rudimentary organization of nerve cells according to frequency to which they respond best exists [17]. This means that frequency tuning is a product of activation of neural plasticity.

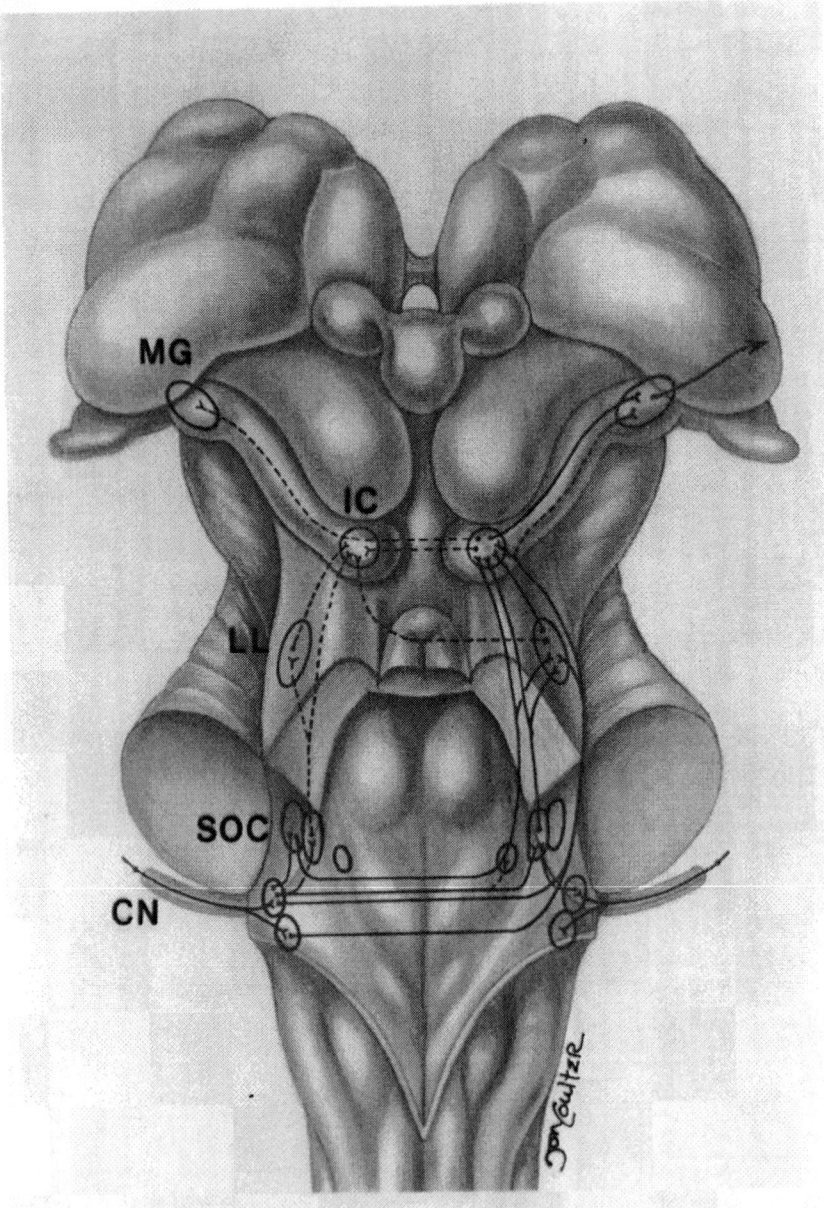

Figure B.2. Simplified drawing of the ascending classical hearing pathways indicating where in the brain the different nuclei and fiber tracts are located. AN: Hearing nerve, SOC: Superior olivary complex; LL: Lateral lemniscus; IC: Inferior colliculus; MG: Medical geniculate body. AN: Hearing nerve, SOC: Superior olivary complex; LL: Lateral lemniscus; IC: Inferior colliculus; MG: Medical geniculate body (From Møller,1988 [7]).

The sharpness of the tuning changes as the information ascends towards the cortex where some nerve cells respond more selectively to sounds than nerve cells of the nuclei or the ascending pathways. The result is that some cells respond to a broader range of frequencies than hearing nerve fibers, while others respond to a narrower range. This is caused by convergence of signals from nerve cells that are tuned to slightly different frequencies and by the interplay between inhibition and excitation.

The convergence of signals onto nerve cells can be altered through activation of neural plasticity. This means that the range of frequencies to which cells respond (broadness of tuning) can be changed by activation of neural plasticity, as can the frequency to which a cell is tuned.

The separation of the parts of the brain that process signals from different senses prevents interaction between the signals that are received by different sense organs. This is why touching or rubbing the skin normally does not affect how we perceive a sound, and the way we hear sounds is not affected by what we see. This separation should not be mistaken from the coordination of what is received by the difference senses, which occurs in higher central regions of the brain, the association cortices.

The primary hearing cortex is not the end station for hearing information. Information travels in several directions from the primary hearing cortex. Some nerve fibers lead to the opposite side's hearing cortex. After passing the primary hearing cortex, the information travels to other parts of the hearing cortex, other parts of the cerebral cortex, and other parts of the brain.

Further processing occurs in the parts of the cerebral cortex, known as association cortices. Different kinds of sounds are processed in different parts of the association cortices (known as *stream segregation)*. One such region is known as Wernicke's area, which is involved in understanding the meaning of speech. It is also involved in production of speech. Understanding of speech is done best by the left side of the brain, whereas music is interpreted mostly on the right side.

Since the hearing cortex on both sides of the brain receives similar information from each (because of the connections between the two side's inferior colliculi), injuries to the primary hearing cortex on one side of the brain has little effect on understanding of normal speech, but understanding of distorted speech is impaired [16].

1.2.2. Non-classical Pathways

The classical hearing pathways described above are only one part of the hearing nervous system, but it is the part described in most detail in books on hearing. In some texts it is the only part that is described. The other part, much less known, has several names such as the extralemniscal pathway, the non-specific pathways, the diffuse pathways, or the polysensory pathways. More recently, these pathways became known as the non-classical pathways [9].

The non-classical pathways mainly travel in parallel with the classical pathways, but there are some distinct differences. The non-classical pathways use other nuclei on the way to the cerebral cortex [1,9].

While the classical hearing pathways use the central nucleus of the inferior colliculus, the non-classical pathways use nuclei that surrounds the central nucleus, known as the dorsal cortex, and the external nucleus of the inferior colliculus (see Figure B.3).

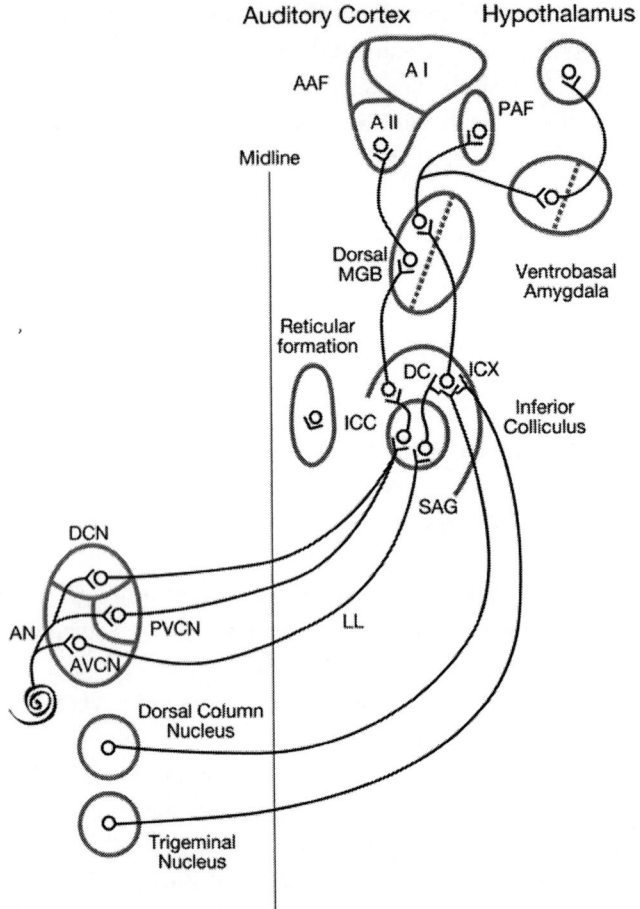

Figure B.3. A schematic diagram of the non-classical hearing pathways from one ear. AN: Auditory (hearing) nerve; DCN: Dorsal cochlear nucleus; PVCN: Posterior ventral cochlear nucleus; AVCN: Anterior ventral cochlear nucleus; LL: Lateral lemniscus; ICX: external nucleus of the inferior colliculus; DC: Dorsal cortex of the inferior colliculus; ICC: Central nucleus of the inferior colliculus; SAG: Sagulum; MGB: Medial geniculate body (of thalamus); PAF: Posterior auditory field; AAF: anterior auditory field; AI: Primary hearing cortex; AII: Secondary hearing cortex. (Reproduced from: Møller, A.R. 2006. *Hearing: Anatomy, Physiology, and Disorders of the Auditory System*, 2nd Ed. Academic Press, Amsterdam, with permission from Elsevier) [9].

    While the classical pathway makes use of one part (the ventral part of the medial geniculate body, MGB) of the hearing part of the thalamus, the non-classical systems use a different part of the thalamus (the dorsal and medial parts). This is important because these two parts project to different structures. Nerve cells in the ventral part of the nucleus project to the primary hearing cortex, while the cells in the dorsal and medial geniculate body bypass the primary cortex and connect to secondary and association cortices (see Figure B.3).

    The responses from nerve cells in the non-classical pathways to sounds are thus less distinct than the responses from nerve cells in the classical pathways. In general, the nuclei of the non-classical pathways process sounds much less than the classical pathways. The non-classical pathways are probably older phylogenetical (in the evolution of species) than the classical pathways, which offer capabilities of more complex analysis of sounds than the non-classical pathways. Perhaps the non-classical pathways were developed to serve the purpose of warning of imminent dangers through sound, and the classical pathways evolved later when demands of more complex analysis of sensory information became important for survival and reproduction.

The two pathways are sometimes known as the "slow and accurate" and the "fast and dirty".

There are other important differences between these two pathways. While all nerve cells in nuclei of the classical pathways and those of the primary cortices only respond to sound stimulation, many nerve cells in the non-classical hearing pathways also respond to other sensory modalities such as touch [1] and light that reaches the eye [11]. Processing of sounds in the nuclei of the non-classical pathways can be modulated by signals from other senses. This is known as *cross-modal interaction,* and it means that nerve cells in the non-classical hearing pathways receive signals from other sensory systems than hearing. This may seem as a violation of a fundamental law of sensory systems, namely Johannes Müller's law of the specific nerve energies.

The implication of the Müller's law of the specific nerve energies is that any stimulation of the hearing nerve results in a sensation of a sound (only), any stimulation of the optic nerve results in an experience of light, and so on. The reason for that is that the nerves from our sense organs, ear, eye, nose, and skin deliver their message to certain and different parts of the brain. This means sensory stimulation is perceived according to which part of the brain is activated rather than how the sensory nerves are activated (when activated directly). This is why any kind of stimulation of the hearing nerve is always (normally) perceived as a sound of some kind.

There is evidence that the non-classical pathways are not normally active in adults [12,14]. The possible role of the non-classical ascending pathways has been investigated in experimental studies where the effect of electrical stimulation of a peripheral nerve (the median nerve at the wrist) on perception of sounds was evaluated. In adults, such electrical stimulation of the median nerve does not normally affect how sounds are perceived [14], nor does rubbing the skin produce sensation of sound or affect how sounds are perceived. This means that cross-modal interaction normally does not occur in adults, and the conclusion has been that the non-classical pathways are normally not active in adults. Nevertheless, similar studies have shown evidence that cross-modal interaction occurs regularly in children under the age of 15 [15]. Electrical stimulation of the median nerve evokes a tingling sensation in parts of the hand because the median nerve innervates the skin of the hand. It was shown in these studies that in children, such stimulation can change the perception of sounds presented through earphones. That was taken as a sign of involvement of the non-classical pathways because the nerve cells in the non-classical hearing pathways receive signals from other sensory systems, which cells in the classical pathways do not.

There are also signs that non-classical pathways are active in some forms of tinnitus [2,14] and in some autistic individuals [13].

Information about sound can reach the amygdala through two different routes. One is through the classical hearing pathways, which must be regarded as the normal way information reaches the amygdala. The other route is through the non-classical pathways. The parts of the structures that are involved in emotional reactions are foremost is the amygdala.

> The *amygdala* is the structure in the brain that plays an important role in emotional reactions such as fear it is also central to diseases such as depression. The amygdala is a part of the limbic system, also known as the visceral brain. The amygdala consists of three main nuclei the lateral nucleus, the basolateral, and the central nucleus.

Cells in the dorsal and medical nuclei also connect directly to several other parts of the brain, such as the amygdala, while cells in the ventral part of the thalamic nucleus do not have such direct connections to brain structures such as the amygdala. The classical pathways use a much longer route to the amygdala (see Appendix A, Figure A.10).

The route to the amygdala through the classical sensory pathways has been called "slow and accurate", while non-classical pathways have been called "fast and dirty". The non-classical pathways developed early in the evolution of mammals. Classical pathways developed later.

The classical hearing pathways provides signals to the amygdala through a long route (the *"high route"*) [5,10] that takes the information from the hearing cortex through several parts of the association cortices to finally reach the lateral nucleus of the amygdala. This route involves many steps of processing in which information can be transformed in various ways and suppressed or enhanced.

The amygdala can also receive signals directly from the thalamus (*"the low route"*). The lateral nucleus receives signals directly from the nucleus of the thalamus used by the non-classical pathway [4,6,8]. Information that travels to the amygdala through the low route does not need to go through the primary, secondary, and association cortices to reach the amygdala because it can use the direct (subcortical) connection between the thalamus and the lateral nucleus of the amygdala.

When the amygdala receives its signals from the classical hearing pathways, the information passes through a long chain of nerve cells in the hearing cortices and the association cortices (the "high route"). It is assumed that "reasoning" can interrupt the information in the "high route" before it reaches the amygdala. A sound may evoke fear the first time it is heard. However, after it is clear the sound is not dangerous, it will not evoke fear when it is heard again. If the fear reaction is mediated through a direct (subcortical) route provided by the non-classical pathways, it may not be possible to interrupt the signals before they reach the amygdala. Consequently, a fearful sound will continue to evoke fear although the person knows that it is not a sign of danger. Some individuals with tinnitus have signs that the non-classical pathways are active [12]. This may explain why sounds evoke fear (known as phonophobia) in some individuals with tinnitus, who may feel fear from many common sounds although they know that these sounds do not involve any danger. The non-classical pathways, unlike the classical pathways, have a "direct line" (subcortical connection) to the emotional brain, the amygdala.

1.2.3. Descending Hearing Pathways

In addition to these two ascending pathways that connect structures from the hearing nerve to structures at the top of the ascending pathways (cerebral cortices of the brain), there are extensive connections from the top to the bottom (descending pathways) of the hearing nervous system. In fact, these downward aiming pathways may be better described as being pathways that travel in parallel with the two ascending pathways (reciprocal pathways). While the anatomy of these descending pathways may be relatively well known [18], practically nothing is known about their function - perhaps with one exception, known as the olivocochlear system. These descending (efferent) pathways terminate on cochlear hair cells; more on outer hair cells than inner ones [9]. Since these pathways receive their signals from more central parts of the hearing nervous system, it is possible that they provide some control over the sensitivity of the cochlear hair cells by the central nervous system. It is known that sound applied to one ear can modulate the sensitivity of the hair cells in the ear on the opposite side [3], and that is mediated through the olivocochlear part of the descending pathways. The functional importance of that is not known.

REFERENCES

[1]   Aitkin LM. *The auditory midbrain, structure and function in the central auditory pathway*. Clifton, NJ: Humana Press; 1986.

[2]   Cacace AT, Lovely TJ, McFarland DJ, Parnes SM, Winter DF. Anomalous cross-modal plasticity following posterior fossa surgery: Some speculations on gaze-evoked tinnitus. *Hear Res*. 1994;81:22-32.

[3]   Collet L, Kemp DT, Veuillet E, Duclaux R, Moulin A, Morgon A. Effect of contralateral auditory stimuli on active cochlear micro-mechanical properties in human subjects. *Hear Res*. 1990;43:251-62.

[4]   Doron NN, LeDoux JE. Cells in the posterior thalamus project to both amygdala and temporal cortex: a quantitative retrograde double-labeling study in the rat. *J Comp Neurol*. 2000;425:257-74.

[5]   LeDoux JE. Brain mechanisms of emotion and emotional learning. *Curr Opin Neurobiol*. 1992;2:191-7.

[6]   LeDoux JE, Cicchetti P, Xagoraris A, Romanski LM. The lateral amygdaloid nucleus: Sensory interface of the amygdala in fear conditioning. *J Neurosci*. 1990;10:1062-9.

[7]   Møller AR. *Evoked potentials in intraoperative monitoring*. Baltimore: Williams and Wilkins; 1988.

[8]   Møller AR. *Sensory Systems: Anatomy and Physiology*. Amsterdam: Academic Press; 2003.

[9]   Møller AR. *Hearing: Anatomy, Physiology, and Disorders of the Auditory System, 2nd Ed.* Amsterdam: Academic Press; 2006.

[10]   Møller AR. *Neural plasticity and disorders of the nervous system*. Cambridge: Cambridge University Press 2006.

[11] Møller AR. Tinnitus: Present and Future. In: Langguth B, Hajak G, Kleinjung T, Cacace A, Møller A, editors. *Tinnitus, Pathophysiology and Treatment*. Amsterdam: Elsevier; 2007. p. 3-16.

[12] Møller AR, Jho HD, Yokota M, Jannetta PJ. Contribution from crossed and uncrossed brainstem structures to the brainstem auditory evoked potentials (BAEP): A study in human. *Laryngoscope*. 1995;105:596-605.

[13] Møller AR, Kern JK, Grannemann B. Are the non-classical auditory pathways involved in autism and PDD? *Neurol Res*. 2005;27:625-9.

[14] Møller AR, Møller MB, Yokota M. Some forms of tinnitus may involve the extralemniscal auditory pathway. *Laryngoscope*. 1992; 102: 1165-71.

[15] Møller AR, Rollins P. The non-classical auditory system is active in children but not in adults. *Neurosci Lett*. 2002;319:41-4.

[16] Møller MB (Korsan-Bengtsen, M.). Distorted Speech Audiometry. *Acta Otolaryng (Stockholm)*. 1973;Suppl. 310.

[17] Snyder RL, Rebscher SJ, Cao K, Leake PA. Effects of chronic intracochlear stimulation in the neonatally deafened cat: I. Expansion of central spatial representation. *Hear Res*. 1990;50:7-33.

[18] Winer JA, Lee CC. The distributed auditory cortex. *Hear Res*. 2007;229:3-13.

APPENDIX C

1. AUTISM SPECTRUM DISEASES

Autism is not one disease. It is therefore more correct to refer to a class of diseases: "Autism Spectrum Diseases" (ASD), which is one part of a larger group of Pervasive Developmental Diseases (PDD) [4,17]. According to Stedman's Electronic Medical Dictionary, *PDD is any of a group of mental disorders of infancy, childhood, or adolescence characterized by distortions in the acquisition of the multiple basic psychological functions necessary for the elaboration of social skills, language skills, and imagination; also characterized by restricted or stereotypical activities and interests.*

There are five diseases normally included in the group of PDD and they are:

1. Autistic Disease
2. Asperger's Disease
3. Childhood Disintegrative Disease (CDD)
4. Rett's Disease
5. PDD-Not Otherwise Specified (PDD-NOS)

Stedman's Electronic Medical Dictionary defines autism as: *A mental disorder characterized by severely abnormal development of social interaction and of verbal and nonverbal communication skills. Affected people may adhere to inflexible, nonfunctional rituals or routines. They may become upset with even trivial changes in their environment. They often have a limited range of interests but may become preoccupied with a narrow range of subjects or activities. They appear unable to understand others' feelings and often have poor eye contact with others. Unpredictable mood swings may occur. Many demonstrate stereotypical motor mannerisms such as hand or finger flapping, body rocking, or dipping* (Stedman's Electronic Medical Dictionary, Version 7.0).

This definition of autism is based on behavioral criteria described by Kanner in 1943. *"By definition, symptoms are manifested by 36 months of age and are characterized by delayed and disordered language, impaired social interaction, abnormal responses to sensory stimuli, events and objects, poor eye contact, an insistence on sameness, an unusual capacity for rote memory, repetitive and stereotypic behaviour and a normal physical appearance"* [1].

1.1. Symptoms and Signs

The symptoms and signs of autism vary considerably from person to person, but sensory dysfunction is common and it affects all senses [8]. Some autistic children display repetitive behavior and some are seemingly insensitive to pain. Individuals with autism often perceive sounds and other sensory signals differently than non-autistic individuals and often have a lower tolerance for sound, touch, and pain. Some enjoy touch and other forms of bodily stimulation, and sensory stimulation often causes greater emotional reactions than it does in non-autistic individuals; some feel great pleasure from certain sensory stimulation including painful stimulation [4]. Some dislike certain sounds and bright light. Some enjoy deep body stimulation (see Appendix C for further discussions about sensory procession in autistic individuals).

Many autistic individuals have other symptoms. About 30% have epileptic seizures and many have constipation and other digestive diseases. Some 10-15% of autistic children improve over time and as adults can have a normal life with a job and family. On the other end of the scale are individuals who are so severely disabled they cannot take care of themselves and must be institutionalized [6].

1.2. High Performance Autistic Individuals

So-called "high performance" autistic children (also known as Asperger's syndrome) only have few of the symptoms often ascribed to autism. Asperger's disease is defined by Stedman's Electronic Dictionary as

"*a pervasive developmental disorder characterized by severe and enduring impairment in social skills and restrictive and repetitive behaviors and interests, leading to impaired social and occupational functioning but without significant delays in language development; however, constructs of Asperger's disorder other than those in* The Diagnostic and Statistical Manual of Mental Diseases, Fourth Edition (*DSM-IV) include the criteria of less social impairment than in autism and in impaired communications.*

Many will not include Asperger's diseases in the category of autistic diseases but regard it as a separate disease.

1.3. Prevalence of Autism

The prevalence of autism in the US is reported to one in 150 births (CDC 2007), and it is increasing at a rate of 10-17 percent per year. Autism is about 4 times more prevalent in boys than in girls, indicating genetics in one way or another may be involved. Genetics may be a factor in autism, but heredity factors cannot explain the recent increase in the occurrence of autism.

2. ANATOMIC AND FUNCTIONAL ABNORMALITIES

Studies regarding anatomical abnormalities in autistic individuals have been made but very few neurophysiological studies concerning abnormalities in the function of the brain have been published.

2.1. Anatomical Abnormalities

The few neuropathological studies that have been performed on the brains of autistic individuals have shown early abnormalities in many regions of the brain, including the cerebral cortex, cortical nerve fibers (white matter), amygdala, brainstem, and cerebellum [15,16].

Other studies have shown an increased brain volume in autistic individuals and some other anomalies such as an altered gray/white matter ratio. (It is interesting to notice that other diseases such as depression are associated with more nerve cells than normal [19]). Some investigators, especially Dr. E. Courchesne and his group at the Neuropsychology Research Laboratory at the Children's Hospital Research Center in San Diego, have focused on anomalies in the cerebellum for explaining some of the symptoms of autism [5].

Studies agree that individuals with autism have more nerve cells than individuals who are not autistic, the cells are packed tighter [14] and errors have occurred in the connections between nerve cells in the brain [3]. It is also known that pruning of connections and re-organization of various parts of the brain normally occurs during the first years of life ("midcourse correction" see Chapter III). It has therefore been suggested that this process has not proceeded correctly in individuals with autism, and the different kinds of deficits and abnormalities of behavior that typically occur with autistic children may be caused by deficiencies in the "midcourse correction" [11].

2.1.1. Abnormal Involvement of the Amygdala

The limbic system is important for learning and memory, and the amygdala nuclei especially play an important role in emotion and many kinds of behavior. Irregularities in limbic structures may therefore explain some emotional and learning abnormalities that are common in autistic individuals.

Further signs of the amygdala's involvement come from some old studies of the behavior of monkeys in which the amygdala was removed. This study by H. Klüver- and P. C. Bucy [9] has been discussed extensively. It supports the suggestion that autism is associated with abnormalities of the amygdala.

2.2. Abnormalities in Sensory Systems

Autistic individuals have symptoms that are related to sensory processing and to emotions. Therefore, let us look at abnormalities in sensory systems in the brain and in the "emotional brain", foremost the amygdala.

2.2.1. Sensory Deficits

Autistic individuals have many signs of abnormal processing of sensory signals [2]. These abnormalities have received little attention and their cause has not been studied much. These abnormalities are likewise not included in the profile of autism as described in the DSM-IV, despite the fact they affect all senses [8].

The abnormalities in the processing of sensory signals indicate that individuals with autism spectrum diseases use their non-classical sensory systems to a greater extent than non-autistic individuals [12]. (The non-classical pathways using dorsal and medial parts of the thalamus were discussed in Chapter II and Appendix B.) This could also be explained by a faulty development after birth where normally the activation of the non-classical hearing pathways decreases [13], probably by turning on neural plasticity or preventing the normal activation of neural plasticity to occur.

The results of a recent study supported the hypothesis that the non-classical pathways are more active in autistic individuals [11,12] than in non-autistic individuals.

We studied autistic individuals to find out if they used their non-classical hearing pathways more than non-autistic individuals. For that we used the finding that non-classical pathways receive signals from more than one sensory modality while classical sensory systems only respond to one sensory modality of stimulation (see Chapter I). In praxis we activated the somatosensory system that normally responds to touch of the skin by electrically activating a nerve (median nerve) in the wrist while the person listened to sounds through earphones [12]. We thought that if the electrical impulses used to stimulate the median nerve could alter the way the sound is perceived it would suggest that signals from touch receptors in the skin could modulate the flow of information in the hearing nervous system. If that would occur, it would be a sign that the non-classical pathways were involved in the perception of the sound because only nerve cells in the non-classical pathway would receive signals from touch receptors. Nerve cells in the classical hearing pathways only receive signals from the ear.

Our studies showed that the perception of sounds by children with autism was affected, often very much, by electrical stimulation of the median nerve, indicating that they used the non-classical ascending hearing pathways for hearing [12]. However, non-autistic children also have signs of non-classical hearing pathways usage [13], but the involvement decreases gradually as children grow and few individuals above the age of 15 have such signs. This means that these studies indicate that autistic individuals use their non-classical pathways to a greater extent than non-autistic individuals, and suppression of the involvement of the non-classical sensory pathways that normally occurs during early childhood [13] has not proceeded normally in children with autism. This is an objective sign of something being wrong with sensory processing in autistic individuals.

The processing performed by the non-classical pathways is less sophisticated ("fast and dirty") than that performed in the classical pathways ("slow and accurate"). In particular, the non-classical pathways send non-processed (raw) sensory signals directly to the emotional brain (amygdala), whereas sensory signals that travel in the classical pathways can only reach the amygdala after having passed large groups of nerve cells in the cerebral cortex where extensive processing occurs. That would explain the abnormal feeling of pleasure and displeasure the autistic children experience from all senses [8]. As an example of abnormal perception of sensory stimulation, some autistic individuals who participated in our study of the non-classical pathways [12] enjoyed the electrical stimulation of the skin over the median nerve at the wrist used in these studies. This is just another sign of abnormal sensory processing.

The pleasure from deep body pressure that many autistic individuals experience can be explained by the findings that the non-classical pathways receive signals from receptors deep in the body to a greater extent than the classical pathways. Obviously, the abnormalities in the ascending sensory pathways that suggest that the non-classical pathways are present in individuals with autism spectrum diseases are only a part of the abnormalities that cause the symptoms in these diseases. The abnormalities that cause deficits in social interactions are located on other parts of the brain. The great individual variability of the abnormalities in the sensory systems that can be revealed by simple tests, such as those mentioned above for determining if hearing perception is affected by somatosensory stimulation, only reflect a small part of the variability in the abnormalities in people with autism spectrum diseases.

2.3. Faults in the Immune System

There is increasing evidence that the mother's immune system may be involved in developing at least some forms of autism spectrum disorders. Dr. van de Water's research group at UC Davis, California has especially studied the presence of antibodies against the nervous system. They find that such antibodies seems to be present in many mothers who have given birth to children with autism spectrum disorders [18].

2.4. Environmental Factors

Studies of rat mothers by the Merzenich group in San Francisco have suggested that exposure to certain environmental substances (PCB) may cause serious defects in development of the offspring's' brains [7], and these abnormalities have similarities with abnormalities seen in children with autism.

3. CAUSE OF AUTISM SPECTRUM DISEASES

The focus of most published studies has been on explaining the symptoms and signs of autism. Major efforts have been devoted to find the cause of autism and especially figure out why there has been such a considerable increase in the incidence of autism during the last few years.

Let us see what we know about the cause of autism, and what we believe we know.

Autism is about 4 times more prevalent in boys than in girls, indicating genetics in one way or another may be involved. Some candidates for such genetic predisposition have recently been identified, but it seems obvious that something else is also involved. It has been suggested that childhood developmental diseases such as autism are caused because of errors in the activation of a form of neural plasticity [11].

3.1. Preservatives in Vaccines

Many years ago, it was suggested that the preservatives in childhood vaccines (thimerosal, a preservative containing mercury used in vaccines for measles, mumps and rubella (MMR)) was the cause of autism. Much effort has been devoted to studies about the possibility that this factor caused autism with little attention to other possible causes. Recently, strong evidence has been presented that the mercury preservative cannot be the cause of autism. For example, studies have shown that the rate of new occurrences of autism continued to rise after that these compounds were abandoned and removed from the vaccine, according to a Danish study of more then half a million children [10].

The story about autism and vaccines is a good example that shows, despite overwhelming evidence, it is very difficult to get rid of old concepts. When presenting convincing evidence to the contrary it is often met with the statement: "I believe in the old assumption anyhow" by individuals as well as by some professionals. This particular misconception has caused much suffering and indeed deaths because people have been afraid to have their children vaccinated against common but potentially serious and dangerous diseases.

> Autism is an example of how difficult it is to change people's perception of the cause of a disease. It seems as one can supply all the evidence in world, such as against the vaccine as a cause of autism, and the belief that autism is caused by its mercury based preservatives still occupies professionals and individual parents of autistic children alike. Nobody seems to be concerned about the damaged this erroneous assumption has done. Childhood vaccinations are the most effective way to reduce the risk of serious diseases, and one can only guess how many children have suffered from serious but preventable diseases because the parents were afraid of having their children vaccinated -- some have died.
>
> Nobody seems to be concerned about the damage these unfounded suggestions about vaccines being the culprit have done.
>
> Naturally, the parents suffer when children become sick or die, but few people have thought about the children who have acquired brain damage from preventable diseases because the parents did not allow vaccinations – on the (incorrect) grounds that the vaccinations had serious side effects. How many children have lost quality of life due to this is not known. This is one of the reasons why it is important to find the cause of autism.

3.2. Faults in Development of the Brain after Birth

It may be valid to speculate that the pruning of the nervous system, including programmed cell death, which normally occurs during the first years of life, is not progressing correctly in individuals with autism. Lack of, or incorrect, pruning may cause nerve cells in different parts of the brain to become more tightly packed in autistic children than in non-autistic ones, which may explain why many autistic children have epileptic seizures.

3.2.1. Faults in Midcourse Correction

It seems prudent to assume that developmental events that occur in early childhood are controlled by programs (or rules) that are laid down before birth. Figure C.1 shows a hypothetical flow chart for developmental disorders such as autism [11]. Before birth, genetics and epigenetics are assumed to guide the creation of the programs that will control the development of the nervous system during the first years of life. These programs are assumed to control events during childhood such as the "midcourse correction" discussed earlier (page 87). The programs may be affected during pregnancy by chemicals and other environmental factors, as well as internal effects such as the mother's diet, physical condition (exercise, etc), and habits such as smoking cigarettes, use of narcotics, etc. If this is correct then it can explain why it has been so difficult to find the cause of autistic diseases.

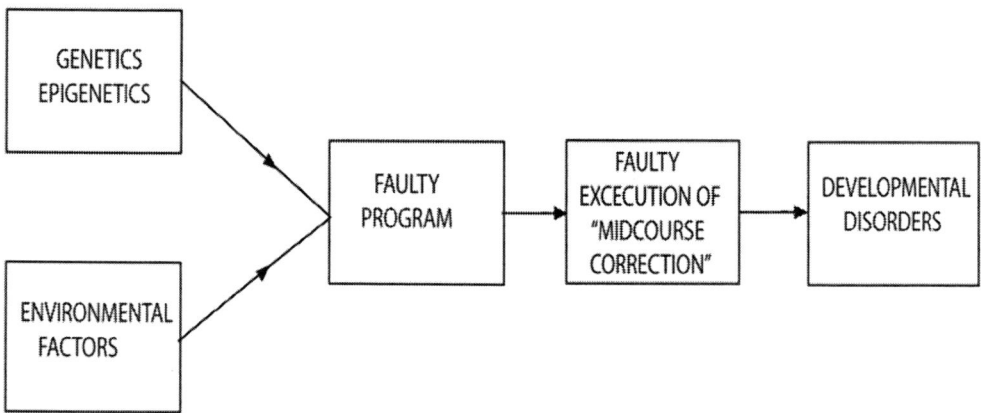

Figure C.1. Hypothetical flowchart of developmental diseases where symptoms are caused by faulty "midcourse correction".

There are reasons to believe that symptoms of autism are at the end of a chain of events that begins before birth and cause the symptoms to debut in the first years of life. Studies of children at the time the symptoms occur will not reveal the cause because the programs that control the development of the disease were established before birth or perhaps more correctly, the corruption of the programs that control the normal development of the brain after birth occurred before birth [11].

If the cause of autism is faulty programs for the "midcourse correction" that were laid down before birth then searching for the cause of the disease in the children who have signs of autism may be an example of looking at the wrong time for the cause. The poor success in treatment of autism is a further indication that the symptoms in childhood are controlled by a program that was laid down earlier, such as before birth.

3.3. Causes of Fault in the Development of the Brain after Birth

The question is naturally, what has caused this error in these programs to occur. It has been suggested that faulty epigenetic modulators are involved in creating developmental diseases such as autism spectrum diseases [20]. Epigenetic changes can be induced by hormones, which affect the regulatory regions on genes. The fact that more boys than girls have autism may support this hypothesis. The structure of DNA is assumed to control how we develop, but the existence of epigenetics confirms that we are not hard-wired by our genes but (internal and external) environmental factors can affect how genetics works. Epigenetics (see page 86) and the effect of environmental factors (intake of or contact with certain chemicals) during pregnancy may be a likely cause of some developmental diseases such as autism.

3.3.1. Environmental Factors

One hint in this direction comes from a recent study by Dr. Michael Merzenich and his group of researchers in San Francisco. As I mentioned earlier in this book, they found that the offspring of rat mothers that had been exposed to the environmental pollutant PCB[69] (polychlorinated biphenyls) during pregnancy had severe abnormalities in the organization of the cerebral cortices that these investigators studied, namely the hearing cortices [7]. However, there were likely similar abnormalities in other parts of their brains that they did not study and which may have an ability to cause other kinds of symptoms and signs.

The rapid increase in the occurrence of autism would indicate a factor that has occurred relatively recently would be suspected. The rapid increase may offer an opportunity to find the cause. One would look for other factors or events that have increased rapidly during the past 20-30 years. These factors could be environmental substances to which mothers might have been exposed. PCB is a valid suggestion, although its use has been terminated. It does not seem to be eliminated or broken down, but it is constantly dispersed in nature so that one can suspect that more and more people are being exposed. Many other environmental factors could affect the programs that are laid down before birth.

Finding these environmental factors would be a challenge that is probably greater than any previous hunt for the environmental factors that caused adverse effects on unborn children.

Other technological developments or changes in lifestyle may also be suspected to be the cause. The suggestion that something in the vaccinations was the cause of autism was a valid suggestion, but it was later proven that the vaccination used for children could not to be involved according to population studies [10] that showed that when the suspected substance,

---

[69] PCB, a chemical, polychlorinated biphenyl, that was used earlier for many purposes such as coolants in transformers. The production of PCB was banned 1970, but it is still widely spread in nature because it does not degrade.

thimerosal, was removed from the vaccine it did not affect the incidence of autism. Of other factors that have increased is the use of cell phones, but the exposure of a fetus in the womb to radiofrequency energy from cell phones seems too small to cause any biological effect.

That exposure to certain chemicals during pregnancy can have disastrous effects on the development of a child became evident from the catastrophes caused many years ago by the medication known as Thalidomide. Thalidomide, a tranquilizer (sedative-hypnotic) and antiemitic medication (medications that are effective against vomiting), was especially recommended for pregnant women to treat "morning sickness", affecting about 10,000 children before the source of these deformities was discovered. (Only 17 children in the US had deformities because the FDA had not approved the medication). The deformations caused by this medication were obvious immediately after birth, and yet it took a long time to find the cause despite the fact it was used worldwide - sold in almost 50 countries during 1956 and 1962. Only with the aid of meticulous records in Germany was it finally possible to find the link between thalidomide and the birth defects.

The deformities caused by Thalidomide were obvious at birth. Autism often does not become diagnosed until 3 years after birth [1]. Finding out what environmental factors mothers who give birth to autistic children would be a formidable detective job.

---

4. REFERENCES

[1]   Bauman ML, Kemper TL. The neuropathology of the autism spectrum disorders: what have we learned? *Novartis Found Symp.* 2003;251:112-22.

[2]   Bauman ML, Kemper TT. *Neurobiology of Autism.* Baltimore: Johns Hopkins University Press; 1994.

[3]   Belmonte MK, Allen G, Beckel-Mitchener A, Boulanger LM, Carper RA, Webb SJ. Autism and abnormal development of brain connectivity. *J Neurosci.* 2004;24(42):9228-31.

[4]   Cohen D, Volkmar F. *Autism and Pervasive Developmental Disorders. 2 ed.* New York: John Wiley & Sons, Inc; 1997.

[5]   Courchesne E, Townsend J, Akshoomof NA, Saitoh O, Yeung-Courchesne R, Lincoln AJ, et al. Impairment in shifting attention in autistic and cerebellar patients. *Behav Neurosci.* 1994;108:848-65.

[6]   Kanner L. Follow-up study of eleven autistic children originally reported in 1943. *J Autism Child Schizophr* 1971;1:119–45.

[7]   Kenet T, Froemke RC, Schreiner CE, Pessah IN, Merzenich MM. Perinatal exposure to a noncoplanar polychlorinated biphenyl alters tonotopy, receptive fields, and plasticity in rat primary auditory cortex. *Proc Natl Acad Sci U S A.* 2007;104(18):7646-51.

[8]   Kern JK, Trivedi MH, Grannemann BD, Garver CR, Johnson DG, Andrews AA, et al. Sensory correlations in autism. *Autism.* 2007;11(2):123-34.

[9]   Klüver H, Bucy PC. Preliminary analysis of functions of the temporal lobes in monkeys. *Arch Neurol Psychiatry.* 1939;42:979-1000.

[10] Madsen KM, Hviid A, Vestergaard M, Schendel D, Wohlfahrt J, Thorsen P, et al. A population-based study of measles, mumps, and rubella vaccination and autism. *N Engl J Med*. 2002; 347(19):1477-82.

[11] Møller AR. Neurophysiologic abnormalities in autism. In: Mesmere BS, editor. *New Autism Research Developments*. New York: Nova Science Publishers; 2007.

[12] Møller AR, Kern JK, Grannemann B. Are the non-classical auditory pathways involved in autism and PDD? *Neurol Res*. 2005;27:625-9.

[13] Møller AR, Rollins P. The non-classical auditory system is active in children but not in adults. *Neurosci Lett*. 2002;319:41-4.

[14] Palmen SJ, van Engeland H, Hof PR, Schmitz C. Neuropathological findings in autism. *Brain*. 2004;127(12):2572-83.

[15] Pickett J, London E. The neuropathology of autism: a review. *Brain Pathol*. 2007;17(4):422-33.

[16] Schmitz C, Rezaie P. The neuropathology of autism: where do we stand? *Neuropathol Appl Neurobiol*. 2007.

[17] Volkmar FR, Pauls D. Autism. *The Lancet*. 2003;362:1133-42.

[18] Wills S, Cabanlit M, Bennett J, Ashwood P, Amaral D, Van de Water J. Autoantibodies in autism spectrum disorders (ASD). *Ann N Y Acad Sci* 2007;107:79-91.

[19] Young KA, Holcomb LA, Yazdani U, Hicks PB, German DC. Elevated neuron number in the limbic thalamus in major depression. *Am J Psychiatry*. 2004;161(7):1270-7.

[20] Zhao X, Pak C, Smrt RD, Jin P. Epigenetics and Neural Developmental Disorders. *Epigenetics*. 2007;2(2):126-34.

GLOSSARY

ABI:	Auditory brainstem implants
Affective disorders:	Mood disturbances
Agonist:	Support an action; opposite to antagonist
Allocortex:	Phylogenetical old parts of the cerebral cortex; has fewer layers than the neocortex.
Allodynia:	pain from light touch of the skin
AMPA:	alpha-amino-hydroxy-5-methylisoxazole-4-propionic acid; a glutamate receptor
Amygdala:	Almond shaped structure in the temporal lobe that consist of three main nuclei.
Analgesics:	Drugs that can reduce pain
Antagonist:	Opposed to something
Anteriorlateral tract:	Pathways for pain, consisting of the spinothalamic tract, the mesencephalic, the spinoreticulo tracts
Apoptosis:	A for of programmed cell death
Apoptosis:	Programmed cell death
Arousal reaction:	awakening of the brain
Ascending sensory pathways:	Pathways that convey sensory information from sense organs to the cerebral sensory cortices
Association cortices:	Cortical areas involved in sensory information processing and multisensory integration
Ataxia:	Inability to coordinate muscle activity
Auditory brainstem implants:	Devices for stimulating nerve cells in the cochlear nucleus electrically. Used in people who have lost function of their hearing nerve.
Auditory:	Pertaining to the sense of hearing
Autism spectrum diseases:	A group of diseases with symptoms and signs related to autism
Autism:	A (developmental) disorder characterized by abnormal verbal and communication skill and inability to have normal social relationships.

Axon:	The inner part of a nerve fiber, may of may not be covered by myelin.
Basilar membrane:	A partition in the cochlea that is set into vibration sound and which separate sounds according to their frequency (spectrum).
BDNF:	Brain derived neurotrophic factor
Bifurcate:	Branch into two. Used about nerve fibers.
BOLD	Blood oxygen level depended
CAM:	Complementary and alternative medicine
CaMKII:	Calcium influx activates a protein kinase II:
Caudal:	A direction towards the tail.
Central nervous system:	Comprising the spinal cord and the brain.
Cerebellum:	Part of the brain that was earlier associated with control of movement but know known to have other functions including memory of cognition.
Chelating:	A way to excrete heavy metal
Classical pathways:	Sensory pathways that use the ventral thalamus and project to primary cortices. Other names are lemniscal, or precise, specific pathways.
CNS:	Central nervous system.
Cochlea:	Part of the inner ear that deals with hearing.
Cognition:	Regards the process of knowing and perceiving; intellectual functions.
Compassion:	Understanding of the emotional state of another and a desire to alleviate suffering.
Cortex:	Bark; cerebral cortex
Critical period:	Term used for the period in life where plastic changes are most easy to activate.
Cross-modal interaction:	Interaction between different kinds of sensory signals such as sounds and touch.
CRPS:	Complex Regional Pain Syndrome I and II.
Dendrite:	The receiving part of a nerve cell.
Dermatomes:	Patches of skin that are innervated by the same spinal nerve.
Descending sensory pathways:	Neural pathways that conduct information from downwards from the cerebral cortex towards nuclei of sensory pathways.
Directional hearing:	The ability to detect the direction to a sound source.
Disease:	Disordered or incorrectly functioning organ.
Disorder:	Disturbance in physical or mental health.
Dizziness:	Common, but imprecise term used to describe various symptoms of the balance system.
DLPT:	Dorsolateral pontomesencephalic tegmentum
DNA:	Deoxyribonucleic acid, the carrier of hereditary

information.

Dormant synapses:	Synapses that cannot activate the cell to which they connect.
DSM-IV:	The Diagnostic and Statistical Manual of Mental Diseases, Fourth Edition (DSM-IV)
Empathy:	The ability to recognize, perceive and feel directly the emotion of another person.
Endoplasmic reticulum:	Part of cells where synthesis of substances occurs.
Epigenesis:	Regulation of expression of genes without the structure of the genes being altered.
EPSP:	Excitatory post synaptic potentials.
Excitability:	Ability to respond to a stimulus
Extralemniscal:	Another name for non-classical pathways, meaning pathways that do not use the lemniscal tracts.
Fiber tracts:	Bundles of nerve fibers in the brain and the spinal cord.
Fibromyalgia:	A disease that is characterized by non-specific muscle pain.
Firing (of nerve fibers or nerve cells):	Nerve discharges.
Functional MRI (fMRI):	Imaging technique based on MRI technologies in connection with measurements of measurements of blood oxygen level (BOLD).
GABA:	Gamma amino butyric acid, common inhibitory transmitter substance in the nervous system.
Ganglion:	Collection of cell bodies of nerve fibers (such a dorsal root ganglia). Also used for collections of cell bodies in the autonomic nervous system.
Genetics:	The science of heredity.
Glia cells:	Cells in the brain that are between nerve cells, role poorly known.
Glycine:	A common excitatory neural transmitter substance.
Gray matter:	Regions of the spinal cord and the brain that are mainly composed of nerve cells.
Hallucinations:	Perceptions of often meaningful sensory event s in the absent of physical stimuli. Occur in connection with psychiatric disorders and from administration of chemical. Hallucinations are common after having undergone anesthesia such as for surgical operations.
Hearing cortex:	End station of ascending hearing pathways.
Hebb's principle:	"Neurons that fire together wire together".
Hyperalgesia:	Decreased threshold for painful activation.
Hyperexcitability:	Increased ability to respond to a stimulus.
Hyperpathia:	Lowered tolerance for painful activations.
Hypertension:	Abnormally high blood pressure (defined as above 140/90).

Idiopathic (disease):	Disease of unknown cause.
Ketamine:	A drug that has similarities to PCP.
Kindling:	Lighting a fire, used to describe the effect of some forms of neural plasticity.
Limbic system:	Part of the old brain including the amygdala, hippocampus, part of the thalamus and limbic cortex. Also known as the emotional brain because of itd involvement in emotion, behavior and memory.
LTD:	Long term depression.
MEG:	Magnetoencephalograpic (recordings).
MK801:	An experimental drug that is an NMDA receptor antagonist.
Morphological:	Study of structure.
Motonucleus:	Cluster of nerve cells the axons of which innervate muscles.
MRI:	Magnetic resonance imaging.
MVD:	Microvascular decompression (operation).
Myelin:	Fatty (insulating) substance covering axons.
Myofascial pain:	Muscle pain characteristic by affecting certain individual muscles and having trigger points.
Neocortex:	New part of the cerebral cortex; has six layers, compared with the old cortex that has 3 layers.
Nerve cell:	A cell in the nervous system that serve to transmit and process signals (information) of various kinds and origin. Other name is neuron.
Nerve fiber:	Extension of a nerve cell, consisting of an axon that may be covered with myelin.
Neural plasticity:	The ability of the brain and the spinal cord to change the way they function.
Neuroma:	Any swelling of a nerve, but often used to describe abnormal growth (benign and malign tumors).
Neuropathy:	Disorder of the nervous system, mostly used for disorders of peripheral nerves.
NMDA:	N-methyl-D-aspartate; a glutamate receptor.
Nociceptors:	Receptors the activation of which give painful sensations.
Non-classical pathways:	Sensory pathways that use the dorsal and medial thalamus and bypass primary cortices. Other names are extralemniscal, diffuse or non-specific pathways.
NSAID:	Non-steroidal anti-inflammatory drugs.
Nucleus:	Cluster of nerve cells in the brain.
Opiates:	Natural substances (alkaloids) found in opium.
Opioids:	Chemical (synthetic) substances with similar effects as morphine.
PAG:	Periaquaductal gray; a structure in the brain that is especially involved in processing painful signals.
Paresthesia:	Abnormal body sensations.

Pathology:	The science or the study of the origin, nature, and course of diseases.
Patient:	A person who is under medical or surgical treatment.
PCB:	Polychlorinated biphenyl, chemical substances that are suspected to cause birth defects and cancer.
PCD:	Programmed cell death.
PCP:	Phencyclidine, and anesthetic drug, also known as angle dust.
Peripheral nerves:	Nerves in the body and the face.
Phantom sensations:	Sensations that are referred to a different place on the body that where they are caused, often pain and tingling that is felt in an amputated limb.
Phonophobia:	Fear of sound.
Physiological:	Has to do with function.
PKA:	Protein kinase A.
Placebo effect:	Latin meaning "I will please". The beneficial effect of a medication with no (known) effect.
Plasticity diseases:	Symptoms and signs caused by changes in the function of the central nervous system.
PNS:	Peripheral nervous system (nerves of the body, divided into the somatic and autonomic nervous systems).
Primary cortex:	The first part of the cerebral cortex to receive information from classical sensory pathways.
Purkinje cell:	Nerve cells with very large dendritic trees, abundant in the cerebellum.
Receptors:	Specialized structures that are sensitive to specific physical modalities such as mechanical deformation, light, specific chemicals.
Referred pain:	Pain that is felt at a different place than where it is caused.
RNA:	Ribonucleic acid; controls synthesis of proteins in cells.
Rostral:	A direction towards the head (actually the beak).
RSD:	Reflex sympathetic dystrophy (now known as CRPS I).
SAMe:	S-adenosyl-l-methionine.
Sensory cortices:	Parts of the cerebral cortex that receive and process sensory information.
Sensory receptor:	A structure that is sensitive to a specific stimulus.
Serotonin:	A transmitter substance, also known as 5-hydroxytryptamine (5-HT).
Shingles:	Painful rash and blisters caused by the same virus that causes chickenpox. Usually appear in dermatomes.
Signs of disease:	Objective measures of abnormalities.
SMP:	Sympathetic maintained pain.
Somatosensory:	Body sense.
Spasm:	Involuntary contractions of one of several muscles

Spasticity:	A form of uncontrolled contraction of muscles.
Stimulus (sensory physiology):	Something that activates sensory receptors
Sympathetic nervous system:	Part of the autonomic nervous system.
Symptom:	Patient's description of signs of a disease.
Synapse:	Termination of an axon on a nerve cell (cell body, dendrite or axon).
Synaptic efficacy:	The ability of a synapse to engage the receiving cell.
Syndrome:	A group of symptoms that characterizes a certain disease or disorder.
Synkinesis:	Involuntarily contractions of other muscles than those anticipated.
Telencephalon:	Frontal part of the brain including the cerebral hemispheres.
TENS:	Transderm electric nerve stimulation.
Thalamus:	Part of the brain through which sensory information is transformed and motor command are modified.
Tic doulouroux:	Trigeminal neuralgia.
Tinnitus:	Ringing in the ears, hearing meaningless sounds that do not come from the environment
Transmitter substances:	Chemicals that conveys neural activity by being shuttled over the synaptic clef into the receiving cell.
Tremor:	A form of uncontrollable rhythmic muscle activity.
Trigeminal neuralgia:	Occasional intensive shooting pain in parts of one side of the face, may resemble toothache.
Vertigo:	A feeling that the surroundings turn (rotate).
Vestibular schwannoma:	Benign growth on the balance or hearing nerve.
Vestibular:	Related to the balance organ.
Viscera:	Internal organs.
White matter:	Parts of the brain and spinal cord that are composed of nerve fibers, fiber tracts.

INDEX

B

C

F

G

H

T